FIFTH EDITION

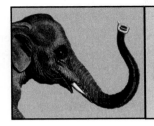

LANGE Q&A™

SURGERY

C. Gene Cayten, MD, FACS, MPH
Editor-in-Chief
Professor of Surgery and Senior Associate Dean
New York Medical College
Residency Program Director of General Surgery
Our Lady of Mercy Medical Center
Bronx, New York

Max Goldberg, MBBCh, MD, FRCSI, FACS
Clinical Assistant Professor of Surgery
Stonybrook University Hospital and
Medical Center
Stonybrook, New York
Director Emeritus,
Department of Surgery Long Beach
Medical Center,
Long Beach, New York

Nanakram Agarwal, MD, MPH, FACS
Professor of Surgery
New York Medical College
Chief of Surgical Intensive Care Unit
Our Lady of Mercy Medical Center
Bronx, New York

**Simon Wapnick, MBChB, MD, FRCS (Eng),
FACS (Deceased)**
Director of Postgraduate Clinical
Anatomy Courses
Department of Cell Biology and Anatomy
New York Medical College
Valhalla, New York

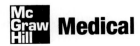

New York Chicago San Francisco Lisbon London Madrid Mexico City Milan
New Delhi San Juan Seoul Singapore Sydney Toronto

Lange Q&A™: Surgery, Fifth Edition

1 2 3 4 5 6 7 8 9 0   QPD/QPD   0 9 8 7

ISBN-13: 978-0-07-147566-2
ISBN-10:   0-07-147566-4

Notice

Medicine is an ever-changing science. As new research and clinical experience broaden our knowledge, changes in treatment and drug therapy are required. The authors and the publisher of this work have checked with sources believed to be reliable in their efforts to provide information that is complete and generally in accord with the standards accepted at the time of publication. However, in view of the possibility of human error or changes in medical sciences, neither the author nor the publisher nor any other party who has been involved in the preparation or publication of this work warrants that the information contained herein is in every respect accurate or complete, and they disclaim all responsibility for any errors or omissions or for the results obtained from use of such information contained in this work. Readers are encouraged to confirm the information contained herein with other sources. For example and in particular, readers are advised to check the product information sheet included in the package of each drug they plan to administer to be certain that the information contained in this work is accurate and that changes have not been made in the recommended dose or in the contraindications for administration. This recommendation is of particular importance in connection with new or infrequently used drugs.

This book was set in Palatino by International Typesetting and Composition.
The editors were Marsha S. Loeb, Katherine Bemesderfer, and Midge Haramis.
The production supervisor was Catherine H. Saggese.
Project management was provided by International Typesetting and Composition.
Quebecor World/Dubuque was the printer and binder.

The book is printed on acid-free paper.

Library of Congress Cataloging-in-Publication Data

Lange Q & A. Surgery / [edited by] C. Gene Cayten ... [et al.].—5th ed.
    p. ; cm.
    Rev. ed. of: Appleton & Lange review of surgery / Simon Wapnick ... [et al.]. c2003.
    ISBN-13: 978-0-07-147566-2 (pbk. : alk. paper)
    ISBN-10: 0-07-147566-4 (pbk. : alk. paper)
    1. Surgery—Examinations, questions, etc.   I. Cayten, C. Gene.   II. Appleton & Lange review of surgery.   III. Title: Lange Q and A. Surgery.   IV. Title: Surgery.
    [DNLM: 1. Surgical Procedures, Operative—Examination Questions. WO 18.2 L269   2007]
2. Surgery—Examination Questions. WO 18.2 L269   2007]
RD37.2.W37   2007
617.0076—dc22

2007001650

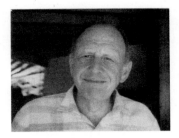

Simon Wapnick, MBChB, MD, FRCS (Eng), FACS, 1937–2003

This book is dedicated to Simon Wapnick, MD, a distinguished and skilled surgeon, clinical anatomist, and medical researcher who wrote and edited the first four editions of Review of Surgery. *He was a professional dedicated to bringing his scientific excellence to humanity for the common good. Simon led a life of profound dedication to the God of his fathers, a life imbued with the spirituality and values of the Torah. His students at New York Medical College in the dedication of their yearbook to him said, "The spirit, enthusiasm, and commitment of Dr. Simon Wapnick will live on in our lives because he played a key role from the very beginning of our professional training. He was someone with the will of a lion and the heart of a lamb, a teacher who was always ready to explain anything and a gentleman who was interested in so many neat things. He was an avid marathoner and was constantly 'looking for improved time and efficient stride.' He encouraged us to keep up the good race for a good life. He validated our choice of the noble profession of medicine."*

James Michener could readily have been thinking about Simon Wapnick when he wrote, "The master in the art of living makes little distinction between his work and his play, his labor and his leisure, his mind and his body, his information and his recreation, his love and his religion. He hardly knows which is which. He simply pursues his vision of excellence at whatever he does, leaving others to decide whether he is working or playing. To him he's always doing both."

As his wife, Isabelle, I shall always carry within my heart so many loving and proud memories of Simon Wapnick.

Contents

Contributors

Andrew Ashikari, MD, FACS
Assistant Professor of Surgery
New York Medical College
Westchester Medical Center
Valhalla, New York

Nilesh N. Balar, MD, RVT, FACS
Assistant Professor of Surgery
New York Medical College
Chief of Vascular Surgery
Our Lady of Mercy Medical Center
Bronx, New York

Nicholas A. Balsano, MD, FACS
Clinical Associate Professor of Surgery
New York Medical College
Our Lady of Mercy Medical Center
Bronx, New York

James E. Barone, MD, FACS, FCCM
Professor of Clinical Surgery
Weill Medical College of Cornell University
Chairman, Department of Surgery
Lincoln Medical and Mental Health Center
Bronx, New York

Alan S. Berkower, MD, PhD
Assistant Professor of Otolaryngology
New York Medical College
Chief of Otolaryngology
Attending, Department of Surgery
Our Lady of Mercy Medical Center
Bronx, New York

E. A. Bonfils-Roberts, MD, FACS
Associate Professor of Surgery
New York Medical College
Section Chief of Thoracic Surgery
Lincoln Medical and Mental Health Center
Bronx, New York

Akella Chendrasekhar, MD, FACS
Medical Director, Trauma
Medical Director, Emergency Department
Wyckoff Heights Medical Center
Brooklyn, New York

Sean Fullerton, MD
Department of Urology
Our Lady of Mercy Medical Center
Bronx, New York

Evelyn Irizarry, MD, FACS, FACRS
Assistant Clinical Professor of Surgery
Weill Medical College of Cornell University
Bronx, New York

Rao R. Ivatury, MD, FACS
Professor of Surgery, Physiology, and Emergency
    Medicine
Chief, Division of Trauma, Critical Care, and
    Emergency Surgery
Medical College of Virginia
Virginia Commonwealth University
Richmond, Virginia

Valerie L. Katz, MD, FACS
Assistant Professor of Clinical Surgery
Weill Medical College of Cornell University
Section Chief, Department of General Surgery
Lincoln Medical and Mental Health Center
Bronx, New York

Marshall D. Kramer, MD
Associate Professor of Surgery
New York Medical College
Chief, Thoracic Surgery
Our Lady of Mercy Medical Center
Bronx, New York

Meno Lueders, MD, FACS
Assistant Professor of Clinical Surgery
Weill Medical College of Cornell University
Lincoln Medical and Mental Health Center
Bronx, New York

Mayank V. Patel, MD
Department of Surgery
Our Lady of Mercy Medical Center
Westchester Square Medical Center
Bronx, New York

Soula Priovolos, MD, FACS
Assistant Professor of Clinical Surgery
Weill Medical College of Cornell University
Lincoln Medical and Mental Health Center
Bronx, New York

Prakashchandra M. Rao, MD, FACS
Clinical Associate Professor of Surgery
New York Medical College
New York, New York

Albert Samadi, MD
Assistant Professor of Urology
New York Medical College
Department of Urology
Our Lady of Mercy Medical Center
Bronx, New York

Aloysius Smith, MD
Assistant Professor of Surgery
New York Medical College
Director, Hand and Plastic Surgery
Lincoln Medical and Mental Health Center
Our Lady of Mercy Medical Center
Bronx, New York

Kamran Tabaddor, MD
Clinical Professor and Chairman
Department of Surgery
Our Lady of Mercy Medical Center
Clinical Professor of Neurosurgery
Albert Einstein College of Medicine
Bronx, New York

Tyr Ohling Wilbanks, MD, FACS
Assistant Clinical Professor of Surgery
Columbia University College of Physicians
    and Surgeons
Associate Chief of Surgery
Lincoln Medical and Mental Health Center
Bronx, New York

Preface

The popularity of the previous editions of *Appleton & Lange Review of Surgery* has encouraged this revised fifth edition. The questions have been selected from the most current pertinent topics, facets, and principles of the wide range of general surgery and its specialities.

The main format of question presentation has been extensively revised to coincide with that recommended by the United States Medical License Examination (USMLE) guidelines. The material is presented in the form of clinical cases with appropriate answers to mirror the focus of the USMLE Step 2. *Lange Q&A: Surgery, Fifth Edition,* will also help equip and familiarize students preparing for the Surgery Miniboard Examinations. Surgical residents have found both the questions and the annotated answers useful in preparation for various inservice examinations leading to the qualifying and certifying exams of the American Board of Surgery and equivalent examinations in other parts of the world. Surgeons in practice and those preparing for recertification in their specialty have found this book to be a useful addendum to their armamentarium of surgical knowledge.

The types of questions have been arranged into two major groupings: one best answer out of five possible answers and the selection of one possible answers chosen from a given list of seven or more items. These question types are explained further in the introduction.

The questions are divided into 14 chapters including the practice test. The reader is encouraged to tackle each chapter in full before referring to the corresponding answer section. Each question should be completed in less than 1 minute. When correcting a chapter, the reader should review the answer and refer back to the question to consolidate knowledge gained during test preparation. Incorrect answers should be reviewed and attempted at a later date.

In many questions in the exam there is a lot of information in the stem of the question, much of it irrelevant. A number of our student consultants suggest that it is useful to look at the question and possible answers at the bottom of the question before reading the question through. This will assist you in deciding what information is pertinent. The examination developed by the USMLE contains 100 questions and the persons taking the test are given 2 hours to complete the exam. Many of our student consultants have indicated that they felt rushed with the examination. Another strategy is to answer the one best answer matching set of questions first. Such questions are usually placed at the end of the examination. These are generally done more quickly and usually help the test taker to complete the 100-question exam within the 2 hours of the allotted time.

If you have any comments as to the contents or usefulness of this book, e-mail gcayten@olmhs.org.

Acknowledgments

I would like to acknowledge the hard work and expertise of our authors. We had considerable input by medical students that had taken the USMLE Step 2 recently. These medical students helped us in assuring the content was pertinent to the exam. They also helped us in assuring the format of our questions was consistent with the exam. These medical students include James Wyss, Memba Penn, Christina Lemoine, Daniel Morello, William So, Keli Mabbott, and Alexandra Stark. We also had several young physicians assist in various editorial functions: Ravi Kumar Pasupuleti, and Cesar A. Mora. Dr. Ravikumar was particularly diligent and meticulous in his assistance.

I also would like to acknowledge the contributors to the fourth edition: Drs. Kenneth A. Falvo, Jaroslaw Bilaniuk, Haroon H. Durrani, John A. Savino, Zahi E. Nassoura, Scott I. Zeitlin, Jose A. Torres-Gluck, Khawaja Azimuddin, and Virany Huynh Hillard.

Special acknowledgement goes to Adriane Pratt, our Surgical Residency Coordinator at Our Lady of Mercy Medical Center. Very special acknowledgement goes to Marsha Loeb from McGraw-Hill who was thorough, patient, and insightful in her editorial functions.

Introduction

This book has been designed to help you review surgery for both examination and patient management. Here in one package is a comprehensive review with over 1000 multiple-choice questions with paragraph-length discussions of each answer. The whole book has been designed to help you assess your areas of relative strength and weakness.

Lange Q&A: Surgery, Fifth Edition, is divided into 14 chapters. Thirteen chapters provide a review of the major areas of surgery. The last chapter, a Practice Test, integrates diverse specialities into one simulated examination.

This introduction provides information on question types, question-taking strategies, various ways you can use this book, and specific information on the USMLE Step 2.

QUESTIONS

The USMLE Step 2 now contains only two different types of questions. In general, most of these are "one-best-answer–single-item" questions; whereas, the remainder require selection of one answer from a list of seven or more items. "Multiple true–false item" and "comparison–matching set" questions have been excluded. Questions that are negatively phrased ("All of the following are correct EXCEPT . . .") have been disposed of in accordance with current USMLE guidelines. In some cases (in both types of questions), a group of two or three questions may be related to a situational theme. Certain questions have illustrative material (diagrams and x-rays) that require understanding and interpretation on your part. Some illustrations, however, are included mainly for their instructive value in clinical surgical practice.

Questions are stratified into three levels of difficulty: (a) rote memory questions; (b) memory questions that require more understanding of the question; and (c) questions that require understanding and judgement. Because the National Board of Medical Examiners (NBME) and other examination bodies are moving away from the rote memory questions, we have tried to emphasize judgement cases throughout this text.

One-Best-Answer–Single-Item Question

This type of question presents a problem or asks a question and is followed by five or more choices, only one of which is entirely correct. The directions preceding this type of question will generally appear as follows:

DIRECTIONS: (Questions 1 through 82): Each of the numbered items in this section is followed by answer. Select the ONE lettered answer is BEST in each case.

An example for this item type is:

1. An obese 21-year-old woman reports increased growth of coarse hair on her lip, chin, chest, and abdomen. She also notes menstrual irregularity, with periods of amenorrhea. What is the most likely cause?

    (A) Polycystic ovary disease
    (B) An ovarian tumor
    (C) An adrenal tumor
    (D) Cushing's disease
    (E) Familial hirsutism

In this type of question, choices other than the correct answer may be partially correct, but there can only be one *best* answer. In the question above the key word is "most." Although ovarian tumors, adrenal tumors, and Cushing's disease are causes of hirsutism (described in the stem of the question), polycystic ovary disease is a much more common cause. Familial hirsutism is not associated with the menstrual irregularities mentioned. Thus, the *most* likely cause of the manifestations described can only be "(A) Polycystic ovary disease."

TABLE 1. STRATEGIES FOR ANSWERING ONE-BEST-ANSWER–SINGLE-ITEM QUESTIONS*

1. Remember that only one choice can be the correct answer.
2. Read the question carefully to be sure that you understand what is being asked.
3. Quickly read each choice for familiarity. (This important step is often not done by test takers.)
4. Go back and consider each choice individually.
5. If a choice is partially correct, tentatively consider it to be incorrect. (This step will help you lessen your choices and increase your odds of choosing the correct answer.)
6. Consider the remaining choices and select the one you think is the answer. At this point, you may want to quickly scan the stem to be sure you understand the question and your answer.
7. Select the appropriate answer. (Even if you do not know the answer, you should at least guess. Your score is based on the number of correct answers, **so do not skip any questions.**)

*Note the steps 2 through 7 should take an average of 50 seconds total. The actual examination is timed for an average of 50 seconds per question.

One-Best-Answer–Matching-Set Questions

These questions are usually accompanied by the following general directions.

DIRECTIONS: (Questions 83 through 100): Each set of matching questions in this section consists of a list of lettered options followed by several numbered items. For each numbered item, select the appropriate lettered option. Select only one answer.

An example for this item type is:

Questions 83 through 84

In each condition listed, select the most appropriate antibiotics.

- (A) Tetracycline
- (B) Chloramphenicol
- (C) Clindamycin
- (D) Vancoymcin
- (E) Fluconazole
- (F) Metronidazole
- (G) Ciprofloxacin
- (H) Chloroquine
- (I) Fluconazole

83. Bone marrow suppression. SELECT ONLY ONE.

84. A 34-year-old woman complains of lower abdominal pain and vaginal discharge due to gonorrhea. SELECT ONLY ONE.

Table 2 lists strategies for answering one-best-answer-matching-set questions.

TABLE 2. STRATEGIES FOR ANSWERING ONE-BEST-ANSWER–MATCHING-SET QUESTIONS*

1. Remember that the lettered choices are followed by the numbered questions.
2. Apply steps 2 through 7 in Table 1 but select EXACTLY ONE ANSWER as stated.
3. Consider covering this section first in the beginning of the test, you'll likely be less rushed and thus the probability of answering these questions correctly when you have time is increased vs. answering them at the end when you're rushed and you must reuse answer choices A–M.

*Remember, you only have an average of 60 seconds per question.

ANSWERS, EXPLANATIONS, AND REFERENCES

In each of the sections of *Lange Q&A: Surgery, Fifth Edition,* the question sections are followed by a section containing the answers and explanations for the questions. This section: (a) tells you the answer to each question; and (b) gives you an explanation and review of why the answer is correct, background information on the subject matter, and/or why the other answers are incorrect. We encourage you to use this section as a basis for further study and understanding.

If you choose the correct answer to a question, you can then read the explanation: (a) for reinforcement; and (b) to add to your knowledge about the subject matter. If you choose the wrong answer to a question, you can read the explanation for an instructional review of the material in the question.

PRACTICE TEST

The 100-question Practice Test at the end of the book covers and reviews all the topics covered in Chapters 1 through 13. The questions are integrated according to question type (one-best-answer–single item, one-best-answer–matching sets.)

HOW TO USE THIS BOOK

There are two logical ways to get the most value from this book. We call them Plan A and Plan B.

In **Plan A**, you go straight to the Practice Test and complete it. Analyze your areas of strength and weakness. This will be a good indicator of your initial knowledge of the subject and will help to identify specific areas for preparation and review. You can now use the first 13 chapters of the book to help you improve your relative weak points.

In **Plan B**, you go through Chapters 1 through 13 checking off your answers, and then comparing your choices with the answers and discussions in the book. Once you have completed this process, you can take the Practice Test and see how well prepared you are. If you still have a major weakness, it should be apparent in time for you to take remedial action.

In Plan A, by taking the Practice Test first, you get quick feedback regarding your initial areas of strength and weakness. You may find that you have a good command of the material, indicating that perhaps only a cursory review of the first 13 chapters is necessary. This, of course, would be good to know early in your examination preparation. On the other hand, you may find that you have many areas of weakness. In this case, you could focus on these areas in your review—not just with this book, but also with textbooks.

However, it is unlikely that you will not do some studying before taking the USMLE (especially because you have this book). Therefore, it may be more realistic to take the Practice Test after you have reviewed the first 13 chapters (as in Plan B). This will probably give you a more realistic type of testing situation, because very few of us sit down to a test without study. In this case, you will have done some reviewing (from superficial to in-depth), and your Practice Test will reflect this study time. If, after reviewing the first 13 chapters and then taking the Practice Test, you still have some weaknesses, you can then go back through Chapters 1 through 13 and supplement your review with your texts.

SPECIFIC INFORMATION ON THE STEP II EXAMINATION

The official source of all information with respect to the USMLE is the NBME, 3750 Market Street, Philadelphia, PA 19104. Established in 1915, the NBME is a voluntary, nonprofit, independent organization whose sole function is the design, implementation, distribution, and processing of a vast bank of question items, certifying examinations, and evaluative services in the professional medical field.

To be eligible to sit for the USMLE Step 2, a person must be either officially enrolled in or a graduate of a U.S. or Canadian Medical School accredited by the Liaison Committee on Medical Education (LCME); officially enrolled in or a graduate of a US osteopathic medical school accredited by the American Osteopathic Association (AOA); or officially enrolled in or a graduate of a foreign medical school and eligible for examination by the Educational Commission for Foreign Medical Graduates (ECFMG) for its certificate. It is not necessary to complete any particular year of medical school in order to be a candidate for Step 2; neither is it required to take Step 1 before Step 2.

SCORING

Because there is no penalty for guessing, you should answer every question. Do not skip any questions. Each question answered correctly counts as one point, and partial credit may be given to partially correct answers.

Information on the USMLE is posted on the NBME's web page, www.usmle.org.

CHAPTER 1

Surgical Critical Care / Pre- and Postoperative Care

Nanakram Agarwal and Akella Chendrasekhar

Questions

DIRECTIONS (Questions 1 through 108): Each of the numbered items in this section is followed by five answers. Select the ONE lettered answer that is BEST in each case.

1. A 35-year-old man is admitted with systolic blood pressure (BP) of 60 mm Hg and a heart rate (HR) of 150 bpm following a gunshot wound to the liver (Fig. 1–1). What is the effect on the kidneys?

    (A) They tolerate satisfactorily ischemia of 3–4 hours duration.

    (B) They undergo further ischemia if hypothermia is present.

    (C) They can become damaged, even though urine output exceeds 1500 mL/d.

    (D) They are affected and cause an increased creatinine clearance.

    (E) They are prevented from further damage by a vasopressor.

2. Twenty-four hours after colon resection, urine output in a 70-year-old man is 10 mL/h. Blood chemistry analysis reveals sodium, 138 mEq/L; potassium, 6 mEq/L; chloride, 100 mEq/L; bicarbonate, 14 mEq/L. His metabolic abnormality is characterized by which of the following?

    (A) Abdominal distension

    (B) Peaked T waves

    (C) Narrow QRS complex

    (D) Cardiac arrest in systole

    (E) J wave or Osborne wave

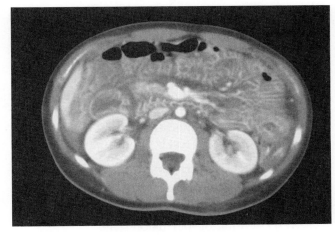

Figure 1–1.
Axial image of **Computed tomography** (CT) scan of abdomen at level of both kidneys shows dense nephrogram, which is attributed to decrease in renal perfusion. *(Reproduced, with permission, from Wapnick S et al.: Appleton and Lange Review of Surgery, 4th ed. 31. McGraw-Hill, 2003.)*

3. A 24-year-old woman has acute renal failure following postpartum hemorrhage. Laboratory studies showed serum glucose, 150 mg/dL; sodium, 135 mEq/L; potassium, 6.5 mEq/L; chloride, 105 mEq/L; and bicarbonate, 15 mEq/L. Therapy should include which of the following?

    (A) Decrease potassium chloride to 10 mEq/L

    (B) Intravenous 0.9% sodium chloride

    (C) 100 mL of 50% glucose water with 10 U insulin

    (D) Intravenous calcitonin

    (E) Intravenous magnesium sulfate

4. A 55-year-old man with Crohn's disease had undergone resection of small bowel and anastomosis. Ten days later, he is found to have bilious drainage of 1 L/d from the drains. He is started on total parenteral nutrition (TPN). Four days later, his arterial blood gases (ABGs) are pH, 7.25; PO_2, 98 mm Hg; and PCO_2, 40 mm Hg. His anion gap is 10. The most likely cause is which of the following?

(A) Diabetic ketoacidosis
(B) Renal failure
(C) Hypovolemic shock
(D) Small-bowel fistula
(E) Uncompensated metabolic alkalosis

5. A 55-year-old man sustains numerous injuries involving the abdomen and lower extremities. During the intra- and postoperative periods, he is resuscitated with 10 L of Ringer's lactate and 2 U of packed red blood cells (RBC). After initial improvement, he has severe dyspnea on the second postoperative day. The most useful initial diagnostic test is which of the following?

(A) Electrocardiogram
(B) Analysis of arterial blood gas
(C) Insertion of a central venous line
(D) Ventilation-perfusion scan
(E) Computed tomography (CT) scan of abdomen

6. A 20-year-old man involved in a car crash sustained severe injuries to the chest, abdomen, and lower extremities. He is intubated and requires increasing concentration of oxygen to maintain his PO_2. The pathologic changes do which of the following?

(A) They cause the alveolar capillary membrane to become more impermeable.
(B) They most frequently occur after severe injuries.
(C) They are associated with low compliance.
(D) They show a characteristic localized pattern on x-ray.
(E) They involve a decrease in dead-space ventilation.

7. A 24-year-old woman is scheduled for an elective cholecystectomy. The best method of identifying a potential bleeder is which of the following?

(A) Platelet count
(B) A complete history and physical examination
(C) Bleeding time
(D) Lee-White clotting time
(E) Prothrombin time (PT)

8. A 24-year-old man who is admitted to the intensive care unit (ICU) following severe head injury develops seizures on the fourth day of hospitalization. His urine output is 500 mL over 24 hours, sodium is 115 mEq/L, and serum and urine osmolality are 250 and 800 mOsm, respectively. The metabolic abnormality is due to which of the following?

(A) Administration of D_5W (5% dextrose in water) and 0.33 normal saline
(B) Syndrome of inappropriate secretion of antidiuretic hormone (SIADH)
(C) Decreased antidiuretic hormone (ADH) secretion
(D) Nasogastric suction
(E) Renal insufficiency

9. A 40-year-old man who weighs 65 kg is being observed in the ICU. Twenty-four hours postoperatively, he develops convulsions. His serum sodium is 118 mEq/L. Appropriate management includes which of the following?

(A) Administration of normal saline (0.9%)
(B) Administration of hypertonic saline (3%)
(C) Emergency hemodialysis
(D) Administration of vasopressin
(E) Administration of Lasix, 40 mg intravenously (IV)

10. A 30-year-old man who weighs 60 kg has the following laboratory values: hemoglobin, 10 g/dL; serum sodium, 120 mEq/L; serum potassium, 4 mEq/L; serum chloride, 90 mEq/L; and serum CO_2 content, 30 mEq/L. What is his sodium deficit approximately?

(A) 20 mEq
(B) 200 mEq
(C) 400 mEq
(D) 720 mEq
(E) 120 mEq

11. A 65-year-old man has urine output of 10 mL/h following abdominal aortic aneurysmectomy. Acute tubular necrosis is suggested by the presence of which of the following?

(A) Urine osmolality of more than 500 mOsm/kg
(B) Urine sodium of more than 40 mEq/L
(C) Fractional excretion of sodium of <1%
(D) Blood urea nitrogen (BUN)-to-serum creatinine ratio (SCR) of more than 20
(E) Urine-to-plasma creatinine ratio (PCR) of more than 40

12. A 30-year-old man with a history of Crohn's disease of the small bowel is admitted with enterocutaneous fistula. The daily output from the fistula is 2 L. The approximate composition of the fluids in mEq/L is which of the following?

	Na	K	Cl	HCO3
(A)	10	26	10	30
(B)	60	10	130	0
(C)	140	5	104	30
(D)	140	5	75	115
(E)	60	30	40	40

13. A 70-year-old woman has a small-bowel fistula with output of 1.5 L/d. Replacement of daily losses should be handled using the fluid solution that has the following composition in mEq/L.

	Na	K	Cl	HCO3
(A)	130	4	109	28
(B)	154	0	154	40
(C)	77	0	77	0
(D)	167	0	0	167
(E)	513	0	513	0

Questions 14 and 15

A 70-year-old man has undergone anterior resection for carcinoma of the rectum. He is extubated in the operating room (OR). In the recovery room, he is found to be restless with an HR of 136 bpm and a BP of 144/80 mm Hg. ABG analysis on room air reveals pH, 7.24; PCO_2, 60 mm Hg; PO_2, 54 mm Hg; HCO_3, 25 mEq/L; and SaO_2, 90%.

14. The physiologic status can best be described as which of the following?

(A) Respiratory alkalosis
(B) Respiratory acidosis
(C) Metabolic acidosis
(D) Metabolic alkalosis
(E) Combined respiratory and metabolic acidosis

15. Appropriate management for this patient should be which of the following?

(A) To administer 40% oxygen by mask
(B) Morphine, 2 mg IV
(C) Ringer's lactate, 250 mL over 1 hour
(D) Intubation and ventilatory support
(E) Deep breathing and coughing

16. A 60-year-old woman with mild hypertension is admitted for elective hysterectomy. On preoperative evaluation, she is found to have osteoarthritis; over the previous 6 months, she had noted watery diarrhea that was becoming progressively worse. The serum potassium is 3 mEq/L. Which is the most likely cause of hypokalemia?

(A) Myoglobinemia
(B) Villous adenoma of colon
(C) High-output renal failure
(D) Massive blood transfusion
(E) Spironolactone (Aldactone)

Questions 17 and 18

A 64-year-old man underwent major abdominal surgery to remove a ruptured aortic aneurysm. Four days after the operation, an attempt was made to wean him off the ventilator. ABG analysis reveals pH, 7.54; PCO_2, 30 mm Hg; PO_2, 110 mm Hg; HCO_3, 30 mEq/L; and SaO_2, 99%.

17. Blood gas analysis reveals which of the following?

    (A) Respiratory acidosis
    (B) Metabolic alkalosis
    (C) Respiratory alkalosis
    (D) Compensated respiratory acidosis
    (E) Combined respiratory and metabolic alkalosis

18. What will be the most likely complication due to the metabolic changes experienced by the patient?

    (A) Hypokalemia
    (B) Shift of oxyhemoglobin dissociation to the right
    (C) Hyperkalemia
    (D) Hypercalcemia
    (E) Hyperchloremia

19. A 42-year-old man with small-bowel fistula has been receiving TPN with standard hypertonic glucose-amino acid solution for 3 weeks. The patient is noticed to have scaly, hyperpigmented lesions over the acral surfaces of elbows and knees, similar to enterohepatic acrodermatitis. What is the most likely cause of the condition?

    (A) Copper deficiency
    (B) Essential fatty acid deficiency
    (C) Excess glucose calories
    (D) Hypomagnesemia
    (E) Zinc deficiency

Questions 20 through 22

A 27-year-old man is involved in a car crash while traveling in excess of 70 mi/h. He sustains an intra-abdominal injury and a fracture of the femur. The BP is 60/40 mm Hg, and the hematocrit is 16%.

20. Which physiologic changes will ensue?

    (A) Peripheral vasodilation
    (B) Inhibition of sympathetic tone
    (C) Temperature rise to 103.8°F
    (D) Eosinophilia
    (E) Lactic acidosis

21. There is likely to be a proportionately greater increase in blood flow to which of the following?

    (A) Kidneys
    (B) Liver
    (C) Heart
    (D) Skin
    (E) Thyroid gland

22. Initial resuscitation is best done by administration of which of the following?

    (A) D_5W
    (B) D_5W and 0.45% normal saline
    (C) Ringer's lactate solution
    (D) 5% plasma protein solution
    (E) 5% hydroxyethyl starch solution

23. A 30-year-old man is brought to the emergency department following a high-speed car accident. He was the driver, and the windshield of the car was broken. On examination, he is alert, awake, oriented, and in no respiratory distress. He is unable to move any of his four extremities; however, his extremities are warm and pink. His vital signs on admission are HR 54 bpm and BP 70/40 mm Hg. What is the diagnosis?

    (A) Hemorrhagic shock
    (B) Cardiogenic shock
    (C) Neurogenic shock
    (D) Septic shock
    (E) Irreversible shock

Questions 24 through 28

A 48-year-old man with severe vomiting as a result of gastric outlet obstruction is admitted to the hospital. There is marked dehydration, with urine output 20 mL/h, and the hematocrit is 48%.

24. Clinical confirmation of pyloric obstruction is most readily established by which of the following?

   (A) Observation of peristalsis from left to right
   (B) Observation of peristalsis from right to left
   (C) Percussion of the upper abdomen
   (D) Succussion splash
   (E) Auscultation of the upper left abdomen

25. What is the predominant metabolic abnormality?

   (A) Aspiration pneumonia with respiratory alkalosis
   (B) Hypochloremic alkalosis
   (C) Salt-losing enteropathy
   (D) Intrinsic renal disease
   (E) Metabolic acidosis

26. Initial treatment for this patient should include which of the following?

   (A) Administration of 10% dextrose ($D_{10}W$) in one-third saline solution IV
   (B) Antiemetic
   (C) Hemodialysis to correct azotemia
   (D) Saline fluid replacement with appropriate potassium administration
   (E) Ringer's lactate solution

27. Severe hypochloremic metabolic alkalosis fails to respond to standard therapy. His metabolic abnormality can be corrected by infusing which of the following?

   (A) Normal saline
   (B) Ringer's lactate solution
   (C) Hypertonic saline
   (D) 0.1 N hydrochloric acid
   (E) 1 N hydrochloric acid

28. In the absence of malignancy, further treatment after appropriate resuscitation should include which of the following?

   (A) Jejunostomy feeding
   (B) Vagotomy and drainage
   (C) Steroids
   (D) No foods given orally (PO) for 6 weeks
   (E) Pyloromyotomy alone

Questions 29 through 31

During cholecystectomy in a 67-year-old woman, there is severe bleeding from accidental injury to the hepatic artery. The patient requires transfusion of 2000 mL of blood. After the operation, 24-hour urine output varies between 1250 and 2700 mL/d. She was adequately hydrated, but BUN levels continue to rise 10–12 mg daily over a 5-day period.

29. What is the main finding?

   (A) Progressive bleeding
   (B) High-output renal failure
   (C) Postcholecystectomy syndrome
   (D) Glomerulonephritis
   (E) Obstructive jaundice

30. Metabolic changes likely to occur include which of the following?

   (A) Hyperkalemia
   (B) Hyponatremia
   (C) Hypophosphatemia
   (D) Metabolic alkalosis
   (E) Hypomagnesemia

31. Management includes which of the following?

   (A) Restriction of fluids to 750 mL/d
   (B) 8 L of fluid daily to remove urea
   (C) Replacement of fluid loss plus insensible loss
   (D) 80 mEq potassium chloride (KCl) per 12 hour
   (E) Ammonium chloride IV

Questions 32 and 33

A 14-year-old boy with a known bleeding tendency since infancy has severe epistaxis. Examination reveals an equinus contracture of the right leg and a large hemarthrosis.

32. What is the most likely diagnosis?

    (A) Diethylstilbestrol (DES) was taken by the mother during pregnancy
    (B) Aplastic anemia
    (C) Henoch-Schönlein purpura
    (D) Hemophilia
    (E) Wilson's disease with cirrhosis

33. Treatment should include which of the following?

    (A) Penicillamine
    (B) Transfusion of factor VIII to 30% of normal factor levels
    (C) Transfusion of factor VIII to 10% of normal factor levels
    (D) Platelet transfusion
    (E) Exploration of joint

34. A 10-year-old boy with history of prolonged bleeding after minor injury is scheduled for tonsillectomy. The bleeding time, PT, and fibrinogen are normal. What would be the most helpful investigation?

    (A) Fibrinolysis (euglobulin clot lysis time)
    (B) Platelet count
    (C) Thrombin time
    (D) Partial thromboplastin time (PTT)
    (E) Factor VII assay

Questions 35 to 37

A 22-year-old man is brought into the emergency department in profound shock after a fall from the fourth floor of a building. After resuscitation, small-bowel resection and hepatic segmentectomy are performed at laparotomy. He receives 15 U of packed RBCs, 4 U of fresh-frozen plasma, and 8 L of Ringer's lactate. On closure, diffuse oozing of blood is noted.

35. What is the most likely cause?

    (A) Hepatic failure
    (B) Hypersplenism
    (C) Platelet deficiency
    (D) Factor IX (Christmas factor) deficiency
    (E) Congenital hypoprothrombinemia

36. Which test is most likely to be helpful in management of this patient?

    (A) Platelet count
    (B) Bone marrow biopsy
    (C) Liver-spleen scan
    (D) Factor VIII assay
    (E) Smear for Howell-Jolly bodies

37. Bleeding persists despite all appropriate blood coagulant replacement, and laparotomy reveals multiple sites of bleeding from the liver and the rest of the abdomen. Treatment should include which of the following?

    (A) Hepatic artery ligation
    (B) Packing with laparotomy towels
    (C) Immediate closure
    (D) A large dose of heparin
    (E) Solu-Medrol, 1 g IV

38. A 50-year-old suffering from chronic alcoholism is admitted to the hospital. He has muscle tremors and hyperactive tendon reflexes. Serum magnesium is 1.8 mEq/L (normal 1.5–2.5 mEq/L). Concerning magnesium, which of the following statements is true?

    (A) It is mainly extracellular
    (B) Excess may cause a positive Chvostek's sign (carpopedal spasm)
    (C) Deficiency is treated with parenteral bicarbonate
    (D) Symptoms are due to deficiency of magnesium
    (E) It may become elevated in acute pancreatitis

Questions 39 and 40

A 30-year-old man with multiple injuries has severe renal insufficiency. On the third day of hospitalization, he is lethargic with generalized weakness and decreased deep tendon reflexes. An electrocardiogram (ECG) reveals a widened QRS complex with elevated T waves.

39. What is the most likely cause of the patient's condition?

   (A) Hypokalemia
   (B) Hyponatremia
   (C) Hypermagnesemia
   (D) Hypocalcemia
   (E) Hypophosphatemia

40. What should be the immediate management of the patient?

   (A) Administration of potassium chloride
   (B) Administration of calcium chloride
   (C) Restriction of fluid intake
   (D) Use of Kayexylate enemas
   (E) Administration of hypertonic saline

41. A 45-year-old male with a known history of alcoholism is admitted with acute pancreatitis. His serum calcium is 7 mg/dL. Management is based upon which of the following?

   (A) One-fourth of calcium in serum is ionized
   (B) Alkalosis increases the ionized calcium component
   (C) Hypocalcemia may cause polyuria and polydypsia
   (D) Determination of serum albumin is necessary
   (E) Treatment should involve intravenous administration of calcium chloride

42. A 36-year-old diabetic woman develops metabolic changes following salpingo-oophorectomy. Serum osmolality of the blood can be calculated from serum values of which of the following?

   (A) Sodium, potassium, chloride, and bicarbonate
   (B) Sodium, potassium, urea, and hemoglobin
   (C) Sodium, potassium, glucose, and urea
   (D) Sodium, albumin, urea, and glucose
   (E) Sodium, potassium, albumin, and glucose

43. In a 12-year-old boy who sustained severe head injury caused by a fall from the third floor of a building, the syndrome of diabetes insipidus is characterized by which of the following?

   (A) Low serum sodium
   (B) High urinary specific gravity or osmolality
   (C) High serum osmolality
   (D) Low urine output
   (E) Expanded extracellular fluid volume

44. In a 40-year-old woman receiving TPN for small-bowel fistula, what finding can be attributed to hypophosphatemia?

   (A) Increased cardiac output
   (B) Diarrhea
   (C) Increased energy production
   (D) Rhabdomyolysis
   (E) Increased white blood cells (WBC) function

Questions 45 and 46

A 60-year-old woman who underwent a mastectomy for breast cancer 2 years earlier presents to the emergency department with headache, backache, and frequent vomiting. She is extremely thirsty and stuporous.

45. Which test is most likely to identify the cause?

   (A) CT scan of the head
   (B) X-ray of spine
   (C) Serum sodium determination
   (D) Serum calcium determination
   (E) Serum glucose determination

46. What should be the initial management of the patient?

   (A) Restrict fluid intake
   (B) Normal saline infusion
   (C) D_5W infusion
   (D) Thiazide
   (E) Hemodialysis

47. A 40-year-old man is found to have severe metabolic acidosis with a high anion gap. What is the most likely cause?

    (A) Diarrhea
    (B) Methanol ingestion
    (C) Proximal renal tubular acidosis
    (D) Distal renal tubular acidosis
    (E) Ureterosigmoidostomy

48. An 18-month-old boy slipped and hurt his right knee while walking. He presents with a tender, swollen, warm knee with significant hemarthrosis. His PT is 12 (normal, 13 seconds), PTT is over 100 (normal, 25 seconds), platelet count is 300,000/mm³, and bleeding time is normal. Initial management should consist of which of the following?

    (A) Fresh-frozen plasma
    (B) Aspiration of knee
    (C) Factor VIII concentrate
    (D) Passive exercise
    (E) Long-leg cast

49. A 30-year-old woman with a history of an uneventful tonsillectomy at age four is scheduled for exploratory laparotomy. Preoperative assessment that identifies the risk of intraoperative bleeding is which of the following?

    (A) Bleeding time
    (B) Platelet count
    (C) PT and PTT
    (D) Complete blood cell count
    (E) Obtaining a detailed history

50. A 43-year-old woman with von Willebrand's disease is scheduled for cholecystectomy. It can be stated that preoperative evaluation will reveal which of the following?

    (A) Normal bleeding time, PT, and PTT
    (B) Platelet aggregate with restocetin
    (C) Increased bleeding time and PTT, and normal PT
    (D) Increased bleeding time and PT, and normal PTT
    (E) Increased bleeding time, and normal PT and PTT

51. Following admission to the emergency department, a 26-year-old woman with severe menorrhagia states that both her father and sister have a bleeding disorder. The hemostatic disorder transmitted by autosomal-dominant mode is which of the following?

    (A) Factor X deficiency
    (B) von Willebrand's disease
    (C) Factor VIII deficiency (true hemophilia)
    (D) Factor IX deficiency (Christmas disease)
    (E) Factor V deficiency (parahemophilia)

52. A 75-year-old man is found to have prolonged bleeding from intravenous puncture sites. Platelet aggregation is inhibited by which of the following?

    (A) Adenosine diphosphate (ADP)
    (B) Calcium
    (C) Magnesium
    (D) Aspirin
    (E) Serotonin

53. A 45-year-old woman with deep vein thrombosis is taking warfarin (Coumadin), 5 mg/d. Seven days after initiation of therapy, she has warfarin-induced skin necrosis. Which of the following statements regarding this condition is true?

    (A) It commonly occurs after warfarin therapy.
    (B) It usually involves the upper extremities.
    (C) It improves with an increase in the dose of Coumadin.
    (D) It improves with a decrease in the dose of Coumadin.
    (E) It requires cessation of Coumadin and infusion of heparin.

54. A 50-year-old man with atrial fibrillation is taking warfarin (Coumadin). The effect of Coumadin is decreased by which of the following?

    (A) The presence of vitamin K deficiency
    (B) Phenylbutazone
    (C) Quinidine
    (D) Barbiturates
    (E) Thyrotoxicosis

55. After undergoing a transurethral resection of the prostate, a 65-year-old man experiences excessive bleeding attributed to fibrinolysis. It is appropriate to administer which of the following?

(A) Heparin
(B) Warfarin (Coumadin)
(C) Volume expanders and cryoprecipitate
(D) Aminocaproic acid (Amicar)
(E) Fresh-frozen plasma and vitamin K

Questions 56 and 57

A 64-year-old woman undergoing radical hysterectomy under general anesthesia is transfused with 2 U of packed RBCs.

56. A hemolytic transfusion reaction during anesthesia will be characterized by which of the following?

(A) Shaking chills and muscle spasms
(B) Fever and oliguria
(C) Hyperpyrexia and hypotension
(D) Tachycardia and cyanosis
(E) Bleeding and hypotension

57. The specific test to identify the cause of transfusion reaction for the patient is which of the following?

(A) PT
(B) PTT
(C) Platelet count
(D) Bleeding time
(E) Free plasma hemoglobin

58. A 41-year-old woman has an episode of mild right upper quadrant (RUQ) pain associated with jaundice that resolves completely with antibiotics. Workup reveals numerous large stones in the gallbladder. The patient has polycythemia vera, a hematocrit of 58%, and a platelet count of 1.8 million. What is the preferred course of treatment for this patient?

(A) She should be referred to the medical clinic for follow-up care and be observed.
(B) She should undergo phlebotomy and then be scheduled for cholecystectomy.

(C) She should be treated with chlorambucil for 6 weeks and then undergo cholecystectomy.
(D) She should receive miniheparin and urgent cholecystectomy.
(E) She should undergo cholecystectomy.

59. A 56-year-old man underwent prostatectomy. He bled excessively and urgently required blood over and above what had been requested before surgery. In deciding on an appropriate blood transfusion protocol, what should be kept in mind?

(A) Group AB is the universal donor.
(B) Serum from the recipient stored for 1 week is suitable for testing.
(C) Hypothermia is indicated if cryoglobulin is found.
(D) Cross-matching should be done before dextran administration.
(E) Fresh-frozen plasma can be given instead of 4 U of packed cells.

60. A 60-year-old man with carcinoma of the esophagus is admitted with severe malnutrition. Nutritional support is to be initiated. What should be his daily caloric intake?

(A) 1 kcal/kg body weight/day
(B) 5 kcal/kg body weight/day
(C) 15 kcal/kg body weight/day
(D) 30 kcal/kg body weight/day
(E) 100 kcal/kg body weight/day

61. TPN is initiated in a 44-year-old woman with Crohn's disease. In parenteral alimentation, carbohydrates should be provided in an optimal ratio of which of the following?

(A) 1 kcal/g nitrogen
(B) 5 kcal/g nitrogen
(C) 10 kcal/g nitrogen
(D) 100 kcal/g nitrogen
(E) 1000 kcal/g nitrogen

62. After undergoing subtotal gastrectomy for carcinoma of the stomach, a 64-year-old woman is receiving peripheral parenteral nutrition. To increase calories by the peripheral route, what should be prescribed?

(A) D_5W in normal saline
(B) Multivitamin infusion
(C) $D_{25}W$ (25% dextrose in water)
(D) Soybean oil
(E) Lactulose

63. A 35-year-old man with duodenal stump leak after partial gastrectomy is receiving central parenteral nutrition containing the standard $D_{25}W$, 4.25% amino acid solution. Which is TRUE of essential fatty acid deficiency seen after hyperalimentation?

(A) It occurs if soybean oil is given only once weekly.
(B) It is usually noted at the end of the first week.
(C) It causes dry scaly skin with loss of hair.
(D) It is accompanied by hypercholesterolemia.
(E) It is treated with insulin.

64. In metabolic alkalosis, there is which of the following?

(A) Gain in fixed acid
(B) Loss of base
(C) Hyperkalemia
(D) Rise in base excess
(E) Hyperchloremia

65. Following urinary tract infection associated with extraction of a bladder stone, a 64-year-old woman developed gram-negative septicemia. Which statement is true for gram-negative bacterial septicemia?

(A) *Pseudomonas* is the most common organism isolated.
(B) Many of the adverse changes can be accounted for endotoxin release.
(C) The cardiac index is low.
(D) Central venous pressure (CVP) is high.
(E) Endotoxin is mainly a long-chain peptide.

66. In septic shock, which of the following is true?

(A) The mortality rate is between 10% and 20%.
(B) Gram-negative organisms are involved exclusively.
(C) The majority of patients are elderly.
(D) The most common source of infection is the alimentary tract.
(E) Two or more organisms are responsible in most cases.

67. A 68-year-old man has a history of myocardial infarction. He undergoes uneventful left hemicolectomy for carcinoma of the colon. In the recovery room, he is hypotensive and given a fluid bolus of 500 mL Ringer's lactate over 30 minutes. He is intubated, and his neck veins are distended. His HR is 130 bpm, his BP is 80/60 mm Hg, and his urine output is 20 mL over the last hour. What should be the next step in his management?

(A) Administration of Ringer's lactate, 500 mL over 1 hour
(B) Administration of dopamine
(C) Insertion of a Swan-Ganz catheter
(D) Administration of Lasix
(E) Extubation of the patient

68. A 75-year-old woman who is in the ICU after undergoing cholecystectomy for acute cholecystitis is hypotensive and tachycardic. Pulmonary capillary wedge pressure (PCWP) is elevated to 18 mm Hg, and cardiac output is 3 L/min. She is in shock best described as which of the following?

(A) Hypovolemic shock
(B) Septic shock
(C) Cardiogenic shock
(D) Anaphylactic shock
(E) Neurogenic shock

69. A 40-year-old woman with deep vein thrombosis is being treated with IV heparin, 1000 U/h. On the seventh day of treatment, her laboratory values are hemoglobin, 14 g/dL; WBC count, 7600/mm³; platelet count, 30,000/mm³; PT, 13 seconds (control, 12.5 seconds); and PTT,

50 seconds (control, 26 seconds). What management would be appropriate?

(A) Continue with heparin at the same dosage

(B) Increase heparin

(C) Decrease heparin

(D) Discontinue heparin

(E) Continue heparin and start warfarin (Coumadin)

70. A 55-year-old man involved in an automobile accident is unresponsive and is intubated at the scene. On arrival in the emergency department, he responds to painful stimulation. His systolic BP is 60 mm Hg, his HR is 140 bpm, his neck veins are distended, and his breath sounds are absent on the left side. Immediate management should involve which of the following?

(A) Insertion of a central venous line on the right side

(B) Insertion of an 18-gauge needle in the left second intercostal space

(C) Pericardiocentesis

(D) Peritoneal lavage

(E) CT scan of head

71. A 25-year-old man sustained laceration of the liver and rupture of the spleen in an automobile accident. He was hypotensive for more than 1 hour and received 10 L of crystalloids and 10 U of blood. On the second postoperative day, he is intubated, his HR is 120 bpm, his BP is 110/60 mm Hg, his urine output is 40 mL/h, and his CVP is 13 cm H_2O. His ABGs on 70% oxygen reveal a pH of 7.42, a PO_2 of 58 mm Hg, and a PCO_2 of 35 mm Hg. What is the most appropriate management?

(A) Increase the fraction of inspired oxygen (FiO_2).

(B) Increase the tidal volume (VT).

(C) Administer Lasix, 20 mg IV.

(D) Institute positive end-expiratory pressure (PEEP).

(E) Decrease FiO_2.

72. A 40-year-old paraplegic is taken to the OR for cholecystectomy for acute cholecystitis. She is given succinylcholine before intubation. Immediately after induction of anesthesia, she develops cardiac arrest. What is the most likely cause?

(A) Esophageal intubation

(B) Hyperkalemia

(C) Perforation of gallbladder

(D) Hypovolemic shock

(E) Myocardial infarction

73. A 70-year-old woman has low cardiac output with increased PCWP and increased systemic vascular resistance. What should be the drug of choice?

(A) Dopamine

(B) Norepinephrine

(C) Dobutamine

(D) Epinephrine

(E) Phenylephrine

74. A 60-year-old man had undergone exploratory laparotomy for perforated gastric ulcer with severe peritoneal contamination. Six hours after surgery, he is tachycardic, hypertensive, and has shallow respirations. Intubation and institution of ventilatory support is indicated in the presence of which of the following?

(A) Respiratory rate of 23 breaths/min

(B) $PaCO_2$ of 45 mm Hg

(C) PaO_2 of 55 mm Hg on room air

(D) HR of 140 bpm

(E) BP of 150/100 mm Hg

75. A 60-year-old man is being weaned from a ventilator in the ICU. The likelihood that weaning is going to fail is suggested by the presence of which of the following?

(A) A respiratory rate of 24 breaths/min

(B) A PaO_2 of 80 mm Hg on FiO_2 of 40%

(C) A vital capacity (VC) of 5 mL/kg body weight

(D) A minute ventilation of 8 L/min

(E) A maximum negative inspiratory pressure of –30 cm H_2O

76. A patient is being weaned from mechanical ventilation. Weaning parameters are obtained prior to deciding on extubation. Successful weaning from a ventilator is suggested by the presence of which of the following?

    (A) An alveolar arterial gradient of more than 350 mm Hg
    (B) A PaO_2/FiO_2 ratio of <200
    (C) A $PaCO_2$ over 55 mm Hg
    (D) A tidal volume of over 5 mL/kg
    (E) A minute ventilation of 12 L/min

77. A 55-year-old man with oat cell carcinoma of the lung is suspected to have SIADH. This is characterized by which of the following?

    (A) Decreased total body water (TBW)
    (B) Low serum sodium
    (C) Increased urine output
    (D) Urine sodium of <10 mEq/L
    (E) Low urinary specific gravity

78. Following surgery for a perforated appendix with generalized peritonitis and multiple intra-abdominal abscess, a 25-year-old man is admitted to the ICU. On the third postoperative day, he continues to be febrile and has a nasogastric tube. What is the metabolic characteristic seen in him?

    (A) A decrease in energy expenditure
    (B) Fat as his primary fuel
    (C) Respiratory quotient of 0.6–0.7
    (D) Proteolysis
    (E) Decreased hepatic synthesis of protein

79. Increase in energy expenditure by 100% over normal, or two times greater than normal, is seen in a patient with which of the following?

    (A) Pyloric obstruction from chronic duodenal ulcer
    (B) Fractured femur
    (C) Perforated diverticulitis of colon
    (D) Severe thermal burns of more than 30% total body surface area (BSA)
    (E) Right inguinal herniorrhaphy for incarcerated inguinal hernia

80. A 30-year-old man with a gunshot wound to the abdomen has severe injuries involving the liver, duodenum, pancreas, and colon. Why is parenteral nutrition support preferred over enteral nutrition support?

    (A) It is less expensive.
    (B) It preserves gut mucosal mass and mucosal immunity.
    (C) It prevents gut permeability and translocation.
    (D) It is easy to start and administer nutrient requirement rapidly.
    (E) It attenuates hypermetabolic response to surgery.

81. A 24-year-old man with multiple injuries is receiving standard TPN. The following is true regarding glutamine.

    (A) It is a major fuel for the brain.
    (B) It is an essential amino acid.
    (C) It is a major fuel for the gut.
    (D) It is synthesized de novo in the kidney.
    (E) It is a component of TPN solutions.

82. A 50-year-old man with small-bowel fistula has been receiving TPN for the previous 3 weeks through a single-lumen central venous catheter. He is scheduled for exploratory laparotomy and closure of fistula. On the morning of the day of surgery, TPN is discontinued and intravenous infusion with balanced salt solution (Ringer's lactate) is started. An hour later, the patient is found to be anxious, sweating, and tachycardic. What is the most likely cause?

    (A) Anxiety
    (B) Hypoglycemia
    (C) Hypovolemia
    (D) Unexplained hemorrhage
    (E) Hyperglycemia

83. A 40-year-old woman with inflammatory bowel disease has been receiving TPN for over 3 weeks. Workup reveals pelvic abscess. She undergoes exploratory laparotomy, resection of small bowel with anastomosis, and drainage of pelvic abscess. During surgery, TPN is maintained at the original rate of 125 mL/h. In the recovery

room, the patient is found to have a urine output of 200 mL/h. CVP is 1, and laboratory results are Na, 149; K, 3.5; Cl, 110; HCO_3, 18; BUN, 40; and creatinine, 1 mg/dL. Which of the following statements is true regarding this condition?

(A) The patient's urine output is secondary to fluid overload during surgery.
(B) The patient is in high-output renal failure.
(C) Hyperosmolar-nonketotic coma will develop if the condition is not aggressively treated.
(D) Diuresis is a normal response to stress of surgery.
(E) Potassium supplementation is not indicated.

84. A 42-year-old man who weighs 60 kg is receiving 3 L of standard hypertonic 25% glucose-amino acid solution. He has no history of smoking or bronchial asthma. In the ICU, he is alert, afebrile, and hemodynamically stable, but he remains intubated and attempts to wean him off the ventilator have been unsuccessful. What is the most likely cause?

(A) Copper deficiency
(B) Excess fat calories
(C) Excess glucose calories
(D) Excess amino acids
(E) Inadequate glucose calories

85. An 85-year-old male is admitted to the ICU in septic shock. A pulmonary artery (PA) catheter is placed. The PA catheter does not directly measure which one of the following?

(A) PA systolic pressure
(B) PCWP
(C) Systemic vascular resistance
(D) Right ventricular diastolic pressure
(E) Right atrial pressure

86. A 50-year-old woman with adult respiratory distress syndrome (ARDS) is intubated. The oxyhemoglobin curve is shifted to the right with increased oxygen delivery by which of the following?

(A) Metabolic acidosis
(B) Older age
(C) Decreased 2,3-diphosphoglycerate (DPG)
(D) Decreased thyroid hormone level
(E) Hypothermia

87. A 70-year-old man was administered 20,000 U of heparin before femoral artery embolectomy. Following surgery, he is noted to have generalized bleeding from the wound margins. Immediate management should consist of administration of which of the following?

(A) Fresh-frozen plasma
(B) Cryoprecipitate
(C) Platelet transfusion
(D) Intravenous protamine sulfate
(E) Intravenous sodium bicarbonate

88. A 70-year-old female has been admitted to your ICU in shock. You determine that a PA catheter is needed. Which of the following is not a known complication associated with the insertion of PA catheter?

(A) Transient arrhythmias such as ventricular tachycardia
(B) Right bundle branch block
(C) Pneumothorax
(D) Mural thrombus
(E) Cardiac perforation

89. A 34-year-old male has serum sodium of 114 mEq/L. Correction of hyponatremia can be done by raising serum sodium by what amount?

(A) 1 mEq/L/h
(B) 3 mEq/L/h
(C) 5 mEq/L/h
(D) 7 mEq/L/h
(E) 10 mEq/L/h

Questions 90 and 91

A 47-year-old woman with chronic renal failure has been maintained on chronic dialysis for several years. She had undergone kidney transplantation but because of rejection, she was placed back on dialysis. She had repeated bouts of pain in the RUQ and was intolerant to fatty meals. Ultrasound showed cholelithiasis.

90. Following elective cholecystectomy, severe bleeding occurred. This was most likely attributed to which of the following?

    (A) Elevated PT
    (B) Elevated PTT
    (C) Low platelet count
    (D) Decreased platelet aggregation
    (E) Sepsis

91. The most appropriate management of this patient is the administration of which of the following?

    (A) Heparin
    (B) Protamine sulfate
    (C) Fresh-frozen plasma
    (D) Desmopressin
    (E) Factor VIII concentrate

92. A 70-year-old man, who weighs 70 kg, is admitted with acute cholecystitis. His calculated daily fluid requirement for maintenance is approximately which of the following?

    (A) 1 L
    (B) 2 L
    (C) 2.5 L
    (D) 3 L
    (E) 4 L

93. A 90-year-old woman with a fractured neck of femur is receiving low-molecular-weight heparin (LMWH). Which of the following statements regarding LMWH is true?

    (A) It has molecular weight below 4000 d.
    (B) Its anticoagulant effect is by binding to antithrombin III.
    (C) It should be administered two to three times a day.

    (D) It has lower bioavailability than standard heparin.
    (E) It has a greater rate of heparin-associated thrombocytopenia.

DIRECTIONS (Questions 94 through 100): Each set of matching questions in this section consists of a list of lettered options followed by several numbered items. For each numbered item, select the appropriate lettered option(s). Each lettered option may be selected once, more than once, or not at all.

Questions 94 through 96

    (A) Copper deficiency
    (B) Chromium deficiency
    (C) Zinc deficiency
    (D) Manganese deficiency
    (E) Vitamin A deficiency
    (F) Vitamin D deficiency
    (G) Vitamin E deficiency
    (H) Vitamin K deficiency
    (I) Vitamin C deficiency

94. A 45-year-old man receiving TPN has signs of retarded wound healing. SELECT ONLY THREE.

95. A 40-year-old woman with no previous history of diabetes is receiving TPN. After 4 weeks, she is hyperglycemic, and it is difficult to control her glucose despite insulin therapy. SELECT ONLY TWO.

96. A 42-year-old man with small-bowel fistula has been receiving TPN with standard hypertonic glucose-amino acid solution for the previous 3 weeks. The patient is noticed to have scaly, hyperpigmented lesions over the acral surfaces of elbows and knees, similar to enterohepatic acrodermatitis. What is the most likely cause of this condition? SELECT ONE.

Questions 97 through 99

    (A) Factor II (prothrombin)
    (B) Factor V
    (C) Factor VII
    (D) Factor VIII
    (E) Factor IX

(F) Factor X

(G) Factor XII

(H) Calcium

(I) Fibrin split products

97. A 72-year-old man requires blood transfusion. He was initially given stored plasma. He is most likely to show a deficiency of what? SELECT TWO.

98. What is the coagulation factor involved exclusively in the extrinsic coagulation system? SELECT ONE.

99. A 48-year-old man with severe liver cirrhosis is admitted to the hospital with hematemesis. What coagulation factors are not synthesized in the liver? SELECT TWO.

Question 100

A 20-year-old man has undergone appendectomy for perforated appendicitis with generalized peritonitis. Seven days postoperatively, his temperature continues to spike to 103.8°F despite antibiotic therapy with ampicillin, gentamicin, and metronidazole. A CT scan reveals a large pelvic abscess. Soon afterward, he has bleeding from the mouth and nose with increasing oozing from the surgical wound and all intravenous puncture sites. What is the most likely diagnosis?

(A) Anaphylactoid reaction to intravenous dye

(B) Disseminated intravascular coagulation (DIC)

(C) Antibiotic-induced coagulopathy

(D) Liver failure

(E) Congenital bleeding disorder

101. During the treatment of septic shock, a 28-year-old male remains hypotensive despite adequate volume replacement; PA occlusion pressure is 18 mm Hg. When dopamine is started , ventricular tachycardia develops and this is unresponsive to lidocaine. The V-tach converts back to sinus rhythm once the dopamine is stopped.

At this point, which of the following treatments are most appropriate for this hypotensive patient?

(A) Amrinone

(B) Dobutamine

(C) Epinephrine

(D) Phenylephrine

(E) Intra-aortic balloon pump

102. A 65-year-old male is resuscitated using hydroxyethyl starch (hetastarch). Which of the following is associated with the use of hetastarch ?

(A) Thrombotic thrombocytopenia

(B) Elevated levels of factor VIII

(C) Elevation of serum creatinine

(D) Hyperbilirubinemia

(E) Hyperamylasemia

103. A 28-year-old female several minutes after receiving an intravenous dose of ampicillin for dental prophylaxis against endocarditis develops diffuse pruritis, cutaneous erythema, and hypotension (BP = 60/40 mm Hg). All of the following hemodynamic parameters are typical of this type of shock initially, except

(A) Increased HR

(B) Intravascular hypovolemia

(C) Vasodilation

(D) Increased cardiac output

(E) Decreased preload

104. A 55-year-old male presents to the emergency room (ER) with a history suggestive of myocardial infarction, but without a diagnostic ECG pattern of ST-segment elevation. Which of the following ECG patterns strongly suggests that thrombolytic therapy should be administered.

(A) Right bundle branch block

(B) Left bundle branch block

(C) Second-degree AV block (Wenckebach type)

(D) Complete artrioventricular (AV) block

(E) Runs of V tachycardia

105. You are called to the emergency department to evaluate a 55-year-old woman following motor vehicle crash with associated head trauma. She withdraws to pain and is intubated for airway protection. In order to calculate the Glasgow Coma Scale score, which of the following components of the neurologic examination are necessary?

   (A) Motor response, verbal response, corneal reflexes
   (B) Motor response, eye opening, verbal response
   (C) Eye opening, pupillary light reflexes, motor response
   (D) Pupillary light reflexes, motor response, verbal response
   (E) Corneal reflexes, pupillary light reflexes, motor response

106. A 40-year-old woman is given a routine injection of ragweed allergen immunotherapy by her family physician. She developed a shortness of breath and a sensation of throat swelling. She was taken to the emergency department where she was noted to be flushed and sweating profusely and in moderate distress. She was also noted to be wheezing, tachycardic and hypotensive. Which of the following interventions is most appropriate at this time?

   (A) Ranitidine 50 mg PO
   (B) Diphenhydramine 50 mg PO
   (C) Ringer's lactate, 250 ml over 1 hour
   (D) Methylprednisolone 125 mg PO
   (E) Epinephrine 0.5 mL intramuscular (IM)

107. A 67-year-old man with severe ARDS is receiving pressure assisted control ventilation. He is requiring an FiO_2 of 100% to maintain the following blood gas levels: pH = 7.26, PCO_2 = 60, PO_2 = 58. You decide to put the patient in prone position. Fifteen minutes later, on the same vent settings, the patient's tidal volume is now decreased and his blood gas values are pH = 7.09, PCO_2 = 76, PO_2 = 89. He is hemodynamically unchanged and his chest x-ray (CXR) is also unchanged. The most likely cause of his worsening respiratory acidosis in the prone position is

   (A) Pneumothorax
   (B) Increased dead space
   (C) Decreased cardiac filling
   (D) Reduced chest wall compliance
   (E) Pulmonary edema

108. You are asked to see a 70-year-old male admitted to the ICU with anterior chest pain radiating to the back described as "a tearing sensation." The pain reached maximum intensity within 30 minutes. The patient has a history of hypertension (noncompliant with medications). His BP in the ICU is 170/110 mm Hg, HR = 110/min. Physical examination reveals a 2/6 diastolic murmur and unequal femoral pulses. A CXR of this patient was normal and the CT chest, which was obtained, is shown in Fig. 1–2. Which of the following statements regarding his treatment and prognosis are correct?

   (A) The patient will require nitroprusside and beta blockade, but will not require surgical intervention.
   (B) The patient will require only nitroprusside but will not require surgical intervention.
   (C) The patient will require nitroprusside and β-blockade prior to emergency surgical intervention.
   (D) Neither nitroprusside nor β-blockade is required prior to surgical intervention.
   (E) Nitroprusside and β-blockade are required initially, but surgery may be done electively within 4–6 weeks.

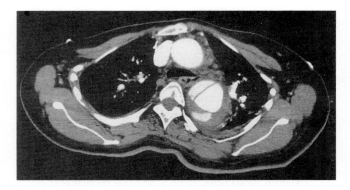

Figure 1–2.
Computed tomography (CT) scan demonstrating aortic dissection. *(Reproduced, with permission, from Brunicardi FC et al.: Schwartz's Principles of Surgery, 8th ed. 706. McGraw-Hill, 2005.)*

Answers and Explanations

1. **(C)** High-output renal failure should be suspected if the BUN continues to rise with urine output >1000–1500 mL/d. It is associated with mild-to-moderate renal insufficiency; in comparison, severe renal injury results in oliguric renal failure. The kidneys do not tolerate ischemia for more than 30–90 minutes. Hypothermia is protective. There is a decrease in creatinine clearance. Vasopressors aggravate the deleterious effects of shock.

2. **(B)** Hyperkalemia can manifest by GI or cardiovascular signs. GI symptoms include nausea, vomiting, intestinal colic, and diarrhea. Abdominal distension as a result of paralytic ileus is due to hypokalemia. An ECG is useful to monitor potassium levels. Hyperkalemia is characterized by peaked T waves. ECG changes also include ST-segment depression, widened QRS complex, and heart block. Cardiac arrest occurs in diastole with increasing levels of potassium. Osborne (J) wave is seen in hypothermia.

3. **(C)** In hyperkalemia, all oral and intravenous potassium must be withheld. Sodium chloride worsens the metabolic acidosis. Sodium bicarbonate intravenously is given to divert potassium intracellularly by causing alkalosis. Calcium gluconate (1 g [10 mL of 10% solution]) is given to counteract the effect of potassium on the myocardium. The hypertonic glucose solution stimulates the synthesis of glycogen, which causes cellular uptake of potassium. Small amounts of insulin (1 U/5 g of glucose) is helpful. The usual recommended dose is 100 mL of 50% glucose with 10 U of insulin. Calcitonin is used for treating hypercalcemia. Serum magnesium is also elevated in renal failure.

4. **(D)** This patient has metabolic acidosis with normal anion gap. The normal value of anion gap is 10–15. Loss of bicarbonate (e.g., small-bowel fistula, pancreatic fistula, or diarrhea) and gain of chloride (e.g., administration of ammonium chloride or HCl and decreased excretion as in distal renal tubular acidosis) result in metabolic acidosis with normal anion gap. In contrast, in acidosis due to increased production of an organic acid (e.g., ketoacids in diabetes, sulfur and phosphoric acid in renal failure, and lactic acid in shock), the anion gap is increased.

5. **(B)** The patient has acute respiratory distress syndrome (ARDS). Measurement of ABGs provides initial evaluation of pulmonary function in terms of oxygenation and ventilation. ECG is valuable for diagnosing myocardial ischemia or cardiac arrhythmias. Ventilation perfusion scanning is used for diagnosing pulmonary embolism. A central venous line provides information regarding the volume status of the patient, which may be low to normal in ARDS.

6. **(C)** Increased airway resistance (stiff lung) may be noted early in shock lung. The alveolar capillary membrane becomes more permeable. There is a leak of a high-protein fluid from the capillary to the interstitial tissues and then into the alveoli. This is commonly called ARDS. Sepsis syndrome is the most frequent cause of ARDS (39%), followed by aspiration, multiple transfusion, massive soft-tissue injury, multiple trauma, near drowning, fat embolism, DIC, and pancreatitis.

ARDS is associated with ventilation–perfusion imbalance. In some areas of lung, there is ventilation with no perfusion, whereas, in other areas, nonventilated alveoli are being perfused. The net result is decrease in functional residual capacity, shunting, and increased dead space ventilation. Chest x-ray reveals diffuse alveolar infiltration, and findings are normal in the initial stage.

7. **(B)** A history of bleeding should alert the clinician to evaluate the underlying cause. The bleeding time is influenced by those factors affecting platelet and capillary integrity. Prolongation of the PT may be attributed to decreased absorption of fat-soluble vitamin K, liver impairment, or decrease in the blood components because of consumption.

8. **(B)** Possible causes of this syndrome include head injury, central nervous system (CNS) disorders, neoplastic diseases, pulmonary diseases, drugs, and idiopathic. It results in impaired water excretion characterized by oliguria, hyponatremia, significantly decreased serum osmolality, and increased urinary osmolality. Administration of a hypotonic solution(D5/0.33 NS) would not result in decreased urine output. Decreased ADH secretion would result in an increased urine output as opposed to a decreased urine output. Naso-gastric suction while it can result in a hypo-kalemia, hyponatremia is less likely. Renal insufficiency would likely result in a decreased urine osmolality.

9. **(B)** Hyponatremia occurs because of overhydration and/or inadequate sodium replacement. When serum sodium is <130 mEq/L, acute symptomatic hyponatremia is manifested by CNS symptoms due to increased intracranial pressure. Muscle twitching and increased tendon reflexes seen in moderate hyponatremia progress to convulsions, loss of reflexes, and hypertension with severe hyponatremia. Oliguric renal failure may become irreversible if not immediately treated. Mild asymptomatic hyponatremia is treated with fluid restrictions. In the presence of CNS symptoms, the patient should be given hypertonic saline.

10. **(D)** Sodium deficit is estimated by multiplying the decrease in serum sodium times the total body water, which is 60% of body weight:

(normal serum sodium − observed serum sodium) × 0.6 × (total body weight)
= (140 − 120) × 0.6 × 60 = 720 mEq

Half of this amount should be administered over 12–18 hours.

11. **(B)** Oliguria may be prerenal or renal. The following table characterizes findings in prerenal failure versus those observed in intrinsic renal failure (acute tubular necrosis).

TABLE 1–1. PRERENAL VS. INTRINSIC RENAL FAILURE

	Prerenal Failures	Intrinsic Renal Failures
Urine osmolality (mOsm/kg)	>500	<350
Urine sodium (mEq/L)	<20	>40
Fractional excretion of sodium	<1%	>2%
BUN/SCR	>20	<10
Urine/PCR	>40	<20

12. **(C)** The composition of various GI secretions is different. They are as follows: **A**, saliva; **B**, gastric; **C**, ileal; **D**, pancreatic; and **E**, colonic. The composition of intestinal fluid is the closest to that of plasma.

13. **(A)** The composition of small intestinal fluid is sodium, 140 mEq/L; potassium, 5 mEq/L; chloride, 104 mEq/L; and bicarbonate, 30 mEq/L. Daily losses are best replaced by administration of balanced salt solution (Ringer's lactate) whose composition is depicted in **A**. **B** represents normal saline (0.9%), **C** is half normal saline (0.45%), **D** is M/6 sodium lactate, and **E** is 3% sodium chloride.

14. **(B)** A decrease in pH below 7.4 indicates acidosis. PCO_2 is increased over 40 mm Hg, suggesting respiratory acidosis. To differentiate *pure* from *combined* acidosis, pH is calculated based on changes in CO_2. A change of 10 mm Hg from 40 mm Hg changes pH by 0.08 from 7.4. In this

case, there is a 20 mm Hg increase in PCO_2, which would decrease pH by $2 \times 0.08 = 0.16$ from 7.4 or 7.24. The measured pH is 7.24. Therefore, the patient has pure respiratory acidosis.

15. **(D)** Respiratory acidosis in the immediate postoperative period is due to inadequate ventilation. Adequate ventilation needs to be restored by prompt intubation and ventilatory support. Use of morphine will further depress the respiration.

16. **(B)** Villous adenoma of colon can result in watery diarrhea and hypokalemia. Massive tissue injury producing myoglobinemia is associated with significant release of intracellular potassium. Massive blood transfusion results in release of large amounts of potassium. The ability to excrete potassium is impaired in high-output renal failure. Spironolactone is a potassium-sparing diuretic.

17. **(E)** A change in PCO_2 of 10 mm Hg from the normal value of 40 mm Hg produces a 0.08 change in pH (from 7.4). A PCO_2 of 30 mm Hg, representing a decrease of 10 mm Hg, can account for an increase in pH by 0.08 (i.e., 7.4–7.48). The patient's measured pH is 7.54. The additional increase in pH is due to metabolic alkalosis.

18. **(A)** Alkalosis is associated with hypokalemia. Hypokalemia can be sudden and severe. It is related to (a) intracellular shift of potassium in exchange for hydrogen and (b) excessive urinary potassium loss. The oxyhemoglobin dissociation curve is shifted to left, and a decrease in levels of ionized calcium can result in tetany and convulsions.

19. **(E)** Zinc is one of the metalloenzymes involved in lipid, carbohydrate, protein, and nucleic acid metabolism. Skin lesions similar to enterohepatic acrodermatitis are the most common sign seen in zinc deficiency. Other manifestations include hypogonadism, diminished wound healing, and immunodeficiencies. Copper deficiency is characterized by microcytic hypochromic anemia.

20. **(E)** The fall in pressure will signal changes via baroreceptors located in the arch of the aorta and carotid sinus and will cause sympathetic stimulation with tachycardia, peripheral vasoconstriction, and hypothermia. Eosinopenia rather than eosinophilia is more likely to be present. There is a switch from aerobic to anaerobic metabolism. Lactic acid accumulation indicates an adverse prognosis in shock. There is a progressive deterioration in prognosis as the blood lactate level increases from 1 to above 3 mm/L.

21. **(C)** The fall in cardiac output results in a relatively larger proportion of blood to be distributed to the heart. The changes are mediated mainly by sympathetic stimulation. There is increased arteriolar and precapillary sphincter tone in the skin and in the renal and splanchnic circulation. In the heart, coronary artery vasodilation occurs, which is brought about partly by local release of vasodilator substances (due to hypoxemia and acidosis).

22. **(C)** Initial resuscitation of a trauma patient is best done by administering Ringer's lactate, because it is isotonic, and it is similar to plasma in electrolyte composition. There is no conclusive evidence that colloid solutions (albumin, plasma protein solution, or hydroxyethyl starch solution) improve the rate of resuscitation or eventual outcome. D_5W and D_5W and 0.45% normal saline are hypotonic. Use of crystalloid solutions also aids in the resuscitation of the interstitial compartment.

23. **(C)** Neurogenic shock (not to be confused with spinal shock, which is defined by loss of reflexes below the area of spinal cord injury, a neurologic phenomena) is secondary to high spinal cord injury as evidenced by inability to move all four extremities. Neurogenic shock is clinically manifested by warm skin, bradycardia, and hypotension. In septic shock, while the skin is warm, the patient usually has tachycardia. In all other types of shock, the skin is cold. Treatment consists of volume replacement with balanced salt solution (lactated Ringer's solution). On rare occasions, some patients may need vasoconstrictors (e.g., phenylephrine hydrochloride).

24. **(D)** Succussion splash is elicited by placing one hand behind and the other in front of the left abdomen and rib cage and rocking the patient gently between the two hands. In pyloric obstruction, one can feel the fluid hitting the fingers (succussion). Peristalsis is likely to be observed in infants with congenital pyloric stenosis.

25. **(B)** Duodenal ulcer and gastric carcinoma are the most likely causes of pyloric obstruction in adults. Metabolic alkalosis results from loss of fixed acids from the stomach. The bicarbonate content of the blood accompanies the elevation in pH. In severe metabolic alkalosis, paradoxical loss of acid (hydrogen) in the urine occurs in an attempt to conserve potassium. Hypokalemia worsens the metabolic consequences of metabolic alkalosis.

26. **(D)** Potassium should not be given initially until moderate hydration has been achieved, and urine flow is adequate. Normal saline is required initially to correct the hypochloremia.

27. **(D)** Initial management of hypochloremic metabolic alkalosis includes administration of isotonic sodium chloride solution with replacement of potassium chloride. In patients refractory to standard therapy use of 0.1 N and 0.2 N hydrochloric acid has been shown to be safe and effective therapy. Ammonium chloride solution has also been used, but this can lead to ammonia toxicity, especially in patients with hepatic insufficiency.

28. **(B)** The actual surgical treatment for obstruction caused by peptic ulcer is controversial. Appropriate gastric surgery with drainage usually is required if pyloric stenosis is severe. Drainage procedures include pyloroplasty, gastrojejunostomy, or antrectomy. An alternative to vagotomy and drainage would be vagotomy, antrectomy with gastrojejunostomy, or a Billroth II subtotal gastrectomy with gastrojejunal anastomosis. It is important to be certain that a gastric carcinoma is not the cause of the pyloric outlet obstruction.

29. **(B)** The presence of an adequate urine output does not preclude a diagnosis of high-output renal failure. The mechanism is based in part on prior ischemia to the nephron structure of the kidneys. There may be an initial period of oliguria. Urea, potassium, and acids are still partly excreted in the urine, and lactate or bicarbonate is given to avoid development of acidosis.

30. **(A)** Potassium should not be given, and potassium levels must be monitored carefully to avoid hyperkalemia. Phosphorous and magnesium levels may be increased, and hypernatremia is likely to occur when fluid is restricted and a solute-poor urine is excreted. Autopsy in patients dying early shows that the distal nephron is affected more than the proximal nephron. Although mortality figures are high, if the patient survives the postoperative period, satisfactory renal function can be anticipated.

31. **(C)** Marked fluid restriction may result in hypernatremia. If the condition is treated appropriately, urea nitrogen usually falls after 1 or 2 weeks. In elderly and cardiac patients, pulmonary edema occurs more readily, and diuretics may be contraindicated because azotemia may be made more severe. Ammonium chloride would make the acidosis worse. Potassium has to be monitored carefully, because severe hyperkalemia is readily induced.

32. **(D)** Hemophilia (factor VIII deficiency) usually occurs during infancy. It is sex-linked, recessive, and affects males almost exclusively. DES administered during the mother's pregnancy has not been incriminated in coagulation disorders but is associated with vaginal carcinoma in adolescent girls. Henoch-Schönlein purpura usually occurs about 3 weeks after a streptococcal infection and includes joint pain, purpura, and nephritis. Wilson's disease is associated with a disturbance in copper metabolism.

33. **(B)** Spontaneous bleeding occurs when factor VIII is reduced below 2–3%. Once serious bleeding occurs, a higher factor VIII activity—probably approaching 30%—is required for adequate hemostasis. The half-life of factor VIII is 8–12 hours. In minor lesions, 10 U/kg body weight of factor VIII is administered. For severe lesions, the dosage is 40–50 U/kg body weight

of factor VIII. After major surgical procedures, factor VIII must be given daily for 7–10 days. Penicillamine is used to inhibit excess copper deposition (e.g., in Wilson's disease).

34. **(D)** The clinical picture is suggestive of hemophilia. The normal bleeding time excludes capillary fragility or platelet deficiency. If fibrinolysis was evident, the fibrinogen level would be reduced. In the presence of a normal PT, a prolonged PTT indicates a deficiency of factor VIII, IX, XI, or XII. The PT evaluates the extrinsic coagulation pathway. The normal PT excludes factor VII deficiency. The thrombin time evaluates fibrinogen to fibrin conversion with an external source of thrombin and will be normal as fibrinogen levels are normal.

35. **(C)** Thrombocytopenia is the major hemostatic disorder in massive blood transfusion. Platelet transfusion usually is indicated when more than 6–8 U of blood is transfused rapidly. There is the risk of causing hepatitis. Stored blood is deficient in factors V and VIII; as such, PT and PTT may be slightly prolonged after massive blood transfusion. Fresh-frozen plasma is the source of factors V and VII, which would be deficient in banked blood. Unless there is previous liver cirrhosis, the procedures enumerated are unlikely to lead to liver failure. Hypersplenism occurs in patients with enlarged spleens.

36. **(A)** Platelet deficiency is likely to be evident, but tests to exclude other causes of bleeding are indicated. The possibility of defibrinogenation, intravascular coagulopathy, or fibrinolysis must be excluded by appropriate coagulation studies. Bleeding from a vein or artery, incompatible blood transfusion, DIC, acidosis, and hypothermia are other considerations to explain any unusual bleeding after a major surgical procedure.

37. **(B)** In desperate cases where bleeding persists despite all other measures, packing the abdomen with laparotomy packs may offer temporary control. The patient is taken to the OR 24–48 hours later for removal of packing after stabilization of hemodynamic status and correction of coagulopathy.

38. **(D)** Symptoms are due to magnesium deficiency. Magnesium is mainly intracellular. Magnesium deficiency occurs in the presence of starvation, malabsorption syndrome, acute pancreatitis, and chronic alcoholism. Symptoms are characterized by neuromuscular and CNS hyperactivity, such as muscle tremors, hyperactive tendon reflexes, and tetany with a positive Chvostek sign. The syndrome of magnesium deficiency can exist in the presence of normal serum magnesium levels. Magnesium deficiency is treated with parenteral magnesium sulfate or magnesium chloride.

39. **(C)** Symptomatic hypermagnesemia is seen after early thermal injury, massive trauma, surgical stress, and in the presence of severe renal insufficiency. ECG changes resemble those seen with hyperkalemia. Hypokalemia and hypophosphatemia can cause symptoms of generalized weakness, but potassium and phosphorus are increased in renal failure. Hypokalemia is characterized by flattening of T waves and U waves. Hypocalcemia is characterized by hyperactive tendon reflexes. Hyponatremia is characterized by nervous irritation as restlessness and convulsions with no specific ECG changes.

40. **(B)** Administer calcium chloride. Management of hypermagnesemia involves correction of extracellular volume deficit and acidosis and withholding exogenous magnesium. Calcium chloride should be administered to reverse the ECG changes temporarily. Peritoneal dialysis or hemodialysis is necessary for persistent symptoms or toxicity. Calcium chloride stabilizes the cardiac cell membrane and thereby reduces the risk of dysrhythmias.

41. **(D)** Determination of serum albumin or protein level is necessary for proper determination of serum calcium level. For every 1 g decrease of serum albumin, the serum calcium level is corrected by 0.8. Intravenous administration of calcium chloride is indicated in the presence of symptoms. Approximately 45% of serum calcium is ionized and responsible for neuromuscular stability. Half of the calcium in the blood is bound to protein, and an additional 5% is

attached to substances other than protein. Alkalosis decreases the ionized component. Hypercalcemia causes polydypsia and polyuria.

42. **(C)** Serum osmolality is calculated from serum values of sodium, potassium, glucose, and BUN by using the formula 2 (Na + K) + BUN/2.8 + glucose/18.

43. **(C)** Injury to the pituitary stalk in major skull fractures involving the base of the skull can result in decreased secretion of vasopressin (ADH). There is increased urine output that is diluted (osmolality <270 mOsm/kg). The extracellular fluid volume is contracted, resulting in high serum osmolality (>300 mOsm/kg) and increased serum sodium.

44. **(D)** Hypophosphatemia results in decreased synthesis of phosphorylated intermediate metabolites such as adenosine triphosphate (ATP), 2, 3-DPG, and cyclic adenosine monophosphate (cAMP). Deficiency can result in erythrocyte membrane instability, WBC dysfunction, platelet dysfunction, congestive heart failure, arrhythmias, weakening of respiration muscles, hemolysis, and rhabdomyolysis.

45. **(D)** The symptoms are suggestive of hypercalcemia. Major causes of hypercalcemia are cancer with bony metastasis and hyperparathyroidism. Symptoms involve the GI, renal, musculoskeletal, and CNS.

46. **(B)** Patients with hypercalcemia have decreased extracellular fluid volume due to vomiting and polyuria. Vigorous resuscitation with salt solution will lower the serum calcium by dilution and increased renal excretion. Furosemide and not thiazides increase renal excretion of calcium. Additional therapy includes administration of oral or intravenous inorganic phosphates, corticosteroid, mithramycin, and calcitonin.

47. **(B)** Methanol ingestion results in increased production of lactic acid causing an increased anion gap. The other conditions listed are associated with normal anion gap. Diarrhea, proximal renal tubular acidosis, and ureterosigmoidostomy result in loss of bicarbonate, while distal renal

tubular acidosis is associated with decreased acid excretion.

48. **(C)** The boy has hemophilia. Management consists of infusion of factor VIII concentrate. Bed rest and local cold packs are helpful. Aspiration of the knee to remove blood and passive exercise are not recommended for fear of recurrent bleeding. In contrast, active exercise is beneficial because movement beyond the point when bleeding can recur is limited owing to pain. Fresh-frozen plasma has a low level of factor VIII (0.6 U/mL) and is not useful because the required volume is excessive. Patients can use long leg splint.

49. **(E)** Obtaining a detailed history is the most important preoperative information that predicts the risk of unexpected intraoperative bleeding complication. It is even more reliable than laboratory tests.

50. **(C)** von Willebrand disease is characterized by decreased level of factor VIIIc (procoagulant). It has autosomal-dominant inheritance. These patients have prolonged bleeding times and PTT, with normal PTs. In contrast to platelets of normal patients that aggregate when restocetin is added, in von Willebrand's resease, platelets fail to aggregate in presence of restocetin.

51. **(B)** von Willebrand disease is the most common hemostatic disorder transmitted by autosomal-dominant mode. Other disorders transmitted by this mode are hereditary hemorrhagic telangiectasia and factor XI deficiency. Diseases transmitted by an autosomal-recessive mode are factor X, factor V, factor VII, and factor I deficiencies. Factor VIII (true hemophilia) and factor IX (Christmas disease) deficiencies are sex-liked recessive.

52. **(D)** ADP, serotonin, and thromboxane A_2 are important mediators of platelet aggregation. In the presence of calcium, magnesium, and platelet factor 4, they cause release of platelet content and their granules resulting in the formation of a *platelet plug*. This process is inhibited by aspirin.

53. **(E)** Requires cessation of Coumadin and infusion of heparin. Warfarin (Coumadin)-induced skin necrosis is a rare complication with high morbidity and mortality. It usually occurs 3–10 days after initiation of therapy, affects women more commonly than men, and most often involves the skin of thighs, buttocks, abdomen, and breast. The exact mechanism is unknown but may be related to depression of protein C levels in some patients. Management involves immediate cessation of Coumadin and administration of heparin IV.

54. **(D)** Patients receiving barbiturates, oral contraceptive agents, and corticosteroids often require larger amounts of Coumadin to maintain adequate anticoagulation. In patients with vitamin K deficiency or impaired liver function and in those with thyrotoxicosis, there is increased effect of Coumadin. Also, the cholesterol-lowering agent clofibrate, D-thyroxine, and certain antibiotics given concomitantly with Coumadin enhance its anticoagulant effect. It is important to adjust the dose of Coumadin when initiating anticoagulation therapy in such patients.

55. **(D)** Fibrinolysis may be primary or acquired. Primary fibrinolysis is seen after fibrinolytic therapy with streptokinase or urokinase; surgical procedures on the prostate gland (which is rich in urokinase) and severe liver failure. Secondary fibrinolysis is most commonly seen in DIC. If the PT, PTT, and platelet count are normal, DIC is unlikely to be present. Aminocaproic acid inhibits plasminogen activation to plasmin and can be used if there is excessive fibrinolysis. It must not be given in DIC, because serious intravascular clotting may occur.

56. **(E)** In the anesthetized patient, the classic signs of transfusion reaction are masked. The sudden unexplained onset of bleeding and hypotension should include transfusion reaction in the differential diagnosis. In the conscious patient, chills, fever, pain in the lumbar region, a tight sensation over the chest, flushing of the face, and dark-colored urine may be evident.

57. **(E)** Acute hemolytic transfusion reaction due to transfusion of incompatible blood in a patient under general anesthesia usually presents as generalized bleeding due to DIC. PT, PTT, and bleeding time will be abnormally high, and platelets may be decreased because of DIC. The most specific tests to determine hemolysis are free plasma hemoglobin and hemoglobinuria. The laboratory criteria are hemoglobinuria with a concentration of free hemoglobin over 5 mg/dL, a serum hepatoglobin level below 50 mg/dL, and serological criteria to show antigen incompatibility of the donor and recipient blood.

58. **(C)** Patients with polycythemia vera do poorly in general surgery if they have not had appropriate treatment to reduce the RBC and platelet count. With chlorambucil treatment, elective cholecystectomy should be performed to avoid the possible need to perform the operation on an emergency basis when the patient is not fully prepared.

59. **(D)** Cross-matching should be done before dextran administration. Group O is the universal donor, and if there is insufficient time to do appropriate cross-matching of blood, this type of blood should be used. Serum of the recipient should be <24 hours old, because antigenicity may be altered in blood stored for a longer time. Before hypothermia is undertaken, the patient's (recipient's) blood should be tested for cold agglutinin titer. Cryoglobulin may be present in patients with lymphoma or leukemia. Blood must be given at room temperature to such patients.

60. **(D)** In general, total caloric needs for the majority of patients ranges between 25 and 35 kcal/kg/d. An alternative formula for calculating daily caloric requirements is the Harris-Benedict equation, which is based on sex, age, weight, and height. The caloric requirements of humans also varies by amount of activity, degree of stress of surgery, trauma, sepsis, or burns.

61. **(D)** The baseline protein requirements are calculated as 1 g/kg/d. Following stress, there is an increased protein requirement, and protein intake should be 1.5 g/kg/d after surgery, 2 g/kg/d after polytrauma, and after sepsis. Glucose and amino acids must be infused simultaneously to appropriately utilize nitrogen.

The ideal ratio is 100 nonprotein kcal/g of nitrogen. In starvation, the nonprotein calorie-to-nitrogen ratio of 150 kcal/g is adequate.

62. **(D)** Lipid emulsions derived from soybean or safflower oils are widely used. One of the real advantages of lipid emulsion is that a large amount of calories can be provided through a peripheral vein. The 10% solution provides 4.62 kJ/mL and the 20% solution, 9.24 kJ/mL. Dextrose concentration in peripheral route is 10%. Concentrations >10% require administration into a central vein to prevent phlebitis owing to hypertonicity of the solutions. Lactulose is used to treat hepatic encephalopathy.

63. **(C)** Essential fatty acid deficiency usually occurs if hyperalimentation is extended for more than 1 month and when soybean oil is not administered at least twice a week. There is a decrease in linolenic, linoleic, and arachidonic acids and an increase in oleic and palmitoleic acid. In addition to the skin changes, there may be poor wound healing, increased susceptibility to infection, lethargy, and thrombocytopenia. It is characterized by a triene-to-tetraene ratio >0.4.

64. **(D)** In metabolic alkalosis, there may be a loss of fixed acids or excess of base. It is associated with hypokalemia because of renal conservation of H^+ ions and urinary potassium loss. Loss of hydrochloric acid as seen in vomiting in patients with pyloric obstruction results in hypochloremic, hypokalemic, metabolic alkalosis.

65. **(B)** Many of the adverse changes can be accounted for by endotoxin release. *Escherichia coli* is the most common organism involved in gram-negative septicemia, followed by *Klebsiella, Aerobacter, Proteus,* and *Pseudomonas.* The cardiac index is high, peripheral resistance is decreased, and CVP is low to normal. The most common conditions leading to gram-negative sepsis are those of the urinary tract, followed by respiratory and biliary tract and abdominal visceral infections. Endotoxins are lipopolysaccharide complexes. The lipid A portion is probably responsible for the toxicity.

66. **(C)** Most patients are elderly. The underlying conditions leading to septic shock occur more commonly in elderly patients. The mortality is higher in this patient population. The overall mortality rate exceeds 40–50%. Gram-positive organisms, parasites, or fungi also may be responsible. The genitourinary and respiratory tracts are more common sources for initiating sepsis. Two or more organisms are found in 10–20% of cases.

67. **(C)** The patient's clinical picture is suggestive of cardiogenic shock. However, he may still be hypovolemic, because distension of neck veins does not accurately reflect the filling pressures of the heart. A Swan-Ganz catheter should be inserted for appropriate assessment of hemodynamic status and institution of appropriate therapy. Fluid therapy will worsen cardiogenic shock, and Lasix will make the patient hypovolemic. Dopamine will increase BP but is deleterious to the heart. The patient should not be extubated until he is stable.

68. **(C)** Low cardiac output in the presence of elevated filling pressures is characteristic of cardiogenic shock. PCWP is decreased in all the other types of shock.

69. **(D)** Thrombocytopenia is a common complication of heparin therapy. The most common form, type I (seen in up to 30% of patients), is a milder form that occurs after 2–3 days of heparin therapy. The platelet count remains over 50,000/mm^3 and has no clinical significance. Type II, seen in 1–2%, usually occurs 7–10 days after heparin treatment. It is immune mediated and can be caused by heparin therapy in any form, in any dose, including heparin flushes and heparin-bonded intravenous catheters. Treatment consists of immediate cessation of heparin administration in any form.

70. **(B)** The patient has tension pneumothorax, as evidenced by distended neck veins and absent breath sounds. Increased intrathoracic pressure interferes with venous return to the heart, resulting in shock. Immediate management should be insertion of a large-bore needle in the left second intercostal space, followed by

insertion of a chest tube. In a trauma patient, venous access should be achieved by inserting two large-bore (16-gauge) angiocatheters in the cubital veins. Insertion of a central venous line on the right side should not be done, because it carries the risk of producing pneumothorax in the opposite side.

71. **(D)** Institute positive end-expiratory pressure (PEEP). This patient has developed ARDS, which is associated with a significant decrease in functional residual capacity (FCR) of the lungs from collapse of alveoli and increased shunt from perfusion of unventilated alveoli. The most appropriate way to improve his oxygenation is by instituting PEEP.

72. **(B)** Administration of a depolarizing anesthetic agent such as succinylcholine in quadriplegics, in paraplegics, or after burns and severe trauma can result in life-threatening hyperkalemia from release of intracellular potassium.

73. **(C)** Dobutamine is the drug of choice for improving cardiac function. It is a β_1-receptor agonist and increases myocardial contractibility and also reduces afterload by β_2 effect. Dopamine at low doses (1–3 mg/kg/min) stimulates dopaminergic receptors and increases renal blood flow. At moderate doses (3–10 mg/kg/min), it stimulates β-receptors, resulting in a positive inotropic and chronotropic effect. Systolic and mean BP are increased; whereas, diastolic BP is usually unchanged. At higher doses (10–20 mg/kg/min), stimulation of α-receptors occurs and it significantly increases systemic vascular resistance. Norepinephrine, epinephrine, and phe-nylephrine are powerful vasoconstrictors.

74. **(C)** The criteria for need for ventilatory support are apnea, respiratory rate >30 breaths/min, PaO_2 <60 mm Hg on room air, and $PaCO_2$ >55 mm Hg (except in patients with chronic obstructive pulmonary disease [COPD]).

75. **(C)** Vital capacity (VC) of 5 mL/kg body weight. See Answer 76.

76. **(D)** Successful weaning from the ventilator is suggested by the presence of

   (a) PaO_2 of 70 mm Hg or more with an FiO_2 of 0.35 or less
   (b) An alveolar arterial gradient of <350 mm Hg
   (c) A PaO_2-to-FiO_2 ratio of >200
   (d) A $PaCO_2$ of over 30 mm Hg and <55 mm Hg
   (e) A VC of more than 10–15 mL/kg
   (f) A maximum negative inspiratory force of more than -25 cm H_2O
   (g) A minute ventilation of <10 L/min
   (h) A tidal volume of over 5 mL/kg
   (i) A respiratory rate of <30 breaths/min

77. **(B)** Patients with SIADH have low urinary output with hyponatremia. Urine-specific gravity or osmolality is increased, urinary excretion of sodium is increased (>20 mEq/L), and TBW is increased as manifested by low serum osmolality. SIADH is seen after various CNS disorders, in neoplastic disease, pulmonary diseases, and with some drugs and may be idiopathic.

78. **(D)** The metabolic response to stress is different to that seen following starvation, as illustrated in Table 1–2.

TABLE 1–2.

	Starvation	Stress
Resting energy expenditure	Decreased	Increased
Respiratory quotient	(0.6–0.7)	(0.8–0.9)
Mediator activation	NA	+++
Primary fuels	Fat	Mixed
Proteolysis	+	+++
Branched-chain oxidation	+	+++
Hepatic protein synthesis	+	+++
Ureagenesis	+	+++
Urinary nitrogen loss	+	+++
Glucogenesis	+	+++
Kelone body production	++++	+

(Reproduced, with permission, from Brunicardi FC et al.: Schwartz's Principles of Surgery, 8th ed. 31. McGraw-Hill, 2005.)

79. **(D)** Resting energy expenditure is decreased following starvation (e.g., in the patient with pyloric obstruction) and increased after the stress of surgery, trauma, or sepsis. The increase in energy

expenditure correlates with the severity of insult being 1.2 times greater after minor operation (e.g., right inguinal herniorrhaphy), 1.35 times greater after skeletal trauma (e.g., fractured femur), 1.6 times greater after major sepsis (e.g., perforated diverticulitis), and 2 times greater after severe thermal burns.

80. **(D)** It is easy to start and administer nutrient requirements rapidly. Parenteral nutrition should be administered when enteral access cannot be obtained, when enteral nutrition support fails to meet nutritional requirements, or when feeding into the GI tract is contraindicated. Current evidence suggests that in addition to safety, convenience, and cost, enteral feeding is well tolerated, preserves gut mucosal mass and normal gut flora, prevents increased gut permeability to bacteria and other toxins, maintains mucosal immunity, and attenuates the hypermetabolic response to surgery. As compared to parenteral nutrition, enteral nutrition is also associated with significantly reduced septic complications. Therefore, enteral feeding is preferred over TPN when feasible.

81. **(C)** It is a major fuel for the gut. It is readily synthesized de novo in skeletal muscle, lung, and liver. Glutamine is a nonessential amino acid. It is not a component of presently available TPN solutions because of its lack of stability. Glutamine is a major fuel for the small intestinal mucosa and other replicating cells such as lymphocytes, macrophages, fibroblasts, and endothelial cells. Glucose is the primary source of fuel for the brain.

82. **(B)** Patients on TPN with hypertonic glucose solutions have elevated islet-cell production of insulin. Sudden cessation of TPN can lead to rebound hypoglycemia, because pancreatic islet-cell insulin secretion is not immediately downregulated. Symptoms are attrbutable to high catecholamine release secondary to hypoglycemia. In general, the TPN rate should be reduced to 50 mL/h during surgery. This prevents both hypoglycemia and the hyperglycemia seen with higher infusion rates. Weaning from TPN should be done gradually over 24–48 hours. In instances where TPN is discontinued suddenly, a solution of $D_{10}W$ should be administered in the interim.

83. **(C)** Hyperosmolar-nonketotic coma is a serious complication seen when an excessive amount of glucose is given, especially in the presence of sepsis, steroids, or inadequate insulin. Furthermore, the combination of surgery and sepsis results in an increased insulin-resistant state. The increased urine output is secondary to osmolar load from blood glucose. Low CVP, hypernatremia, and BUN-to-creatinine ratio over 20 suggest hypovolemia and not fluid overload. Normal creatinine level and BUN-to-creatinine ratio over 20 rules out high-output renal failure. The stress of surgery is characterized by water retention and not diuresis. Management consists of aggressive hydration, discontinuation of TPN, and insulin drip. Insulin drives the potassium intracellularly and potassium must be replaced.

84. **(C)** Glucose infusion should not exceed 4–5 mg/kg/min, equivalent to 365–432 g for this patient. The patient is receiving 750 g of glucose. Glucose has a respiratory quotient of 1. Excess glucose results in increased production of CO_2, making it difficult to wean the patient off ventilator. Treatment consists of reducing glucose load and providing fat calories (up to 40% of total calories). Fat has a respiratory quotient of 0.7, resulting in decreased production of CO_2.

85. **(C)** Systemic vascular resistance (an approximation of afterload) is a calculated value. All the other choices are directly measured.

86. **(A)** The oxyhemoglobin dissociation curve is a convenient method to study the affinity of hemoglobin for oxygen. It is S-shaped, which provides an efficient method of uptake and release of oxygen. It holds on to the oxygen at high concentrations and as the blood enters the lower pressures encountered in the capillaries, it releases the oxygen. Hemoglobin is 75% saturated at a PO_2 of 40 mm Hg and 50% saturated at a PO_2 of 27 mm Hg. At the peripheral tissues, a right or left shift does have a real impact on the affinity of hemoglobin for oxygen. If the S-curve

is shifted to the right, there is a decreased affinity of hemoglobin for oxygen (more oxygen is released). A right shift occurs with increase in 2,3-DPG, acidosis, increase in temperature, and increase in hormones (cortisol, thyroid, or aldosterone). A left shift occurs with a decrease in temperature, alkalosis, low DPG, carboxyhemoglobinemia, and old age.

87. **(D)** Intravenous protamine sulfate. The cause of bleeding is circulating heparin. The anticoagulative effect of heparin can be immediately neutralized by intravenous protamine sulfate. One milligram of protamine sulfate usually neutralizes 100 U of heparin. Fresh-frozen plasma is given to counteract the effect of warfarin (Coumadin). Cryoprecipitate is useful in treating patients with hemophilia. Intravenous sodium bicarbonate is indicated after mismatched blood transfusion to alkalinize the urine. Platelet transfusions are necessary to correct dilutional thrombocytopenia seen after massive blood transfusion.

88. **(D)** Transient arrhythmias and right bundle branch block are seen during the insertion of the PA catheter as it may hit the wall of the right ventricle causing these electrical disturbances. Pneumothorax is a risk associated with the insertion of the introducer for the PA catheter. Cardiac perforation is certainly a risk anytime a catheter is being placed through the heart. Mural thrombus is not a known complication.

89. **(A)** Rapid correction of hyponatremia >1–2 mEq/L/h can lead to central pontine myelinolysis. Serum sodium level should not be raised >25 mEq/L within 48 hours of starting therapy. Only symptomatic hyponatremia requires treatment with hypertonic saline, otherwise fluid restriction is sufficient.

90. **(D)** Abnormal hemostasis, common in chronic renal failure, is characterized by prolongation of bleeding time, decreased activity of platelet factor 3, abnormal platelet aggregation, and adhesiveness. The prolonged bleeding time is related to failure of platelet interaction with von Willibrand's factor (factor 8-VWF)

This interaction can be corrected by using desmopressin or by transfusing cryoprecipitate.

91. **(D)** The coagulation changes can be reversed with desmopressin or cryoprecipitate.

92. **(C)** Daily maintenance fluid requirements are calculated on the basis of 100 mL/kg for the first 10 kg of body weight, 50 mL/kg for the second 10 kg of body weight, and 20 mL/kg for each additional kg of body weight (i.e., $100 \times 10 + 50 \times 10 + 20 \times 50 = 2500$ mL). Hourly fluid requirement can be calculated using the 4, 2, 1 rule as follows: 4 mL/kg, for the first 10 kg, 2 mL/kg for second 10 kg, and 1 mL/kg for each additional kg of body weight (i.e., $4 \times 10 + 2 \times 10 + 1 (50 = 110$ mL/h).

93. **(B)** Low molecular weight heparins (LMWH) are fragments of unfractionated standard heparin with mean molecular weights between 4000 and 64,000 d. They bind to and accelerate the activity of antithrombin III. LMWH has greater bioavailability, more effective anticoagulant effect, lower incidence of heparin-associated thrombocytopenia, and can be administered once daily.

94. **(C, E, I)** Zinc deficiency, vitamin A deficiency, and vitamin C deficiency. Zinc is a metalloenzyme involved in protein and nucleic acid metabolism. Deficiency results in diminished wound strength and healing rates. Vitamin A deficiency results in delayed wound healing, specifically epithelization. Vitamin C deficiency results in defective sulfonated mucopolysaccharides and chondroitin sulfate with retarded wound healing.

95. **(B, D)** Chromium is an insulin cofactor. Deficiency state results in hyperglycemia. Manganese is a cofactor of enzyme of energy and protein metabolism and also of fat synthesis. Besides causing glucose intolerance, manganese deficiency also causes hypocholesterolemia.

96. **(C)** Zinc is one of the metalloenzymes involved in lipid, carbohydrate, protein, and nucleic acid metabolism. Skin lesions similar to enterohepatic acrodermatitis are the most common signs seen

in zinc deficiency. Other manifestations include hypogonadism, diminished wound healing, and immunodeficiencies. Copper deficiency is characterized by microcytic hypochromic anemia.

97. **(B, D)** Factor V and VIII are deficient in stored plasma. In contrast, fresh-frozen plasma contains all the coagulation factors. The major disadvantage of plasma administration, however, is the risk of hepatitis.

98. **(C)** There are two coagulation pathways—extrinsic and intrinsic. In the extrinsic system, tissue thromboplastin (a lipoprotein) interacts with factor VII. The intrinsic pathway requires factors XII, XI, IX, and VIII. Factor XII is the initial step in the coagulation cascade. Factor XII, activated by contact with a nonendothelial substance, will activate factor XI (plasma thromboplastin antecedent). However, factor XI can be activated even when factor XII is deficient. Calcium is required for nearly all of the enzyme reactions in both the intrinsic and extrinsic systems. The amount of ionized calcium required for these reactions is extremely small, and clinical hypocalcemia itself is not a cause of abnormal bleeding. Fibrin split products are not part of the normal pathway in either the intrinsic or extrinsic system. The excessive breakdown of fibrinogen results in measurable amounts of the breakdown products of fibrinogen in the blood. Their presence may signal DIC if the PT and platelet count are deranged. In pure fibrinolysis, fibrinogen breakdown product levels also may be increased.

99. **(D, H)** All the coagulation factors except thromboplastin, calcium, and factor VIII are synthesized in the liver. Factors II, VII, IX, and X are vitamin K dependent.

100. **(B)** Disseminated intravascular coagulation is characterized by diffuse intravascular coagulation, thrombosis, and fibrinolysis. It results in thrombocytopenia, hypofibrinogenemia, prolongation of PT and PTT, and increased concentration of fibrin degradation products in plasma. Sepsis is a major factor that can trigger DIC.

101. **(D)** Dopamine activates β_1-receptors and this was probably the reason for the arrhythmia. Amrinone will inhibit phosphodiesterase and result in an increased cyclic AMP level, producing the same result as β-receptor stimulation. Dobutamine and epinephrine also stimulate the β- receptors. The only choice which stimulates only α-adrenergic receptors is phenylephrine. Intra-aortic balloon pump is invasive, therefore, less appropriate as a choice.

102. **(E)** Hetastarch is a synthetic colloid that is metabolically inert and can be infused IV. A 6% solution of hetastarch has the same osmotic properties as 5% albumin. Relatively few complications are associated with hetastarch. Large volumes do cause dilution of plasma proteins as well as coagulation and platelet function disorders. Hetastarch binds to amylase and impairs renal excretion of amylase causing hyperamylasemia.

103. **(D)** In anaphylactic shock, which this patient is showing, the HR would reflexively increase due to the drop in BP. The intravascular hypovolemia and decreased preload are clearly present along with the vasodilation; however, the cardiac output is initially decreased not increased.

104. **(B)** The only ECG rhythm, which can obscure ST-segment changes seen in acute myocardial infarction, is left bundle branch block. All the other rhythms would allow visualization of the ST-segment changes.

105. **(B)** The Glasgow Coma Score scale is made up of eye opening, verbal response, and motor response.

106. **(E)** The patient is suffering from anaphylaxis, and the treatment of choice is epinephrine. Epinephrine IM has been shown to be more effective than SC for the treatment of anaphylaxis.

107. **(D)** The prone positioning reduces the disparity in mechanics between the dependent and nondependent regions of the lungs. This reduces the collapsing of the alveoli in the

dependent portions of the lungs and overdistention in the nondependent portions of the lungs. The prone position also has other effects—it allows a more normal curvature of the diaphragm and allows better function. It also stiffens the chest wall allowing a more even distribution of ventilation and reduction in overventilation of nondependent alveoli.

108. **(C)** The patient has a diagnosis of dissecting aortic aneurysm. This requires emergent medical as well as surgical intervention. The BP needs to be lowered by using nitroprusside as well as a β-blocker to reduce dp/dt (the force with which the heart is pumping). Once BP is controlled the surgical intervention is needed to correct the problem.

CHAPTER 2

Skin, Soft Tissue, and Breast

Aloyious Smith and Andrew Ashikari

Questions

DIRECTIONS (Questions 1 through 50): Each of the numbered items in this section is followed by five answers. Select the ONE lettered answer that is BEST in each case.

Questions 1 through 6

1. A 75-year-old farmer complained of a scaly, plaque like skin lesion on his forearm with recent development of ulceration. Biopsy reveals invasive squamous carcinomas within actinic keratosis negative examination of axillary nodes. Definitive treatment is:

    (A) Local wound care until the ulcer heals; then wide excision and repair
    (B) Excision of the lesion with frozen section determined free margins and repair
    (C) Wide excision; split-thickness skin graft and axillary node dissection
    (D) Wide excision; split-thickness graft and radiation therapy
    (E) Wide excision; split-thickness graft and chemotherapy

2. A 65-year-old light-complexioned male presents with a solitary scaly plaque like lesion on his forearm present for many years. The lesion is 0.5 cm in diameter. Shave biopsy reveals intraepithelial squamous cell carcinoma. (Bowen's disease) incompletely excised. Further treatment includes:

    (A) Wide excision of the lesions and sentinel node biopsy
    (B) Referral for local radiation therapy
    (C) Excision and repair of this area, ensuring clear surgical margins
    (D) No further treatment indicated
    (E) Local application of 5-fluorouracil(5-FU) cream

3. A 45-year-old soccer player presents with a 6-month history of an ulcerative nodular lesion, 1.5 cm in diameter in the region of the right oral comunissure. Biospy reveals basal cell carcinoma. The preferred treatment is:

    (A) Mohs micrographic surgery and subsequent reconstruction
    (B) Excision with a clinical margin and local flap repair
    (C) Topical 5-FU
    (D) Local radiation therapy
    (E) Cryotherapy

Questions 4 and 5

4. A 43-year-old window cleaner fell off a scaffold. He sustained an open wound on the right leg. Debridement was carried out in the emergency department, and the edges of the wound were left open. The wound measures 4 cm × 6 cm. What is TRUE of wound contraction?

   (A) It occurs within 12 hours of injury.
   (B) It is more prominent over the tibia than gluteal region.
   (C) It is accelerated if wound is excised 3 days after injury.
   (D) It accounts for excessive fibrous tissue formation and fixation of tissue around a joint.
   (E) It is experimentally less affected by excision of tissue from center of wound rather than at the periphery.

5. Which factor is least likely to inhibit wound contraction?

   (A) Radiation
   (B) Cytolytic drug
   (C) Transformation growth factor β
   (D) Full-thickness skin graft
   (E) External splints

6. A 43-year-old male undergoes a total proctocolectomy for ulcerative colitis. The terminal ileum is brought out on the anterior abdominal wall as an end (Brooks) ileostomy. What is necessary to obtain optimal healing?

   (A) The ileostomy should be circular rather than square.
   (B) The seromuscular layer is sutured to the epithelium of the skin to avoid inflammatory changes.
   (C) The ileostomy must be constructed to avoid fixing the mesentery.
   (D) The mesentery of the ileal loop should be widely cut to increase its mobility.
   (E) The ileostomy must be constructed on the right side.

Questions 7 and 8

A 64-year-old male is to undergo an elective laparotomy procedure. The proposed wound is considered as "clean-contaminated."

7. This term implies an infection rate of which of the following?

   (A) 1%
   (B) 2%
   (C) 9%
   (D) 15%
   (E) 30%

8. The wound characteristic indicates which of the following?

   (A) Entry of intestinal or urinary tract without significant spillage
   (B) Gross spillage from intestinal tract
   (C) No entry of intestinal tract
   (D) Entry into infected tissue
   (E) Drainage of an abscess

Questions 9 and 10

A 56-year-old male is burned while sleeping in his home. His right upper and lower extremity and the anterior aspect of the upper chest have extensive second-degree burns.

9. A second-degree burn is characterized by which of the following?

   (A) Coagulative necrosis extending to subcutaneous fat
   (B) Pearly white appearance
   (C) Anaesthetic
   (D) Erythema and bullae formation
   (E) Requires immediate skin grafting

10. The extent of the burn is calculated to represent what percentage of body surface area (Fig. 2–1)?

   (A) 10%
   (B) 20%

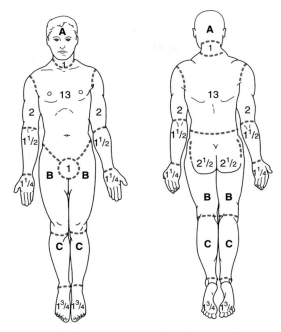

Relative Percentages of Areas Affected by Growth

Area	Age		
	10	15	Adult
A = half of head	5 1/2	4 1/2	3 1/2
B = half of one thigh	4 1/4	4 1/2	4 3/4

Relative Percentages of Areas Affected by Growth

Area	Age		
	0	1	5
A = half of head	9 1/2	8 1/2	6 1/2
B = half of one thigh	2 3/4	3 1/4	4

Figure 2–1.
Table for estimating extent of burns. In adults, a reasonable system for calculating the percentage of body surface burned is the "rule of nines"—Each arm equals 9%, the head equals 9%, the anterior and posterior trunk each equals 18%, and each leg equals 18%; the sum of these percentages is 99%. *(Reproduced, with permission, from Doherty GM: Current Surgical Diagnosis and Treatment, 12th ed. 247. McGraw-Hill, 2006.)*

(C) 30%

(D) 40%

(E) 50%

11. Following initial resuscitation, based upon the Parkland formula, the patient was resuscitated with Ringer's lactate solution at 800 mL/h. Further assessment after 6 hours reveals oliguria. What should the next step in management be?

(A) Continue with increased amount of lactated Ringer's solution

(B) Give Plasma

(C) Give Diuretics to improve urine flow

(D) Colloid solution

(E) Continue initial resuscitation with normal saline

12. After a period of resuscitation, management of this patient should include which of the following?

(A) Tangential excision of all eschar until bleeding is encountered

(B) Split-thickness graft (Fig. 2–2) if wound grows β-hemolytic streptococci

(C) Use of cadaver allograft when required

(D) Avoid use of porcine xenograft

(E) Chest x-ray useful for diagnosis of inhalation injury

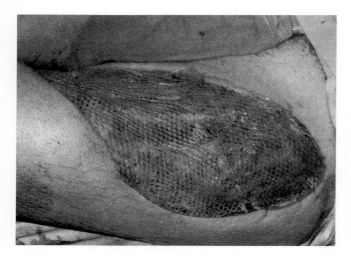

Figure 2–2.
Typical appearance of meshed split-thickness skin graft secured with staples. *(Reproduced, with permission, from Brunicardi FC et al.: Schwartz's Principles of Surgery, 8th ed. 206. McGraw-Hill, 2005.)*

13. A 12-year-old boy has multiple skin lesions that are diagnosed as von Recklinghausen's syndrome (NF-1). What is TRUE of this condition?

   (A) It does not show other malignant lesions.
   (B) It is autosomal recessive.
   (C) It is associated with optic nerve gliomas.
   (D) It is characterized by atrioventricular (AV) malformation.
   (E) It is associated with dermoid.

14. A 29-year-old female swimmer develops a pigmented lesion on the right thigh. With reference to a pigmented lesion, there is an increased risk of developing melanoma if it is identified with which of the following?

   (A) Hutchinson freckle (lentigo maligna)
   (B) Freckle involving basal layer of skin
   (C) Congenital nevocellular nevi
   (D) Hemangioma
   (E) Tophi

15. A 67-year-old business executive and tennis player has a basal cell carcinoma removed from the right cheek. What is TRUE of basal cell carcinoma (Fig. 2–3)?

   (A) It may show a flat ulcer.
   (B) It may metastasize to lymph nodes.
   (C) It may metastasize to remote skin areas.

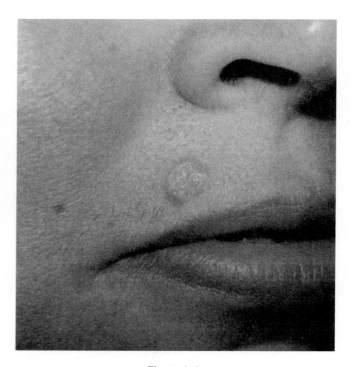

Figure 2–3.
Basal cell carcinoma with rolled, pearly borders. *(Reproduced, with permission, from Brunicardi FC et al.: Schwartz's Principles of Surgery, 8th ed. 440. McGraw-Hill, 2005.)*

   (D) It is found exclusively in the head and neck.
   (E) It is best treated by topical 5-FU.

16. A 38-year-old female undergoes removal of a 2 × 1-cm skin lesion shown to be a melanoma. It is reported as Clark level 1, which implies what?

   (A) It is superficial to the basement membrane.
   (B) It is 1 mm in thickness.
   (C) It has nodal involvement.
   (D) It involves the papillary layer.
   (E) It involves the reticular dermis.

17. A 49-year-old male postman had undergone several operations to excise recurrent infections in both axillary lesions and perianal region. The lesions are hydradenitis supperativa (Fig. 2–4). Which is TRUE of these?

   (A) They arise from stratum corneum of skin.
   (B) They are noninflammatory conditions.

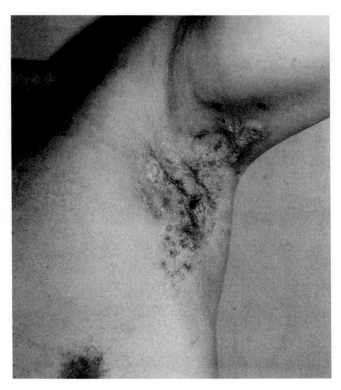

Figure 2–4.
Active hydradenitis suppurative of the axilla. *(Reproduced, with permission, from Brunicardi FC et al.: Schwartz's Principles of Surgery, 8th ed. 435. McGraw-Hill, 2005.)*

(C) They always require surgical intervention.

(D) They frequently involve the scalp.

(E) They are usually caused by staphylococci and streptococci.

18. List the layers of skin from the most superficial to the deepest layer adjacent to the dermis (a) basal layer, (b) granular layer, (c) prickle layer, and (d) stratum corneum.

   (A) a b c d
   (B) d b a c
   (C) d c b a
   (D) c a b d
   (E) c a d b

19. A 12-year-old boy has multiple skin lesions that are diagnosed as von Recklinghausen's syndrome (NF 1). What is TRUE of this condition?

   (A) It does not show other malignant lesions.
   (B) It is autosomal recessive.
   (C) It is associated with optic nerve gliomas.
   (D) It is characterized by AV malformation.
   (E) It is assocated with dermoid.

20. A 35-year-old White male previously diagnosed with basal cell nevus syndrome (Gorlin's syndrome) presents with a new lesion for treatment. Apart from mulitple basal cell lesions other features of this disorder may include:

   (A) The disorder is genetically determined and transmitted as an autosomal dominant.
   (B) Rib abnormalities such as splayed or bifid ribs.
   (C) Skin ribs on the palms and soles.
   (D) A benign clinical course before puberty.
   (E) Normal mental development.

21. A 35-year-old professional dancer presents with a well-defined, tense, smooth mass in the upper outer quadrant of the left breast. She states that the mass becomes larger just before onset of her periods. Aspiration yields a clear yellow fluid and the mass disappears. The most likely diagnosis is:

   (A) Fibroadenoma is a cyst.
   (B) Fibrocystic disease of the breast.
   (C) Carcinoma in a cyst.
   (D) Lipoma.
   (E) Galactocele.

22. An 18-year-old presents with a well-circumscribed 2-cm mass in her right breast. The mass is painless and has a rubbery consistency and discrete borders. It appears to move freely through the breast tissue. What is the likeliest diagnosis?

    (A) Carcinoma
    (B) Cyst
    (C) Fibroadenoma
    (D) Cystosarcoma phyllodes
    (E) Intramammary lymph node

23. Galactorrhea, a milky discharge from the nipple in nonpregnant women, is most likely to be associated with which of the following?

    (A) Fibroadenoma
    (B) Tubular adenoma
    (C) Pituitary adenoma
    (D) Hyperparathyroidism
    (E) Breast abscess

24. A 28-year-old female figure skater presents several weeks after having sustained an injury to her left breast. She has a painful mass in the upper outer quadrant. Skin retraction is noticed, and a hard mass, 3–4 cm in diameter, can easily be palpated. What is the most likely diagnosis?

    (A) Infiltrating carcinoma
    (B) Breast abscess
    (C) Hematoma
    (D) Fat necrosis
    (E) Sclerosing adenosis

25. A 35-year-old patient presents to your office with chronic draining subcutaneous periareolar abscesses, which have been incised and drained many times in the past 5 years but keep recurring. What is the best treatment of choice?

    (A) Repeat incision and drainage (I and D) since the previous procedures were inadequate
    (B) Long-term antibiotics
    (C) Major duct excision
    (D) Complete excision of the drainage tract
    (E) Tell the patient there is nothing to do and that this will eventually resolve with age

26. A patient presents 1 month after a benign right breast biopsy with a lateral subcutaneous cord felt just under the skin and causing pain. The etiology of this condition is?

    (A) Fat necrosis
    (B) Infection
    (C) Superficial thrombophlebitis
    (D) Suture granuloma
    (E) Misdiagnosed breast cancer

27. A 36-year-old woman complains of a 3-month history of bloody discharge from the nipple. At examination, a small nodule is found, deep to the areola. Careful palpation of the nipple-areolar complex results in blood arrearing at the 3 O'clock position. Mammogram findings are normal. What is the likeliest diagnosis?

    (A) Intraductal papilloma
    (B) Breast cyst
    (C) Intraductal carcinoma
    (D) Carcinoma in situ
    (E) Fat necrosis

28. A 35-year-old premenopausal woman whose mother had breast cancer comes into your office and has been told that she has fibrocystic breasts. On examination she has multiple areas of thickening but no discrete mass. Of the following diagnostic tests, which should be performed?

    (A) Re-examination in 6 months
    (B) Bilateral breast ultrasound
    (C) Thermography
    (D) Bilateral breast magnetic resonance imaging (MRI) with gadolinium
    (E) Spot compression views if an area of discrete asymmetry or concerning calcifications is seen

29. During a routine screening mammography, a 62-year-old teacher is informed that she has changes on her mammography, and she should consult her physician. She can be reassured that the findings that indicate a benign condition are which of the following?

    (A) Discrete, stellate mass
    (B) Fine, clustered calcifications

(C) Coarse calcifications

(D) Solid, clearly defined mass with irregular edges

(E) Discrete, nonpalpable mass that has enlarged when compared with a mass shown on a mammogram taken 1 year previously

30. A 40-year-old lawyer comes into your office after seeing some information on the Internet relating to breast cancer. Which of the following factors has not shown to increase a woman's risk for breast cancer?

(A) Smoking

(B) Previous history of benign breast biopsies

(C) Atypia seen on pathology from previous breast biopsy

(D) First-degree relative with history of breast cancer

(E) Increasing age

Questions 31 and 32

A 53-year-old waitress inquires about the implications of positive estrogen receptors (ER+) in an invasive carcinoma that is excised from her left breast.

31. She should be informed of what?

(A) They are more often positive in patients under 50 years of age.

(B) If the receptors are positive, antiestrogen therapy is not indicated.

(C) If the receptors are positive, the prognosis is more unfavorable.

(D) ER and progesterone receptor (PR) status should be determined in all cases of breast carcinoma.

(E) ER are usually negative when PR are positive.

32. The patient is postmenopausal. She should be informed that which of the following hormonal therapy has been shown to be most effective?

(A) Tamoxifen

(B) Raloxifene

(C) Toremifene

(D) Megace

(E) Aromotase inhibitors

33. A 52-year-old undergoes a left modified radical mastectomy for a 2-cm breast cancer. She should be informed that the factor which has the greatest impact on her prognosis is?

(A) The size of the primary tumor

(B) The histological type of the carcinoma

(C) The number of axillary nodes positive for metastasis

(D) Hormonal receptor status of the primary tumor

(E) Positive findings on tests for the presence of the BRCA(breast cancer)1 gene

34. A 46-year-old woman presents with a mammogram that shows a 1-cm cluster of fine calcification in the right breast. Following mammographic wire localization, the lesion is excised and the pathology reported as ductal carcinoma in situ (DCIS) with comedo features and free margins. What advice should be given to the patient?

(A) If untreated, about 30% of such lesions become invasive over a 10-year period.

(B) Comedo DCIS is less aggressive than noncomedo DCIS.

(C) Bilateral mastectomy and radiotherapy are the preferred treatments.

(D) Axillary node dissection is always indicated.

(E) Total mastectomy carries a high (50%) risk of carcinoma recurrence.

35. A 43-year-old premenopausal patient has a biopsy showing focal lobular carcinoma in situ (LCIS) in the area of calcification. With regard to the LCIS, you should tell the patient which of the following?

    (A) She needs a simple mastectomy.
    (B) She must be placed on tamoxifen and chemotherapy.
    (C) This is a premalignant lesion, and she requires additional lumpectomy and radiotherapy.
    (D) She is at increased risk of breast cancer, and she should just be observed closely.
    (E) LCIS often presents with a mass.

36. A partially blind 65-year-old mother presents with a slight change in color of the areola of her left breast. An eczematous rash of the left areola has persisted for the last 3 months. Biopsy of the nipple reveals Paget's disease. In Paget's disease of the nipple which of the following is TRUE?

    (A) Carcinoma of the breast is rarely found.
    (B) Surgical therapy often fails to cure Paget's disease.
    (C) The diagnosis should be made by nipple biopsy when suspected.
    (D) The underlying carcinoma when present is very large.
    (E) Paget's disease of the bone is commonly encountered.

37. A 39-year-old patient presents to your office with a left 3.5-cm breast tumor, which on core needle biopsy, is shown to be an invasive ductal cancer. On left axillary examination, she has a hard nonfixed lymph node. A biopsy of a left supraclavicular node is positive for malignancy. Her stage is currently classified as?

    (A) IIIC
    (B) IV
    (C) IIB
    (D) IIIB
    (E) IIA

38. A 40-year-old patient is diagnosed with a localized 1-cm infiltrating ductal cancer after a needle core biopsy of the lesion. She is clinical node negative; a lumpectomy and sentinel lymph node biopsy are performed. The patient develops an anaphylactic response during the case. Which of the following substances was the likely causative agent?

    (A) Fluorescein
    (B) 99 Tc radiolabeled colloid
    (C) Isosulfan blue dye
    (D) Methylene blue dye
    (E) Indigo carmine

39. A 65-year-old woman undergoes a lumpectomy and sentinel lymph node biopsy and is found to have a 5-mm tubular cancer ER and PR positive and a negative sentinel lymph node. What adjuvant treatment should be recommended?

    (A) Chemotherapy and radiation
    (B) Radiation treatment only
    (C) Hormonal therapy only
    (D) Radiotherapy and hormonal therapy
    (E) Partial breast irradiation

40. A 41-year-old patient presents to your office with a biopsy proven invasive ductal cancer in the upper outer aspect of her left breast, a suspicious palpable left axillary lymph node, and diffuse calcifications throughout the rest of the breast proven to be DCIS on stereotactic biopsy. The best surgical option is:

    (A) Modified radical mastectomy
    (B) Simple mastectomy
    (C) Lumpectomy with sentinel lymph node biopsy
    (D) Radical mastectomy
    (E) Total mastectomy with sentinel lymph node biopsy

41. A premenopausal 44-year-old woman undergoes a quadrantectomy and node dissection for a 2-cm infiltrating carcinoma of the left breast. The margins are clear, and 5 out of 15 lymph nodes are involved. ER and PR are positive. Recommended adjuvant therapy should include which of the following?

    (A) Radiotherapy alone
    (B) Estrogen therapy alone

(C) Modified radical mastectomy

(D) Chemotherapy alone

(E) Chemotherapy, radiotherapy, and tamoxifen

42. An 18-week pregnant, 35-year-old woman presents after undergoing a modified radical mastectomy for a 2-cm ductal cancer with one out of fifteen positive axillary lymph nodes. What should she be informed of regarding breast cancer during pregnancy?

(A) She cannot undergo chemotherapy until after she delivers.

(B) She should have a therapeutic abortion in order to proceed with radiotherapy.

(C) Breast cancer is the most common cancer during pregnancy.

(D) Radiotherapy is indicated.

(E) Most of these cancers are ER+.

43. After undergoing modified radical mastectomy for cancer of the right breast, a 52-year-old female teacher becomes aware that the medial end of her scapula becomes prominent in protraction movements at the shoulder. She also complains of some weakness in complete abduction of the same shoulder. What nerve was injured?

(A) Long thoracic

(B) Thoracodorsal

(C) Ulnar

(D) Median

(E) Intercostobrachial

44. A 50-year-old patient has recently undergone a mastectomy for a 2.5-cm multicentric breast cancer with three positive axillary lymph nodes (stage IIB). A metastatic survey is done, and is negative, and she receives adjuvant chemotherapy. The most common site for distant metastasis would be:

(A) Brain

(B) Bone

(C) Lung

(D) Gastrointestinal tract

(E) Liver

45. A 45-year-old premenopausal woman undergoes a left breast lumpectomy for a 1.5-cm, lymph node positive, hormone sensitive invasive breast cancer. She receives chemotherapy, radiotherapy, and is on tamoxifen. Recommended follow-up after therapy should always include:

(A) Blood tumor markers drawn every 3–6 months after treatment.

(B) Routine monitoring of liver function tests (LFTs) every 3–6 months after treatment.

(C) Yearly bone scans.

(D) Routine clinical examination every 3–6 months for the first 5 years after treatment as well as continued yearly mammography.

(E) Yearly breast MRI with gadolinium.

46. A 43-year-old female requests breast augmentation surgery. She has no family history of breast cancer and her clinical examination fails to reveal any evidence of pathology. What should she be informed about the procedure?

(A) In the United States only silicone gel-filled and not saline-filled implants are performed.

(B) Breast implants increase the incidence of malignancy of the breast.

(C) The occurrence of subsequent breast cancer occurs at a later stage than those without implants.

(D) Saline implants have a more natural appearance than silicone gel-filled implants.

(E) Implants in the submuscular plane allow better mammographic findings than those placed in the subglandular position.

47. A 56-year-old male patient develops an accentric hard breast lump over the past few months and a biopsy proves this to be breast carcinoma. Of all breast cancers, the rate of occurrence in males is which of the following?

    (A) <1%
    (B) 4%
    (C) 7%
    (D) 10%
    (E) >10%

48. A 25-year-old nonalcoholic man has noticeable right gynecomastia since age 20. He is most uncomfortable and reluctant to swim or exercise at a gym for fear of being an object of derision. He should be advised to have which of the following?

    (A) Right mastectomy
    (B) Observation
    (C) Needle biopsy of the breast
    (D) Endocrine workup and right subcutaneous mastectomy
    (E) Testosterone therapy by transdermal patch

49. A 36-year-old woman presents with a substantial unilateral breast enlargement. She had presumed that this was normal, but on examination, a large, firm tumor is palpated by the attending physician. There is early erosion on the skin. A favorable outlook can be anticipated if the lesion is which of the following?

    (A) Sarcoma
    (B) Cystosarcoma phyllodes
    (C) Colloid carcinoma
    (D) Infiltrating carcinoma
    (E) Inflammatory carcinoma

50. A 55-year-old postmenopausal woman undergoes a left axillary lymph node biopsy, which turns out to be an adenocarcinoma. Breast examination fails to show any abnormality and mammography, ultrasound, and metastatic workups are all negative. The tumor is ER+/PR+. The following statements are true EXCEPT for which of the following?

    (A) Recurrence and survival results for this patient are worse than those identified with primary tumor in the breast.
    (B) This is most likely a lesion from the larynx or pharynx.
    (C) This is a common site for papillary carcinoma of the thyroid to metastasize.
    (D) The treatment should be a left axillary dissection followed by chemotherapy and radiation therapy.
    (E) A primary breast cancer is only found in 10–20% of mastectomy specimens.

DIRECTIONS (Questions 51 through 54): Each set of matching questions in this section consists of a list of lettered options followed by several numbered items. For each numbered item, select the appropriate lettered option. Each lettered option may be selected once.

Questions 51 to 54

    (A) Tubular
    (B) Medullary
    (C) Colloid
    (D) Inflammatory carcinoma
    (E) Infiltrating ductal carcinoma
    (F) Infiltrating lobular carcinoma
    (G) DCIS
    (H) LCIS
    (I) Paget's disease

51. The histology that shows an intense lympho-plasmacytic reaction around and within the tumor, which is usually poorly differentiated with a high mitotic rate. SELECT ONE.

52. Microscopic examination of this malignancy shows large vacuolated cells. SELECT ONE.

53. Clinical findings of this breast cancer typically includes a rash-like erythema, which spreads throughout the skin of the breast. SELECT ONE.

54. This histologic variant is characterized by a linear ("indian-file") arrangement of tumor cells and a tendency to grow circumferentially around ducts and lobules. SELECT ONE.

Answers and Explanations

1. **(B)** Actinic (solar) keratosis is the most common premalignant lesion usually seen in older, light-complexioned individuals. The incidence of degeneration to invasive squamous carcinoma is 20–25%. These carcinomas, arising from actinic keratosis, metastasize suggesting conservative excision in treating them.

2. **(C)** Bowen's disease represents an intraepithelial squamous cell carcinoma (carcinoma in situ) and is seen in older patients. These lesions tend to have a long clinical course. Adequate excision is the recommended treatment as these lesions can become invasive squamous cell carcinomas and metastatasize.

3. **(A)** Basal cell carcinoma is the most common malignancy in caucasians. The lesion is cured by complete excision and reconstruction (Moh's) surgery.

4. **(E)** Wound contraction refers to the decrease in diameter of an open wound. It commences on about the fourth day after injury and continues at a relatively rapid rate (1/2–1 mm/d). It is maximal in areas where tissue laxity exists. Wound contraction should not be confused with wound contracture where scar formation over a joint interferes with mobility. Experimentally, it less affected by excision of tissue from the center of the wound, rather than at the periphery.

5. **(D)** Following the application of a full-thickness graft, contraction at the site of the recipient site is maximally inhibited by a full-thickness and to a lesser extent by the partial-thickness graft.

6. **(A)** The ileostomy should be circular rather than square to avoid excessive stenosis of the stoma. Wound healing by a square incision results in a greater degree of stenosis than by an equivalent circular stoma. Failure to close the gap between the ileal loop on the abdominal wall may lead to subsequent internal herniation. It is critical to ensure that the ileal stump is not devascularized.

7. **(C)** In a *clean* wound, the anticipated infection rate should be 1.5–5%, in a *contaminated* wound, 15%, and a *dirty* wound, 30–40%.

8. **(A)** If spillage is substantial or infected tissue has entered, the wound is classified as *contaminated*. *Dirty* wounds are used for drainage of an abscess or debridement of infected tissue.

9. **(D)** In a second-degree burn, the skin appendages in the dermis are minimally destroyed (superficial partial thickness) or more extensively destroyed (deep partial thickness). In a third-degree(full-thickness) burn, all of the dermis, with skin appendages, are destroyed, and the lesion extends to the subcutaneous fat layer.

10. **(D)** In calculating burn surface area, the rule of "9's" assigns 9% to each upper extremity, 18% to each lower extremity, and 9% to the head and neck. The trunk and abdomen (36%) is divided into four equal parts (9% each). Thus, upper trunk anteriorly would be 9%.

11. **(A)** Continue with increased amount of lactated Ringer solution. Urine flow should be 0.5–1.0 mL/kg/h. Patients exposed to inhalation on burns, and those admitted following alcoholic intoxication require additional fluids. In general,

for second- and third-degree burns, the Parkland formula is used to administer 4 mL/kg weight of patient × percentage of area of burn. Half of the calculated amount is given within 8 hours and the remainder during the subsequent 16 hours.

12. **(C)** Use cadaver allograft when required. Tangential excision of the skin (to secure a bleeding surface) is done with a guarded dermatome. However, because of possible extensive blood loss, it should be limited to an area <20% of the total body surface area. The presence of bacteria growth $>10^5$ organisms/cm^2 or growth of β-hemolytic streptococci should contraindicate split-skin-thickness grafting.

13. **(C)** It is inherited as a autosomal dominant disorder and noted in nearly 1/5000 births. The NF-1 gene encodes a protein neurofibromin that plays a role in neuroectodermal differentiation and cardiac development.

14. **(C)** Most melanoma arise from nondysplastic nevi. Congenital nevocellular nevi found in about 1/100 births have a 3–5% lifetime risk of undergoing malignant change. Dysplastic (a typical) nevi may be familial and predisposed to malignancy. Hutchinson freckle occurs mainly in older patients.

15. **(A)** The surface of a basal cell carcinoma has a shiny appearance with telangiectasia. Ulcer formation may occur; hence, are named *rodent ulcer.* Although treatments with 5 FU, cryosurgery, or electrodessication are effective in treatment, surgical excision offers the best results and ensures an accurate diagnosis.

16. **(A)** Level II involves papillary layer III between papillar and reticular layer, IV the reticular layer, and V the subcutaneous fat. The Breslow classification utilizes differences in the thickness of the tumor.

17. **(E)** Usually caused by staphylococci and streptococci. Hydradenitis supperativa is an infection of the apocrine glands and surrounding subcutaneous tissue and fascia, which most commonly involves the axilla, groin, perineum, and perianal region. The periumbilical and areola region may be involved. In milder cases, local hygienic measures and tetracycline may be adequate; in more severe cases, wide excision is indicated.

18. **(C)** The stratum corneum consists mainly of dead cells and keratin.

19. **(C)** It is inherited as a autosomal dominant disorder and noted in nearly 1/5,000 births. The NF-1 gene encodes a protein neurofibromin that plays a role in neuroectodermal differentiation and cardiac development.

20. **(E)** Gorlin's syndrome is genetically determined, a disorder of childhood onset. Along with multiple basal cell carcinomas, other abnormalities include skin ribs on the palms and soles, epithelial jaw line cysts, rib abnormalities, ectopic calcifictions in the dura, and mental retardation. The disease is transmitted as autosomal dominant with no sex linkage. Generally the tumors have a benign clinical course until after puberty.

21. **(B)** Breast cysts are often well demarcated and tend to get larger and contain nonbloody fluid, which is usually acellular and cytology is rarely indicated. Galactoceles present in pregnant and nursing women are filled with milky fluid.

22. **(C)** Fibroadenomas are most often found in teenage girls. They are firm in consistency, clearly defined , and very mobile. The typical feature on palpation is that they appear to move freely through the breast tissue ("breast mouse").

23. **(C)** Galactorrhea is fairly common up to old age. The discharge may vary in color from brown to milky. Hormonal causes are associated with elevated prolactin levels or with pituitary or thyroid disorders. Tranquilizers have also been implicated. Simple abscesses do not cause galactorrhea.

24. **(D)** Fat necrosis is a rare condition that follows injury. Diagnosis may be difficult, and mammography and exicision may be necessary to rule out carcinoma. Sclerosing adenosis is a variant of fibrocystic disease and may present

with a hard mass. In a hematoma, evidence of resolving ecchymosis may be present.

25. **(D)** Mammary fistula also known as Zuska's disease is felt to represent dilated laciferous ducts, which develop chronic inflammation presenting with these periareolar draining sinuses. They will continue to recur until completely excised, which may require removal of the terminal duct into the nipple, leaving the wound open.

26. **(C)** This entity is known as Mondor's disease and is caused by superficial thrombophlebitis usually induced by surgery, infection, or trauma. The process is self-limiting and resolves within 2–10 weeks.

27. **(A)** Intraductal papilloma is the most common cause of bloody discharge from the nipple. The lesion is treated by excision and is benign in most cases. Cancer is present in 5% of cases. Preoperative ductography can be used to help locate the offending duct .

28. **(D)** Patients who present with fibrocystic mastopathy at this age should undergo routine screening mammography, either regular film or digital, and ultrasound if no obvious benign etiology is seen on mammography. Spot compression mammography is done for any questionable abnormality. Routine use of screening MRI is not indicated at this time.

29. **(C)** Coarse calicifications are usually benign. Fine, clustered califications are often milignant and require biopsy. Solid tumors of the breast, especially those that have increased in size or have changed in appearance, are suspicious for carcinoma and require biopsy.

30. **(A)** Any history of previous breast biopsy, even benign, does show an increase risk of breast cancer. Atypia, family history, and increasing age also increase a woman's risk. Smoking has not shown an increase risk for breast cancer.

31. **(D)** ER and PR status should be determined in all cases of breast carcinoma. Positive ER and PR are indicative of an improved outlook and likelihood of response with antiestrogen medication. PR+ do not predict negative ER status.

32. **(E)** Recent studies are showing aromatase inhibitors to be more beneficial than tamoxifen in preventing breast cancer recurrence in postmenopausal women. Tamoxifen, raloxifene, and toremifene are all selective ER modulators (SERMS), which act by competitively blocking estrogen binding sites and thus reducing estogen stimulation of breast tissue. Megace (megestrol acetate) has been used for metastatic breast cancer.

33. **(C)** The number of positive axillary nodes remains one of the best prognostic indicators in breast carcinoma. The current American Joint Committee on Cancer (AJCC) staging classification now defines patients with 1–3 positive nodes (N1), 4–9 positive nodes (N2), and 10 or more positive nodes (N3) due to their different prognosis.

34. **(A)** DCIS is a noninvasive lesion. Comedo DCIS is more aggressive than noncomedo DCIS. Axillary disease in uncommon is DCIS, and lymph node staging is generally not required. Breast conserving procedures can be performed as long as extensive or multicentric disease is not present. Radiation therapy is generally indicated after breast conserving therapy for DCIS.

35. **(D)** She is at increased risk for breast cancer and should be followed closely. LCIS is usually in incidental finding. Although multifocal throughout both breasts, it is thought not to be precancerous itself but rather an indicator of increased cancer risk. Therefore, wide resection is not indicated. Careful examinations, every 6 months and yearly mammograms are done to detect invasive carcinoma at the earliest time. Lifetime breast cancer risk is about 30%.

36. **(C)** The diagnosis should be made by nipple biopsy when suspected. Paget's disease represents a ductal carcinoma that has grown along the ducts into the nipple/areolar region. The lesion often presents with an eczematous rash, which does not resolve and can be diagnosed with a small incisional biopsy. Typically swollen

vacuolated Paget's cells are found on histolog-icl examination. Many cases involve small breast cancers, which are missed on clinical examination and mammogram. Surgical therapy is often curative. This is unrelated to Paget's disease of the bone.

37. **(A)** Ipsilateral supraclavicular lymph node disease is stage IIIC in breast cancer. The new AJCC staging system includes ipsilateral supraclavicular nodes as IIIC and not IV. These patients require appropriate metastatic workup and often get neoadjuvant chemotherapy.

38. **(C)** Both methylene blue or isosulfan (lymphazurin) blue dye can be used for sentinel lymph node identification and have been associated with some allergic reactions. Isosulfan blue has been associated with rare anaphylactic reactions in <1% of patients. Methylene blue can cause skin necrosis if injected too superficially. Fluorenscein and indigo carmine are not given in these surgeries. 99 Tc is given for the lymphoscintigraphy and gamma probe isolation of the sentinel node and has no known anaphylactic reactions.

39. **(D)** Generally patients with small (<1 cm) breast cancers, which are pathologically node negative, are spared from chemotherapy. Radiation and hormonal therapy is indicated. Partial breast irradiation can be offered though there is no current randomized data to show the best modality of treatment (currently an ongoing NSABP/RTOG trial).

40. **(A)** This patient has a palpable axillary lymph node making sentinel node biopsy contraindicated. The multicentricity of the disease also makes the use of sentinel lymph node biopsy relatively contraindicated. Radical mastectomies are no longer performed unless gross tumor invasion into the pectoralis muscle is found.

41. **(E)** Current National Institute of Health (NIH) consensus conference advises chemotherapy for all invasive cancers >1 cm as well as for node-positive cancers. Radiotherapy is required whenever breast conserving surgery is undertaken and tamoxifen should be given for all

ER+ and/or PR+ invasive tumors whose patients are premenopausal.

42. **(C)** Breast cancer is the most common cancer during pregnancy. It is usually ER–/PR–. Patients can undergo chemotherapy (nonmethotrexate regimens) starting after the first trimester and continue on with the pregnancy. Radiotherapy cannot be given during pregnancy, so mastectomy is often indicated unless the patient is toward the end of the pregnancy, and the radiotherpy can be given postpartum.

43. **(A)** Axillary dissection during modified radical mastectomy requires exposing the long thoracic and thoracodorsal nerves. Injury to the long thoracic nerve that supplies the serratus anterior muscle causes "winging of the scapula". The intercostobrachial nerve supplies sensory innervation to the skin in the axilla and proximal upper extremity. The medial and ulnar nerves are outside of the usually axillary dissection field.

44. **(B)** Bone metastasis is the most common distant metastatic site for breast cancer. They are typically osteolytic lesions and can be treated by biphosphonates, which inhibit bone demineralization and have been shown to reduce the pathologic fracture frequency and need of radiation.

45. **(D)** Follow-up after breast cancer treatment is very variable. There is no consensus and no follow-up test has shown a survival advantage. Routine 3–6 month clinical examinations and yearly mammography should always be performed. The use of tumor markers such as a CA 15-3 has not shown any proven significant value and may lead to unnecessary worry.

46. **(E)** There is no evidence that long-term insertion of breast implants leads to an increased incidence of breast cancer or detection of the cancer at an inappropriate late stage. Although the use of silicone gel implants is still confined by the Food and Drug Administration (FDA) to select circumstances (e.g., breast reconstruction following mastectomy), retrospective studies to date have failed to demonstrate a significant

increase in the incidence of collagen disease in patients who have had a silicone breast implant.

47. **(A)** Cancer of the breast in males constitutes <1% of total cases. It tends to present at a more advanced stage in men than in women, because it is often overlooked. It may easily be confused with the more commonly occurring condition of gynecomastia. Careful clinical radiological follow-up studies are indicated.

48. **(D)** In general, persistent gynecomastia should be evaluated to rule out endocrine abnormalities. In most cases, none are found. Subcutaneous astectomy is indicated if the patient is self-conscious.

49. **(B)** Cystosarcoma phyllodes is a tumor that is very slow growing and has a good prognosis if treated by mastectomy. It is characterized by large polygonal cells with abundant cytoplasm and lymphoid infiltration.

50. **(D)** Occult primary breast cancer is a rare but well-known entity. Stage for stage these patients have a similar prognosis as other patients with node-positive breast cancer. The primary tumor is often found in the breast (60–70% of mastectomy specimens). Either modified radical mastectomy and chemotherapy or just axillary dissection with radiation and chemotherapy are accepted treatment choices.

51. **(B)** Medullary tumors have an intense surrounding lymphoid reaction and though poorly differentiated, have a favorable prognosis compared to other invasive cancers. They tend to be hormone receptor negative.

52. **(I)** Paget's disease is characterized by these large vacuolated intradermoid cells usually arising from a ductal carcinoma that is thought to have grown along the duct to the nipple.

53. **(D)** Inflammatory breast cancer is a very aggressive form of breast cancer characterized by intradermal lymphatic spread of tumor.

54. **(F)** Infiltrating lobular cancers have this typical linear ("indian-file") arrangement of cells. There is a higher incidence of multifocality and bilaterality with lobular cancers. These cancers have a greater tendency to be hormone sensitive.

CHAPTER 3

Endocrine, Head, and Neck

Alan S. Berkower and Prakashchandra M. Rao

Questions

DIRECTIONS (Questions 1 through 92): Each of the numbered items in this section is followed by five answers or by completions of the statement. Select the ONE lettered answer that is BEST in each case.

1. An 85-year-old ventilator-dependent male was endotracheally intubated 10 days ago. He remains unresponsive and is not a candidate for early extubation. The intensive care unit (ICU) attending elects to perform tracheotomy at the bedside. During the procedure, copious dark blood is encountered. This is most likely due to transection of which of the following:

    (A) Anterior jugular vein
    (B) External jugular vein
    (C) Internal jugular vein
    (D) Middle thyroid vein
    (E) Inferior thyroid vein

2. A 43-year-old teacher underwent left parotidectomy. Upon awakening from surgery, paralysis of the left lower lip was observed. This complication was most likely due to injury to which of the following:

    (A) Parotid duct
    (B) Facial nerve - temporal branch
    (C) Facial nerve - cervical branch
    (D) Facial nerve - main trunk
    (E) Platysma muscle

3. A 70-year-old male complains of progressive weight loss and hoarseness. Ear, nose, and throat (ENT) evaluation reveals right vocal cord paralysis and several right neck masses, which fine needle aspiration reveals to be squamous cell carcinoma. The patient undergoes right hemilaryngectomy and right radical neck dissection. Postoperatively, right hemidiaphragm paralysis is noted. This is due to injury of which of the following:

    (A) Vagus nerve
    (B) Brachial plexus
    (C) Cervical plexus
    (D) Spinal accessory nerve
    (E) Phrenic nerve

4. A 65-year-old woman complains of severe, acute onset left temporal headache and changes in left eye vision. She presents to her physician with sweating, malaise, and temperature of 99°F. Medical evaluation reveals:

    (A) Myocardial infarction (MI)
    (B) Pneumonia
    (C) Diabetes
    (D) Cerebral vascular accident
    (E) Temporal arteritis

5. Tracheotomy is performed uneventfully in a 79-year-old ventilator-dependent encephalopathic male. After several spontaneous breaths, however, the patient stops breathing. The anesthesiologist continues to assist the patient's breathing for several minutes, after which the patient again breathes spontaneously. The most likely cause of apnea is:

(A) A mucus plug blocked the tracheotomy tube.
(B) Bleeding in the trachea.
(C) Preoperative respiration was driven by hypoxia.
(D) The patient was allergic to Latex.
(E) Surgery created a tracheoesophageal fistula.

6. While conversing with admirers at a postconcert cocktail party, a trumpet player complains of acute onset intermittent hoarseness and nonproductive cough. Subsequent medical evaluation reveals:

(A) MI
(B) Vocal cord paralysis
(C) Pneumonia
(D) Vocal cord polyp
(E) Supraglottic prolapse

7. While lecturing to her advanced psychology students, a 55-year-old college professor complains of acute onset strained, raspy fluctuating voice, forcing her to discontinue her lecture and seek urgent ear, nose, and throat (ENT) evaluation. Which diagnosis is most likely:

(A) Vocal cord paralysis
(B) Vocal cord hematoma
(C) Vocal cord polyp
(D) Vocal cord spasm
(E) Vocal cord cancer

8. A 16-year-old high school wrestler complains of difficulty breathing after being held in a tight choke hold. He is rushed to the nearest emergency room, where the ENT consultant performs a fiberoptic laryngoscopy. Most likely finding is:

(A) Unilateral vocal cord paralysis
(B) Thyroid cartilage fracture
(C) Thyroid gland bleeding
(D) Parathyroid gland bleeding
(E) Laryngeal tumor

9. A 60-year-old veteran with a 40-pack year smoking history underwent supraglottic laryngectomy and right radical neck dissection for laryngeal squamous cell cancer. Postoperatively, he complained of difficulty swallowing. The most likely cause of his symptom was which of the following:

(A) Recurrent cancer
(B) Recurrent laryngeal nerve injury
(C) Superior laryngeal nerve injury
(D) Sternocleidomastoid muscle injury
(E) Brain metastasis

10. A 3-year-old child presented to the emergency room with thin, gray pus dripping from her left nostril. Her foster mother stated that the child "always had a cold" for as long as she knew her during the past year. Prior treatment with oral antibiotics failed to relieve the symptoms. What was the most likely source of the chronic discharge?

(A) Sinusitis
(B) Tumor
(C) Foreign body
(D) Polyp
(E) Trauma

11. While shaving, a 45-year-old teacher notices a marble-sized mass beneath his left ear. The mass is eventually excised, revealing which of the following benign parotid gland lesions?

(A) Glandular hypertrophy, secondary to vitamin A deficiency
(B) Cystic dilation
(C) Mikulicz's disease
(D) Pleomorphic adenoma
(E) Papillary cystadenoma (Warthin's tumor)

12. Following a vacation in Florida, a 43-year-old man notes shortness of breath. He is a

nonsmoker. His wife points out that his face has become slightly swollen. On examination, his blood pressure is normal. His pupils are equal and respond to light. Dilated veins are noted around the shoulders, upper chest, and face. An x-ray of the chest reveals an opacity in the superior mediastinum. What is the most likely diagnosis?

(A) Thymoma
(B) Neurogenic tumor
(C) Lymphoma
(D) Teratodermoid tumor
(E) Pheochromocytoma

13. A 64-year-old assistant hair stylist undergoes a vaginal hysterectomy under spinal anesthesia. Bleeding occurs when an attempt is made to separate and exclude the right ureter from the operating field. After a short interval, respiratory arrest occurs and intubation must be instituted. What is the most likely cause of respiratory arrest during this procedure under spinal anesthesia?

(A) Paralysis of the intercostal muscle
(B) Paralysis of the diaphragm (phrenic nerves)
(C) Centrally induced mechanism secondary to decreased cardiac output
(D) Diffusion of anesthetic to the level of the pons
(E) Diffusion of anesthetic to the level of the medulla

14. In the evaluation of a 64-year-old woman with fluctuating neurological signs of ptosis, eleventh and twelfth cranial nerve palsy, and generalized extremity weakness are noted. Edrophonium (Tensilon) given intravenously results in clinical improvement. A computed tomography (CT) scan shows a lesion in the anterior mediastinum, and a biopsy confirms the presence of a thymoma. She should undergo which of the following?

(A) High-dose steroid administration
(B) Irradiation of the anterior mediastinum

(C) Calcium administration
(D) Thymectomy
(E) Pneumococcal vaccination

15. A 54-year-old construction worker has smoked two packs of cigarettes daily for the past 25 years. He notes swelling in his upper extremity and face, along with dilated veins in this region. A computerized tomography (CT) scan and venogram of the neck are performed. What is the most likely cause of the obstruction?

(A) Aortic aneurysm
(B) Metastasis
(C) Bronchogenic carcinoma
(D) Chronic fibrosing mediastinitis
(E) Granulomatous disease

16. During a routine chest x-ray offered by a department store to all its employees, a 42-year-old business manager is found to have a 1.5-cm nodule in the upper lobe of the lung with a central core of calcium. He has no symptoms. The management of this lesion should involve which of the following?

(A) Transbronchial biopsy
(B) Percutaneous needle biopsy
(C) Thoracotomy
(D) Periodic x-ray, follow-up evaluation
(E) Mediastinoscopy

17. A 54-year-old manager of a bank is noted to have a solitary 1.5-cm nodule on a routine chest x-ray. He is asymptomatic. The most suggestive feature of malignancy would be the finding of which of the following?

(A) A lesion in the lingula lobe
(B) Central calcification
(C) A laminated calcium pattern
(D) Indistinct margins
(E) A lesion in the left lobe

18. An asymptomatic 56-year-old man is found on routine chest x-ray to have a 2-cm nodule-central tumor in the upper lobe of the right lung. The lesion is not calcified. No previous x-rays exist. What is the most appropriate initial step toward making a diagnosis?

    (A) Fiberoptic bronchoscopy
    (B) Bone scan
    (C) Thoracotomy
    (D) Observation at follow-up examination in 6 months
    (E) Mediastinoscopy

19. At the age of 46, an accountant has developed hoarseness due to an inoperable cancer of the left upper lung lobe. He has smoked heavily since the age of 14. Which of the following features of cancer of the lung indicates distant spread?

    (A) Hypercalcemia
    (B) Cushing-like syndrome
    (C) Gynecomastia
    (D) Syndrome of inappropriate secretion of antidiuretic hormone (SIADH)
    (E) Brachial plexus lesion (Pancoast's syndrome)

20. Surgery is indicated in the initial management of lung cancer in the presence of which of the following?

    (A) Hypercalcemia
    (B) Vocal cord paralysis
    (C) Superior vena cava syndrome
    (D) Small-cell anaplastic carcinoma
    (E) Chest wall and anterior abdominal wall metastasis

21. Pneumonectomy for carcinoma of the lung is contraindicated with which of the following?

    (A) Total atelectasis of the involved lung
    (B) PCO_2 over 60 mm Hg
    (C) Cardiac index (CI) of 3 L/min
    (D) PO_2 of 80 mm Hg
    (E) Maximal breathing capacity of 75% of predicted value

22. After undergoing a percutaneous needle biopsy, a 49-year-old electrical engineer is found to have small-cell carcinoma. The chest x-ray shows a lesion in the peripheral part of the right middle lobe. The patient should be advised to undergo which of the following?

    (A) Right lobectomy
    (B) Right pneumonectomy
    (C) Excision of lesion and postoperative radiotherapy
    (D) Combination chemotherapy
    (E) Radiotherapy

23. While walking to the train station from college, a sophomore is accosted and stabbed in the chest immediately above the second rib. On admission to the hospital, he is bleeding from the wound and the blade of the knife is protruding from the skin. A chest x-ray reveals that the knife is at the level of the inferior margin of the fourth thoracic vertebra. The patient has a blood pressure of 100/60 mm Hg. Which structure is the most likely cause of bleeding?

    (A) Arch of the aorta
    (B) Left ventricle
    (C) Hemizygous vein
    (D) Vertebral artery
    (E) Right subclavian artery

24. Four years previously, a 56-year-old fisherman underwent thyroidectomy for cancer of the thyroid gland. He is now noted to have a single 4-cm lesion in the upper lobe of the left lung. There is no other evidence of disease, and he is in excellent health. Endobronchial biopsy confirms that the lesion is malignant but the organ of origin cannot be determined. What should he be given?

    (A) Radiotherapy
    (B) Combination chemotherapy
    (C) Attempted curative lung resection
    (D) Exploration of the neck for thyroid recurrence
    (E) Androgen therapy

25. A 72-year-old retired miner complains of progressive dyspnea, chest pain, and a 20-lb weight loss. He is a nonsmoker. Examination reveals clubbing of the fingers. CT scan shows a pleural effusion and nodular, irregular thickening of the right lung and involvement of the celiac lymph nodes. Cytology, repeated on several occasions, is not helpful. Which test will most likely establish the diagnosis?

(A) Laparoscopy

(B) Bronchoscopy

(C) Open pleural biopsy

(D) Repeat cytology

(E) Gastroscopy

26. A 28-year-old bank employee undergoes investigation for infertility that revealed oligospermia. On further inquiry, it is found that he has suffered from repeated bouts of coughing since childhood and episodes of recurrent pancreatitis. Clubbing of the fingers is evident. Which test is most likely to reveal the cause of his chronic lung disease?

(A) Chest x-ray

(B) X-ray of the humerus

(C) Sweat chloride elevated to over 80 mEq/L

(D) Sweat chloride reduced to less than 50 mEq/L

(E) Aspergillus in the sputum

27. A 58-year-old male factory worker scheduled to undergo a left inguinal hernia repair is noted to have a severe chronic cough. Further pulmonary function tests revealed reduction of forced expiratory volume in 1 second (FEV_1) and reduction of FEV_1/FVC (forced vital capacity) ratio associated with emphysema. Before rescheduling surgery, which of the following would improve residual function?

(A) Trial of ipratropium bromide bronchodilator therapy

(B) Cromolyn

(C) Cough suppressants

(D) Bilateral carotid body resection

(E) Intermittent positive-pressure breathing (IPPB)

28. The chest x-ray of a 62-year-old woman who complains of weakness, dyspnea, and hemoptysis shows multiple nodules in the right lung. She states that the dyspnea is worse in the supine position (platypnea) and improves on sitting up. On examination, the physician notes multiple hemorrhagic telangiectasia in the mouth and in the skin of the upper chest wall. There is a mild increase in the erythrocyte count, and the PO_2 is 90. An angiogram shows multiple pulmonary arteriovenous (AV) fistula in both lungs. What should be the next step in treatment?

(A) Needle biopsy of lesion

(B) Irradiation

(C) Therapeutic embolization

(D) Endobronchial biopsy

(E) Sympathomimetic inhalation therapy

29. A 32-year-old male janitor complains of a swollen face during the past week. A CT scan reveals an expanding hematoma in the superior mediastinum. Mediastinal tamponade is most likely to manifest as which of the following?

(A) Hypertension

(B) Increased pulse pressure during inspiration

(C) Paresis of the right arm

(D) Venous congestion in the upper extremity

(E) Hyperhidrosis

30. After returning from vacation, a 67-year-old retired judge is admitted to the emergency department with severe dyspnea. On examination, an inspiratory stridor, ecchymosis in his neck, and swelling of soft tissue and veins in his face and upper extremity veins are evident. The CT scan shows an expanding superior mediastinal hematoma. What is the most common source of mediastinal hemorrhage?

(A) Parotid gland surgery

(B) Trauma

(C) Dissecting thoracic aneurysm

(D) Mediastinal tumor

(E) Hemorrhagic diathesis

31. A 42-year-old man known to have Marfan's syndrome is admitted to the emergency department with severe chest pain radiating to the back. His blood pressure is 190/130 mm Hg. An electrocardiogram (ECG) shows no evidence of myocardial infarction. A type I (ascending aorta) dissecting aneurysm is detected on angiography. What should he undergo?

(A) Percutaneous transluminal coronary angioplasty (PTCA)
(B) Nitroprusside and attempted resection of the ascending aorta
(C) Intra-aortic balloon pumping (IABP)
(D) Immediate thoracotomy
(E) Steroid administration

32. In interpreting a follow-up x-ray to exclude metastatic disease in an elderly man with prostatic cancer, the radiologist reports sclerotic metastasis to all floating rib(s). *Floating rib refers to ribs:*

(A) 1
(B) 2
(C) 3–7
(D) 8–10
(E) 11 and 12

Questions 33 and 34

A 36-year-old man is crossing a bridge when he is suddenly swept by a torrent into the river. After rescue and resuscitation, he is admitted to the ICU of the local hospital with adult respiratory distress syndrome (ARDS).

33. Which of the following associated features would suggest a diagnosis of ARDS?

(A) High lung compliance
(B) Activation of surfactant
(C) Consolidation confined to the lingula
(D) Interstitial edema with normal pulmonary capillary wedge pressure (PCWP)
(E) Hypoxia responding rapidly to oxygen therapy

34. Which is one of the most important principles of treatment of ARDS?

(A) Steroid use
(B) Avoidance of positive end-expiratory pressure (PEEP)
(C) Tracheobronchial toilet
(D) Use of large amount of fluids
(E) Early and vigorous use of PEEP and highest FiO_2

35. On his return from a 3-year visit to India, a United Nations research worker complains of night sweats, cough, weight loss, and tiredness. An x-ray shows an apical radiopaque lesion (Fig. 3–1). Several enlarged glands are palpable in the posterior triangle of the neck. The next step toward establishing the diagnosis should involve which of the following?

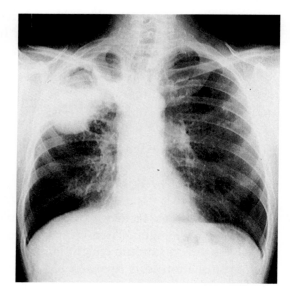

Figure 3–1.
Cavity lesion of the right upper lobe.

(A) Determination of antitrypsin 3 level
(B) Kveim skin test
(C) Examination of sputum for cytology
(D) Thoracotomy and open-lung biopsy
(E) Sputum culture for mycobacterium

36. A student with known human immunodeficiency syndrome (HIV) infection has lost 6 lb in weight and his sedimentation rate is increased to 40. He has no other symptoms. The Mantoux (tuberculin) test results show a change of 7 mm (positive), and x-ray findings reveal a small lesion in the apex of the right lobe of the lung. How should this patient be managed?

    (A) Hospitalized in a public ward
    (B) Hospitalized in an isolated hospital room
    (C) Treated as an outpatient with triple antituberculous drug therapy for 2 weeks
    (D) Treated as an outpatient with multiple antituberculous drug therapy for 2 months and then appropriate antituberculous drugs for 4 more months
    (E) Observed and should undergo repeat skin test after 8 weeks

37. A 12-year-old girl with leukemia develops a lower respiratory tract infection with hemoptysis that is shown to be due to right-sided bronchiectasis. In addition to treatment for the underlying leukemia, the patient should receive which of the following?

    (A) Undergo right pneumonectomy
    (B) Receive selective antibiotics, physiotherapy, and bronchodilator therapy
    (C) Undergo tracheostomy
    (D) Have cough-suppressant medication
    (E) Undergo weekly suction by endotracheal intubation

38. An 18-year-old man develops a severe cough with productive sputum due to *Pseudomonas aeruginosa*. He has had similar episodes in the past, and previous studies revealed bronchiectasis. Which of the following will help elucidate the most likely underlying cause of bronchiectasis?

    (A) Small-intestinal obstruction successfully treated at birth
    (B) Low concentration of deoxyribonucleic acid (DNA) in the bronchial sputum

    (C) Mycobacterium culture from sputum
    (D) Fungus grown from sputum
    (E) Immunodeficiency studies

39. After suffering an episode of hemoptysis, a 14-year-old boy is found, on chest x-ray, to have a well-circumscribed mass that contains both fluid and air. Surgical excision is carried out, and a localized mass adjacent to the carina is excised. What is the most likely diagnosis?

    (A) Tuberculosis
    (B) Bronchogenic carcinoma
    (C) Bronchogenic cyst
    (D) Chronic obstructive pulmonary disease (COPD)
    (E) AV fistula

40. Following thoracotomy, in a 20-year-old man a lesion is detected in the right lower lung lobe and is found to be nonfunctioning lung tissue that is served by vessels separate from those of the adjacent lung tissue. What is the most likely diagnosis?

    (A) Mesothelioma
    (B) Hiatal hernia
    (C) Glomus tumor
    (D) Bronchopulmonary sequestration
    (E) Cystic hygroma

41. A 64-year-old man complains of pain in the lower chest. A CT scan confirms the presence of a tumor of the lung at T10 level to the left of the midline and invading the surrounding left lung base. Because of the structure most likely involved and penetrating the diaphragm at this level, what could be associated?

    (A) Hoarseness
    (B) Latissimus dorsi palsy
    (C) Budd-Chiari syndrome (hepatic venous outlet obstruction)
    (D) Dysphagia
    (E) Tracheobronchial fistula

42. An 8-year-old girl with a prominent chest wall deformity that pushes the sternum inward (i.e., in a posterior direction) is asymptomatic, and she participates fully in athletic activities at school. Surgical correction is recommended. What is the most likely cause of the deformity?

    (A) Funnel chest (pectus excavatum)
    (B) Pectus carinatum (protrusion at the sternum)
    (C) Flail chest
    (D) Cystic hygroma
    (E) Rickets

43. After suffering a respiratory tract infection, a 64-year-old female biochemist develops chronic lung disease requiring intubation in the ICU for an 8-week period. Tracheal stenosis is noted. What is the most likely cause of tracheal stenosis?

    (A) Prolonged intubation
    (B) Tuberculosis
    (C) Scleroderma
    (D) Riedel struma (fibrous thyroiditis)
    (E) Achalasia

44. In evaluating the chest x-ray findings in a 60-year-old man with pleural effusion, which of the following constitutes an abnormal finding of the pleural cavity?

    (A) Communication between the right and left pleural cavities
    (B) Intersection of the twelfth rib posteriorly
    (C) Existence of both a parietal and visceral layer in the upper parts
    (D) Existence of different attachments on the right and left sides
    (E) Extension of the cavity above the levels of the clavicles

45. Because of his involvement in a motor vehicle accident, a 23-year-old football player has a chest wall injury. The only abnormal findings on clinical and radiologic examination are a fracture of the left fifth to seventh ribs and a small hemothorax. What should treatment include?

    (A) Insertion of an intercostal drain to avoid pneumothorax
    (B) Thoracotomy to treat a small hemothorax in the left base
    (C) Insertion of a metal plate to fix the fracture
    (D) Administration of analgesic medication
    (E) Administration of cortisone to prevent callus formation

46. In chest surgery, which is true regarding a thoracoabdominal incision?

    (A) It should be used for most abdominal and thoracic procedures.
    (B) It enters the third to fifth intercostal space.
    (C) It causes less postoperative pain.
    (D) It allows division of the costal margin and the diaphragm.
    (E) It causes severe denervation of the anterior abdominal wall.

47. A rope used to elevate a heavy metal object breaks causing the object to fall on a 55-year-old factory worker and producing chest wall injury. Which is true of associated sternal injury?

    (A) It occurs most commonly at the work site.
    (B) It usually involves the body of the sternum.
    (C) It usually is vertical.
    (D) It involves the hemizygous system.
    (E) It causes miosis of the pupil owing to sympathetic injury.

48. After undergoing an emergency operation for dehiscence of a colon suture line, a 62-year-old patient requires endotracheal intubation. Following prolonged intubation, it is noted that she has tracheal stenosis. What is the most appropriate treatment?

    (A) Administration of steroids
    (B) Resection of segment of tracheal stenosis
    (C) Irradiation
    (D) Treatment with an intrathoracic underwater drain if a tracheoesophageal fistula is present
    (E) Dilatation of the stenotic area

49. A 22-year-old student is scheduled to under go parathyroidectomy for hyperparathryoidism associated with familial multiglandular syndrome. His sister developed peptic ulcer disease secondary to a Zollinger-Ellison (hypergastrinemia) tumor of the pancreas. On examination, a swelling was noted over the posterior aspect of the patient's fifth rib. What is the most likely finding?

    (A) Metastasis from a parathyroid carcinoma
    (B) Osteitis fibrosa cystica (brown tumor) and subperiosteal resorption of the phalanges
    (C) Dermoid cyst
    (D) Eosinophilic granuloma
    (E) Chondroma

50. After suffering a severe bout of pneumonia, a 46-year-old renal transplantation patient develops a lung abscess. She has been receiving immunosuppression therapy since her last kidney transplantation 3 years ago. What is the most appropriate treatment?

    (A) Needle aspiration
    (B) Urgent thoracotomy
    (C) Antituberculous therapy
    (D) Antibiotics and vigorous attempts to obtain bronchial drainage
    (E) Insertion of an intercostal pleural drain

51. An 18-year-old girl developed a neck mass anterior to the right sternum mastoid muscle following a upper respiratory tract infection (URTI). What is most characteristic of branchial cleft cysts?

    (A) They usually appear in the axilla.
    (B) They may become infected after an URTI.
    (C) They may be traced to the stomach.
    (D) They arise from endodermal tissue.
    (E) They frequently cause brachial plexus lesions.

52. A 9-year-old boy complains of a swelling on the left side of his neck in the supraclavicular region. The swelling is translucent; a diagnosis of cystic hygroma (Fig. 3–2) is established. What is true of cystic hygroma?

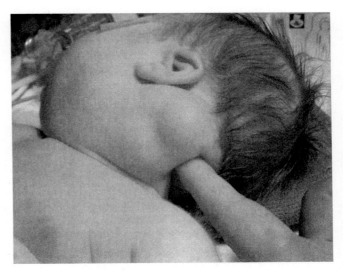

Figure 3–2.
Left cervical cystic hygroma in a 2-day-old baby. *(Reproduced, with permission, from Brunicardi FC et al.: Schwartz's Principles of Surgery, 8th ed. 1476. McGraw-Hill, 2005.)*

    (A) It arises from sweat glands in the neck.
    (B) It is usually an anterior midline structure.
    (C) It may occur in the mediastinum.
    (D) Its lesions are usually easy to enucleate.
    (E) It is premalignant.

53. A 48-year-old woman presents with a 6-month history of intermittent cranial nerve palsy that has become progressively worse in the past 2 weeks. On examination, ptosis and diplopia are evident. Her condition shows a favorable response to the anticholinesterase inhibitory drug prostigmin (neostigmine). What is the most likely diagnosis?

    (A) Cerebral palsy
    (B) Pineal gland tumor
    (C) Adenoma of the pituitary
    (D) Myasthenia gravis
    (E) Tetany

54. Squamous cell carcinoma of the lip is least likely to develop in which of the following?

    (A) Scandinavian fisherman
    (B) Redheaded pornographic actress with a gorgeous year-round tan
    (C) Man from Lohatchie, AL, who smokes a clay pipe
    (D) Brunette secretary who constantly drinks tea
    (E) Mentally defective man who smokes 40 cigarettes a day and keeps the butt in his mouth

55. A 43-year-old male tennis champion develops cancer of the lip. What is true of this condition?

    (A) It involves the upper lip in 90% of patients.
    (B) It is more common at the lateral commissure than in the middle.
    (C) It usually occurs beyond the vermilion border.
    (D) It results in cure in about 60% of cases.
    (E) It requires radical neck dissection.

56. A 58-year-old fisherman has been heavily exposed to the sun for more than 30 years. He develops a thickened, scaly lesion extending over two-thirds of the lower lip. There is no ulceration. Histology reveals hyperkeratosis. What should he undergo?

    (A) Steroid ointment application three times daily
    (B) Antihistaminic medications
    (C) Lip stripping and resurfacing with mucosal advancement
    (D) Radical neck dissection
    (E) Observation and biopsy of any new ulcers

57. A 24-year-old computer technician notes a progressive increase in the size of his left jaw. After x-rays are taken and a biopsy is done, a diagnosis of ameloblastoma is established. What should be the next step in management?

    (A) Radiotherapy
    (B) Laser beam therapy
    (C) Curettage and bone graft
    (D) Excision of lesions with 1–2 cm of normal mandible
    (E) Mandibulectomy with bilateral radical neck dissection

58. A 62-year-old man undergoes excision of a cylindroma of the submandibular gland. He is most likely to have an injury to which of the following?

    (A) Maxillary branch of the trigeminal nerve
    (B) Lingual nerve
    (C) Vagus nerve
    (D) Floor of the maxilla
    (E) Frontozygomatic branch of the facial nerve

59. A 62-year-old alcoholic presents with an indurated ulcer, 1.5 cm in length, in the left lateral aspect of her tongue (not fixed to the alveolar ridge). There are no clinically abnormal glands palpable in the neck, and a biopsy of the tongue lesion reveals squamous cell carcinoma (Fig. 3–3). What should she undergo?

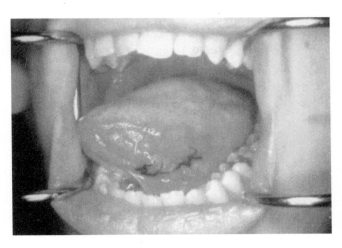

Figure 3–3.
Oral tongue squamous cell carcinoma. *(Reproduced, with permission, from Brunicardi FC et al.: Schwartz's Principles of Surgery, 8th ed. 520. McGraw-Hill, 2005.)*

(A) Chemotherapy

(B) Local excision of the ulcer

(C) Wide excision and left radical neck dissection

(D) Antibiotic therapy and should be encouraged to stop smoking

(E) Wide excision of ulcer and radiotherapy

60. A 59-year-old woman has discomfort in the posterior part of her tongue. A biopsy confirms that the lesion is a carcinoma. What is true in carcinoma of the posterior third of the tongue?

(A) Lymphoid tissue is absent.

(B) Lymph gland spread is often encountered.

(C) There is an excellent prognosis.

(D) The tissue is well differentiated.

(E) The recurrent laryngeal nerve is infiltrated.

61. Adenocarcinoma is the predominant malignant lesion in which of the following?

(A) Hard palate

(B) Lip

(C) Anterior two-thirds of the tongue

(D) Larynx

(E) Esophagus

62. The prognosis for squamous carcinoma of the floor of the mouth is adversely affected by which of the following (Fig. 3–4)?

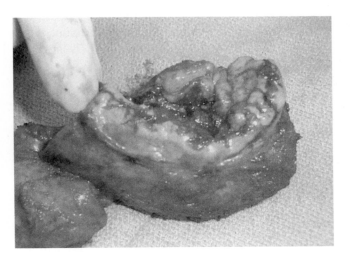

Figure 3–4.
Composite resection specimen of a T4 floor of mouth squamous cell carcinoma. *(Reproduced, with permission, from Brunicardi FC et al.: Schwartz's Principles of Surgery, 8th ed. 522. McGraw-Hill, 2005.)*

(A) Poor differentiation of tumor

(B) Nonverrucous carcinoma

(C) Presence on left side

(D) No tongue involvement

(E) Keratosis of the lower lip

63. A 15-year-old immigrant from China presents with a mass in the left supraclavicular region. He is asymptomatic. Findings on endoscopy and biopsy show that this is a metastatic nasopharyngeal tumor. Clinical evidence of complications of this tumor would most likely be indicated by which of the following?

(A) Decreased growth hormone levels

(B) Bitemporal hemianopsia

(C) Lateral rectus palsy

(D) Hoarseness

(E) Deviation of tongue to the side of lesion

64. A 49-year-old man suffering from depression attempts suicide by jumping out of the window of his third floor apartment. He requires multiple operations during a prolonged, complicated hospital stay. Endotracheal intubation is attempted in the ICU but is unsuccessful because of tracheal stenosis, which is attributed to which of the following?

    (A) Prolonged nasotracheal intubation
    (B) Orotracheal intubation
    (C) Tracheostomy tubes
    (D) High oxygen delivery
    (E) Tracheal infection

65. A 46-year-old Texan develops a lesion in the vestibule of his mouth that on histological examination is revealed to be verrucous carcinoma of the upper aerodigestive tract. What is true of this lesion?

    (A) It is most commonly found on the inside of the cheek.
    (B) It is associated with a high metastatic rate.
    (C) It is ulcerating in appearance.
    (D) It is best treated with radiation.
    (E) It is more common in the northeastern part of the United States.

66. A 16-year-old boy complains of difficulty in breathing through his nose. Endoscopy reveals a tumor infiltrating the nasopharynx. Histology reports this as a juvenile nasopharyngeal hemangiofibroma. The boy's anxious mother requests information concerning the lesion. What should she be told?

    (A) It is a premalignant lesion.
    (B) It usually occurs with laryngeal obstruction.
    (C) It is treated with radiotherapy.
    (D) It may proceed to destroy surrounding bone.
    (E) It is found equally in teenaged girls and boys.

67. A 52-year-old woman has metastatic epidermoid carcinoma on the left side of her neck. Complete head and neck workup fails to identify the primary tumor. What is the recommended treatment?

    (A) Close follow-up monitoring until the primary tumor is found
    (B) Exploratory laparotomy
    (C) Radical neck dissection
    (D) Full course of radiotherapy to the head and neck
    (E) Combination chemotherapy using 5-fluorouracil (5-FU), vincristine, and prednisone

68. A 58-year-old woman undergoes excision biopsy of a tumor in the left posterior triangle of her neck. Histology suggests that this is a metastatic cancer. What is the most likely site of the primary tumor?

    (A) Ovary
    (B) Adrenal gland
    (C) Kidney
    (D) Piriform fossa
    (E) Stomach

69. Arterial infusions via the external carotid artery with methotrexate and 5-FU for head and neck carcinoma have shown a 50% response rate. Widespread use, however, is limited. Why?

    (A) The internal carotid is inadvertently perfused in a large percentage of patients.
    (B) Ipsilateral facial slough has occurred in 3% of patients.
    (C) Blindness occurs in 30% of patients.
    (D) The response is transient, lasting only 2–3 months.
    (E) There is a prohibitive incidence of leukemia.

70. The classic complete neck dissection for palpable adenopathy in the posterior triangle of the neck includes removal of which of the following?

(A) The transverse process, C2–C4

(B) The spinal accessory nerve

(C) Both thyroid lobes

(D) The trapezius

(E) The vagus

71. A 69-year-old endocrinologist complains of progressive facial weakness and loss of taste sensation on the right side of her tongue. What is the most likely structure affected?

(A) Lingual nerve

(B) Middle ear

(C) Ansa hypoglossi

(D) Twelfth cranial nerve

(E) Ninth cranial nerve

72. A 22-year-old female student was found to have an anterior mediastinal mass on a chest x-ray for a persistent cough. What finding is true regarding the thymus gland?

(A) It is located in the posterior mediastinum.

(B) It arises from the first branchial arch.

(C) It controls calcium metabolism.

(D) It is usually excised through an incision along the anterior branch of the sternomastoid.

(E) It results in severe pneumococcal infection when removed in adults.

73. A 29-year-old woman develops difficulty in swallowing. Examination reveals acute pharyngitis. Which organism is most likely to be isolated?

(A) Viral

(B) *Treponema*

(C) Anaerobic

(D) *Staphylococcus aureus*

(E) *Escherichia coli*

74. A 43-year-old man suddenly develops odynophagia. Which organism is most likely to be isolated on throat culture?

(A) Mononucleosis

(B) *S. aureus*

(C) Normal pharyngeal flora

(D) Group A streptococci

(E) Diphtheroid

75. A 72-year-old man presents to the emergency department complaining of frequent nosebleeds. What is the most likely site of acute epistaxis?

(A) Turbinate

(B) Septum

(C) Maxillary sinus

(D) Ethmoid sinus

(E) Sphenoid sinus

76. A 40-year-old woman is suspected of having a carotid body tumor. Which one of the following is most characteristic of such a tumor (Fig. 3–5)?

(A) They secrete catecholamines.

(B) They are more common at sea level.

(C) They arise from structures that respond to changes in blood volume.

(D) They arise from the structures that respond to changes in PO_2.

(E) They are usually highly malignant.

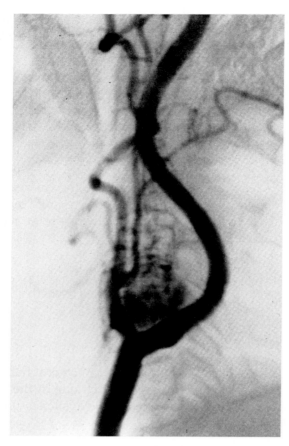

Figure 3–5.
Carotid body tumor. *(Reproduced, with permission, from Doherty GM: Current Surgical Diagnosis and Treatment, 12th ed. 819. McGraw-Hill, 2006.)*

77. A 32-year-old pregnant female presents with a 1-day history of drooping of the right side of her face. A thorough history and physical examination do not reveal an obvious cause of the condition. What is the most likely cause of the patient's facial nerve weakness?

    (A) Labyrinthitis
    (B) Parotid tumor
    (C) Lyme disease
    (D) Herpes zoster
    (E) Idiopathic

78. A 6-year-old girl complains of otalgia, fever, and irritability. Physical examination reveals a stiff, bulging, red tympanic membrane. Previous history of ear infections is denied. Clinical response to amoxicillin is maximized on which of the following durations?

    (A) 1 day
    (B) 5 days
    (C) 7 days
    (D) 10 days
    (E) 2 weeks

79. After undergoing a minor nasal operation, a 65-year-old man is given a neuroleptic agent. Which is the most commonly used neuroleptic?

    (A) Droperidol (inapsine)
    (B) Ketamine
    (C) Fentanyl
    (D) Morphine
    (E) Thiopental (tentothal) be achieved for as long as 4–5 minutes

80. Following surgical resection of a large thyroid mass, a patient complains of persistent hoarseness and a weak voice. What is the most likely cause of these symptoms?

    (A) Traumatic intubation
    (B) Prolonged intubation
    (C) Injury to the recurrent laryngeal nerve
    (D) Injury to the superior laryngeal nerve
    (E) Scar tissue extending to the vocal cords

81. A 9-month-old girl is brought to the physician's office for noisy breathing. The child is otherwise healthy, and her gestation and delivery were uncomplicated. On physical examination, mild inspiratory stridor is heard. What is the most likely cause of stridor in an infant?

    (A) Bilateral vocal cord paralysis
    (B) Laryngomalacia
    (C) Tracheal stenosis
    (D) Epiglottitis
    (E) Arnold-Chiari malformation

82. A 32-year-old teacher presents at her physician's office complaining of hearing loss in her right ear. Physical examination reveals cerumen completely obstructing the ear canal. Ear wax removal is recommended using which of the following?

    (A) Jet irrigation (Water Pik)
    (B) 3% hydrogen peroxide ear drops

(C) Irrigation of the eardrum if perforated

(D) Aqueous irrigation if a bean is present

(E) Aqueous irrigation if an insect is present far in the ear

83. A 4-year-old boy requires prolonged intubation and nasogastric tube placement in an intensive care setting following a closed head injury incurred in a car accident. He develops recurrent fever but is hemodynamically stable. What is the most likely source of sepsis?

(A) Sinusitis

(B) Bacterial tracheitis

(C) Epiglottitis

(D) Small-bowel necrosis

(E) Deep vein thrombosis (DVT)

84. What is the most common site for foreign bodies in the head and neck?

(A) Eye

(B) Ear

(C) Nose

(D) Throat

(E) Esophagus

85. A 25-year-old accountant is seen by her family practitioner for a sore throat. Her physician performs a *Streptococcus* A direct swab test (SADST). What is the specificity of SADST as compared to the standard culture method for the diagnosis of streptococcal pharyngitis?

(A) 25%

(B) 45%

(C) 65%

(D) 80%

(E) 85%

86. A 33-year-old female noted a discharge from a sinus in the overlying skin below the right angle of the mandible. She recalls previous episodes of fullness and mild pain in this region over the past several years. What is the most likely cause?

(A) Thyroglossal duct cyst

(B) Branchial cyst

(C) Teratoma

(D) Myeloma

(E) Trauma to the neck

87. An 85-year-old hypertensive man is evaluated in the emergency department for recent onset epistaxis. His blood pressure is 150/80 mm Hg, and hematocrit is 39%. What is the most likely source of bleeding?

(A) Posterior nasal septum

(B) Anterior nasal septum

(C) Inferior turbinate

(D) Middle turbinate

(E) Floor of nose

88. An elderly man complains of ear pain. During evaluation, the physician asks if the patient has tinnitus. What is tinnitus?

(A) A subjective sensation of noise in the head

(B) A complication of chronic metal ingestion

(C) An audible cardiac murmur

(D) Dizziness with sounds

(E) Nystagmus

89. A 4-year-old girl is diagnosed with bilateral otitis media and is treated for 10 days with an oral broad-spectrum antibiotic. The patient completes the full course of antibiotics and returns for regular follow-up visits. In most children, the appearance of the tympanic membrane returns to normal following a single antibiotic regimen for an episode of otitis media within what period?

(A) 1 week

(B) 2 weeks

(C) 3 weeks

(D) 1 month

(E) 3 months

90. During an examination, the dentist notices a lump between the earlobe and mandible in 6-year-old boy. It feels soft, but it is difficult to distinguish from the rest of the parotid gland. What is the most likely diagnosis?

    (A) Lymphoma
    (B) Squamous cell carcinoma
    (C) Metastatic skin cancer
    (D) Benign mixed tumor
    (E) Hemangioma

91. During a baseball game, the pitcher is hit in the left eye with a hard-hit line drive. He is rushed to the nearest emergency department where CT scan reveals left orbital rim and floor fractures and fluid in the left maxillary sinus. What are physical findings likely to include?

    (A) Exophthalmos
    (B) Lateral diplopia
    (C) Cheek numbness
    (D) Epistaxis
    (E) Blindness

92. A 2-year-old child undergoes tympanostomy tube placement for treatment of chronic bilateral serous otitis media. Which of the following complications is least likely to occur subsequent to surgery?

    (A) Otorrhea
    (B) Chronic perforation
    (C) Cholesteatoma
    (D) Tympanosclerosis
    (E) Scarring of the external auditory canal

DIRECTIONS (Questions 93 through 106): Each set of matching questions in this section consists of a list of lettered options followed by several numbered items. For each numbered item, select the appropriate lettered option. Each lettered option may be selected. EACH ITEM WILL STATE THE NUMBER OF OPTIONS TO SELECT.

Question 93

    (A) Recurrent laryngeal
    (B) Internal laryngeal
    (C) External laryngeal

    (D) Pharyngeal branch of vagus
    (E) Phrenic
    (F) Sympathetic
    (G) Glossopharyngeal
    (H) Ansa hypoglossi

93. After undergoing a left thyroid operation, a 42-year-old opera singer notes no change in speech, but she has difficulty in singing high-pitched notes. Which nerve is most likely to be injured? SELECT ONE.

Question 94

    (A) Scrofula
    (B) Carotid body tumor
    (C) Ganglioneuroma
    (D) Virchow node
    (E) Sternomastoid tumor
    (F) Glomus tumor
    (G) Cervical rib
    (H) Sarcoid

94. A 67-year-old woman has lost weight and complains of night sweats. She had previously undergone treatment for tuberculosis. She has lymph node enlargement in the neck that has broken down to form sinus with overhanging bluish edges. What is the diagnosis? SELECT ONE.

Question 95

    (A) Erysipelas
    (B) Eczema
    (C) Scarlet fever
    (D) Mucor mycosis
    (E) Coccydynia
    (F) Ameba
    (G) Schistosomiasis
    (H) Actinomycosis
    (I) Tuberculosis

95. A 63-year-old man with insulin-dependent diabetes develops a black, crusting lesion in the nose and left maxillary sinus. Biopsy reveals nonseptate hyphae, which confirms the diagnosis of what? SELECT ONE.

Question 96

(A) Cholesteatoma
(B) Dermoid cyst
(C) Glomus tumor
(D) Neurofibroma
(E) Hemangioma
(F) Epidermoid cyst
(G) Mikulicz's lesion
(H) Sarcoma

96. This develops along lines of embryological fusion in the floor of the mouth. SELECT ONE.

Question 97

(A) Optic neuroma
(B) Constricted pupil
(C) Cerebellar dysfunction
(D) Hamartomatous polyps in the small intestine
(E) Diverticulitis
(F) Melanosis coli
(G) Cancer of the breast
(H) Melanoma

97. A 32-year-old man presents with abdominal pain. On examination, he is noted to have pigmented spots in the buccal region. He is diagnosed to have Peutz-Jeghers syndrome, which also results in what? SELECT ONE.

Question 98

(A) Lymphoma
(B) Squamous cell carcinoma
(C) Metastatic skin cancer
(D) Benign mixed tumor
(E) Hemangioma
(F) Neurofibroma
(G) Paget's disease
(H) Ranula

98. A businessman notices a lump in front of his ear while shaving one morning. His wife thinks it has been there for several months. What is the most likely cause of a mass in the parotid gland in this patient? SELECT ONE.

Questions 99 and 100

(A) Foramen cecum
(B) Foramen ovale
(C) Foramen rotundum
(D) Foramen spinosum
(E) Foramen magnum
(F) Foramen jugulare
(G) Foramen of Munro
(H) Foramen of Magendie

99. A 46-year-old accountant notices that he keeps cutting the right side of his lower face while shaving. On self-examination, he notes a loss of sensation of the skin and lower teeth on that side. At his physician's office, a CT scan is ordered. Which structure should be carefully evaluated for this patient's complaint? SELECT ONE.

100. A 4-year-old boy is brought to the physician's office by his father for evaluation of small stature. A thyroid scan is ordered and shows no uptake in the neck. Which structure is embryologically related to the thyroid gland and should be carefully evaluated? SELECT ONE.

Question 101

(A) Human papillomavirus (HPV)
(B) Epstein-Barr virus
(C) HIV
(D) Varicella zoster virus
(E) Herpes type 2 virus
(F) Microcytic anemia
(G) Autoimmune deficiency
(H) Meningioma

101. Mononucleosis in the blood is associated with what? SELECT ONE.

Question 102

(A) Mental status change

(B) Anosmia

(C) Hypopituitarism

(D) Meningitis

(E) Neck mass

(F) Deafness

(G) Bitemporal hemianopsia

(H) Neck stiffness

102. A middle-aged woman from China presents at her physician's office with a history of nasopharynx cancer. A medical history is obtained about her illness. What is the most common complaint of patients presenting with nasopharynx cancer? SELECT ONE.

Question 103

(A) Lymphoma

(B) Squamous cell carcinoma

(C) Metastatic skin cancer

(D) Benign mixed tumor

(E) Hemangioma

(F) Sebaceous cyst

(G) Sjögren's syndrome

(H) Ectopic thyroid

103. A 63-year-old bartender presents at his physician's office complaining of a painful sore on his tongue. On examination, it is found that he has an ulcerated lesion on his tongue and a mass in the submandibular gland triangle. What is the most likely diagnosis? SELECT ONE.

Question 104

(A) Funnel chest (pectus excavatum)

(B) Pectus carinatum (protrusion at the sternum)

(C) Flail chest

(D) Cystic hygroma

(E) Rickets

(F) Sebaceous cyst

(G) Dermoid cyst

(H) Nevi

(I) Lipoma

(J) Tay-Sachs disease

104. Midline swelling causing a double chin appearance is what? SELECT ONE.

Question 105

(A) Metastasis from a parathyroid carcinoma

(B) Osteitis fibrosa cystica (brown tumor) and subperiosteal resorption of the phalanges

(C) Atypical mycobacterium

(D) Eosinophilic granuloma

(E) Chondroma

(F) Dermoid cyst

(G) Thyroglossal duct cyst

(H) Laryngocele

(I) Warthin's tumor

105. A 5-year-old boy is taken to his pediatrician for a laceration on his right knee. A mass on his neck is noticed; his mother states it has been there for several months and is slowly getting larger. The mass is slightly to the left of midline. Ultrasound findings are shown in Fig. 3–6. What is the most likely diagnosis? SELECT ONE.

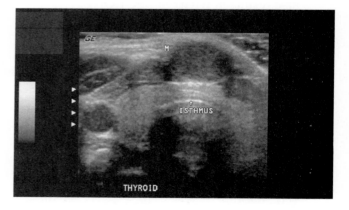

Figure 3–6.
Ultrasound of neck. Midline hypoechogenic mass anterior and superior to the thyroid gland.

DIRECTIONS (Questions 106 through 109): Each of the numbered items in this section is followed by five answers. Select the ONE lettered answer that is BEST in each case.

106. A 60-year-old woman, complaining of joint pains and muscle ache has a normal physical examination. Her routine blood work reveals a normal hemoglobin (Hb). Serum potassium is 4 mEq/L. BUN and creatine are normal. Serum calcium is 11–12 mgm/dL. Which one of the following is not associated with this condition?

   (A) Myoglobin in the urine
   (B) Serum, parathyroid hormones (PTH) is elevated
   (C) Increased urinary excretion of calcium
   (D) Pancreatic tumors may be present
   (E) Pituitary tumors

107. A 5-year-old girl presents with difficulty breathing. On examination, of the oral cavity a 3-cm mass is found in the midline on the posterior aspect of the tongue. The most likely diagnosis is:

   (A) Lingual tonsil
   (B) Lingual thyroid
   (C) Foreign body stuck to the tongue
   (D) Dermoid
   (E) Angioneurotic edema

108. A 40-year-old woman presents with weight loss, palpitations, and exopthalmos. On physical examination, the thyroid gland is diffusely enlarged. Blood tests reveal primary hyperthyroidism. Which one of the following is not the treatment of hyperthyroidism?

   (A) Methimazoli
   (B) Lugols iodine
   (C) I_{131}
   (D) Subtotal thyroidectomy
   (E) Steroids

109. Which one of the following is not part of the management of a patient with hyperparathyroidism

   (A) Hydration with intravenous normal saline
   (B) Steroids
   (C) Exploration of the neck for parathyroidectomy
   (D) Parathyroid scan
   (E) Vitamin D

Answers and Explanations

1. **(A)** The anterior jugular vein can cross the midline overlying the proximal trachea. Midline cervical dissection without adequate visualization can injure the vein and require open surgical repair. The other veins do not cross the midline and are not generally at risk in tracheotomy.

2. **(C)** The cervical branch of the facial nerve innervates the lower lip through the marginal mandibular branch of the nerve (Fig. 3–7). As no cross innervation exits to other branches of the facial nerve, marginal mandibular branch injuries always yield paralysis of the same side of the lower lip. Injuries of the main trunk of the facial nerve or its temporal branch would usually produce upper facial paralysis as well.

3. **(E)** The phrenic nerve is the only component of the cervical plexus, which is not sacrificed during a radical neck dissection. It can be identified as superficial to the anterior scalene muscle (Fig. 3–8) with a nerve stimulator, although direct visualization is usually

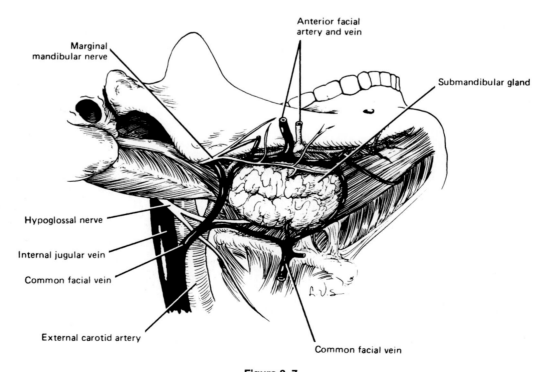

Figure 3–7.
The cervical branch of the facial nerve innervates the lower lip through the marginal mandibular branch of the nerves.

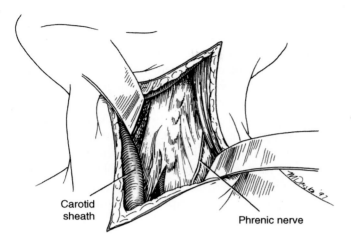

Carotid sheath

Phrenic nerve

Figure 3–8.
The phrenic nerve is the only component of the cervical plescia, which is not sacrificed during a radical neck dissection. *(Reproduced, with permission, from Brunicardi FC et al.: Schwartz's Principles of Surgery, 8th ed. 156. McGraw-Hill, 2005.)*

sufficient. Injury to the phrenic nerve can result in paralysis of the corresponding side of the diaphragm.

4. **(E)** Temporal artery inflammation causes severe throbbing unilateral temporal headache, low-grade fever, visual changes, sweating, and malaise. Acute treatment with prednisone can be followed by temporal artery resection.

5. **(C)** Hypoxia can become the primary stimulation for respiration. Sudden elevation of PO_2 can eliminate the respiratory drive, which will resume by lowering the PCO_2.

6. **(E)** Prolapse of mucosa overlying the true vocal cords (ventricle of Morgagni) can occur in people who routinely elevate air pressure in the chest and larynx. Treatment involves direct laryngoscopy and excision of the protruding mucosa. The other choices, although less likely, must also be considered.

7. **(D)** Spasmodic dysphonia often occurs in both men and women over 40-years old who strain their voices. Fluctuation with normal speech can occur, unlike the other choices presented. The vocal cords appear normal on routine laryngeal exam. Temporary improvement using botulinum toxin is reported.

8. **(A)** Compression of the recurrent laryngeal nerve due to compression of the cricothyroid joint can occur subsequent to choking injury of the neck. Although fracture and internal bleeding can also occur, these are less likely. Acute onset dyspnea secondary to laryngeal tumor is unlikely.

9. **(C)** Dysphagia and aspiration can result from disruption of the internal branch of the superior laryngeal nerve, resulting in sensory loss of the larynx. Contralateral superior laryngeal nerve compensation usually corrects these symptoms.

10. **(C)** Unilateral nasal discharge in a young child is often due to foreign body in the nose. Although the other choices should also be considered in the differential diagnoses of rhinorrhea, nasal foreign body in the child is most likely.

11. **(E)** Papillary cystadenoma lymphomatosum is also called Warthin's tumor. It occurs mainly in men. The epithelial component is interspersed with lymphoid tissue that shows germinal centers. The most common tumor of the parotid gland is a pleomorphic adenoma, with papillary cystadenoma (although much less frequent) as the second most common tumor. Mikulicz's disease involves chronic inflammation and swelling of the salivary glands, which is benign and usually painless.

12. **(B)** The most common cause of primary mediastinal tumor is a neurogenic tumor (20–25%), and 10% are malignant (more likely in children). They usually arise from an intercostal nerve or sympathetic ganglion. Varieties of neurogenic tumors include neurilemmoma (schwannoma), neurofibroma, ganglioneuroma, and neuroblastoma. Next in frequency (of primary mediastinal tumors) are thymoma, congenital cysts, and lymphoma. New diagnostic techniques have resulted in detection of larger numbers of these lesions.

13. **(C)** Spinal anesthesia induces venous vasodilation because of sympathetic blockade. Venous pooling can seriously impair venous return. It is the sympathetic blockade and not somatic nerve blockade that is responsible for the vasomotor and respiratory changes. It is important to

ensure that volume depletion is corrected before spinal anesthesia, because venous return and hence cardiac output are diminished. These changes are aggravated by keeping the head up.

14. **(D)** The role of thymectomy in treating patients with myasthenia gravis who have a thymoma is well established. The thymus gland is located in the anterior mediastinum and can be approached by a cervical or mediastinal approach. It arises from the third and fourth branchial arches. Thymectomy is frequently advised for patients with myasthenia gravis who do not have a thymoma; however, there are some authorities who would treat these patients initially with an anticholinesterase drug such as pyridostigmine (Mestinon). Corticosteroid therapy may be indicated when thymectomy has failed, but it must be undertaken cautiously, because the drug may precipitate severe weakness. Pneumococcal infections (which may occur after splenectomy performed in children) are not a specific complication noted after thymectomy.

15. **(C)** Bronchogenic carcinoma accounts for 70–80% of all cases of superior vena cava (SVC) obstruction; primary mediastinal tumors are the second most common cause. The main bronchial lymphatics are located at the tracheal bifurcation and immediately to the right and left of the trachea. Tuberculosis and mycotic infections are the most likely causes of chronic fibrosing mediastinitis.

16. **(D)** CT is useful, because it delineates the calcification and shows the pattern of the calcification. There is no need for intervention at this stage, because most lesions of this nature are probably benign granulomas.

17. **(D)** By definition, a solitary nodule is one that is 5 cm or less in diameter. In most series, 60% of such lesions are benign, and 40% are malignant. The presence of irregular margins, the absence of calcification, a recent onset of symptoms, or an increase in size of the lesion within a relatively short period (several months) indicate the greater likelihood of malignancy. Thin-section CT scanning may add further information.

18. **(A)** Bronchoscopy is the initial step, particularly if the patient is a smoker and a good risk for surgery. If cancer is confirmed, thoracotomy will probably be undertaken. Patient age is an important consideration in the management of a solitary pulmonary nodule; malignancy occurs in less than 1% of patients under 35 years of age. Benign lesions, such as bronchopulmonary sequestration, which usually affects the posterior aspect of the inferior lobes of the lung, must be considered. Bronchopulmonary sequestration is usually asymptomatic, unless complications occur.

19. **(E)** In apical lung cancers, the malignant tumor may extend above the thoracic inlet, penetrate the suprapleural membrane, and infiltrate the structures found at the root of the neck. The first thoracic nerve and lower trunk of the brachial plexus are most likely to be involved initially, as T1 passes along the inner border of the first rib to reach the neck. If the sympathetic nerve is involved, pupil constriction and ptosis may be evident (Horner syndrome). The other listed items are all features of the paraneoplastic syndrome associated with lung cancer and do not necessarily indicate extranodal metastasis. Cushing's syndrome in lung cancer occurs more frequently in men and in an older age group and has a more rapid downhill course than typical Cushing's syndrome. SIADH should be suspected if the patient with a lung lesion develops unexplained mental changes and an extremely low serum sodium level. Fluid restriction is required. Urine osmolarity is low.

20. **(A)** Hypercalcemia is attributed to the secretion of parahormone from a localized squamous cell carcinoma (paraneoplastic effect); as such, improvement may be seen after surgical resection. Following extension of the tumor into the chest wall, radiotherapy and subsequent extensive resection carried out in selected cases may occasionally be indicated. Small-cell carcinoma (also known as oat-cell carcinoma) accounts for 20–25% of cases of bronchogenic carcinoma, arises centrally and tends to metastasize widely. The initial treatment is combination chemotherapy followed by radiotherapy in those whose cancer responds.

21. **(B)** Uncorrected hypercarbia is the major contraindication to total pneumonectomy. Surgery is the treatment of choice for nonsmall-cell carcinoma of the lung. Although 25% of patients with bronchogenic carcinoma may undergo thoracotomy, many of these patients will have unresectable lesions. Patients with a FEV_1 less than 2 L, a FVC under 70% of predicted value, and maximal voluntary ventilation (MVV) under 50% are likely to tolerate operation poorly. The normal FEV_1/FVC ratio is 0.7 or less; in severe obstructive dysfunction, it is under 0.45. Total atelectasis of the lung may be associated with obstruction of the main bronchus by the tumor.

22. **(D)** Patients with small-cell carcinoma should not be treated initially by thoracotomy. This cancer responds favorably to combination chemotherapy, but few patients survive for more than 1 year. More than 160,000 cases of bronchogenic carcinoma are diagnosed in the United States per year. It accounts for 33% of all cancer deaths in men and 20% of all cancer deaths in women. The most common cancers of the lung are squamous carcinoma, 30% (tumor tends to be central); adenocarcinoma, 30%, (tumor tends to be peripheral) small-cell carcinoma, 20% (tumor tends to be central); and large-cell carcinoma, 15% (tumor tends to be peripheral).

23. **(A)** The arch of the aorta is above the arbitrary line drawn between the manubriosternal joint (angle of Louis) and the lower border of the fourth thoracic vertebra level. Therefore, it is located entirely in the superior mediastinum behind the manubrium. The projected line passing behind the manubriosternal junction and the lower border of T4 is a key surgical anatomic landmark of this region. The ascending aorta (anteriorly), descending aorta (posteriorly), and pulmonary trunk are below this level. The left recurrent laryngeal nerve curves around the ligamentum arteriosus, the arch of the azygous vein enters the SVC, and the upper third of the esophagus are separated arbitrarily from the middle third at this level. On a plain film of the chest, the tracheal bifurcation (carina) is a useful marker of this line.

24. **(C)** Although there is a history of previous thyroid cancer, the presence of a solitary nodule on chest x-ray is more likely to represent a primary carcinoma of the lung than a solitary secondary metastasis. In metastasis, the lesions are more often multiple, they frequently appear bilaterally, and they more commonly present in the lower area of the lungs. A CT scan would be helpful in delineating the pulmonary findings.

25. **(C)** The most likely diagnosis, malignant epithelioma, commonly occurs following chronic exposure (>20–40 years) to asbestos. We need to consider this diagnosis in those employed in milling and construction, as well as in workers in pipe, textiles, gaskets, and other industries in which asbestos (especially crocidolite form) is used. In 75%, the diffuse (malignant) form occurs; less than 25% will survive more than 1 year after the diagnosis is established. In advanced disease, lesions below the diaphragm are frequently encountered.

26. **(C)** Cystic fibrosis is the most common cause of chronic obstructive lung disease (COLD) in children and adolescents. It is an autosomal-recessive disease that affects widespread exocrine glands. COLD is evident in all patients who survive childhood.

27. **(A)** Ipratropium bromide bronchodilator therapy will frequently improve pulmonary function in patients with COPD. Two to four inhalations every 4–6 hours are prescribed. COPD is due to emphysema (COPD type A) or chronic bronchitis (COPD type B). In the early stages, small airway dysfunction (abnormal closing volume) is found. As the disease proceeds, the FEV_1 is reduced, then the FEV_1/FVC ratio (<0.7).

28. **(C)** The presence of multiple masses on a chest x-ray should alert the physician to the possible diagnosis of pulmonary AV fistula. Needle biopsy and endobronchial biopsy of the lesion should not be attempted, because severe hemorrhage may be precipitated. Paradoxical emboli, brain abscess, and hemothorax are recognized complications. If the fistula is localized, resection is undertaken; in multiple lesions,

therapeutic embolization is done. In addition to AV malformation, multiple masses on a chest x-ray could be due to metastasis, granulomatous infection, or sarcoid or rheumatoid arthritis.

29. **(D)** In mediastinal tamponade, hypotension, dyspnea, cyanosis, and a decrease in pulse pressure will be evident. During inspiration, the pulse pressure is further impeded to cause obstruction to transmitted ACV waves in the neck; in congestive cardiac failure, the ACV waves recorded in the neck are more prominent. Paresis of the arm is unlikely to occur, because the lower part of the brachial plexus (T1) passes along the inner border of the first rib to reach the neck.

30. **(B)** Mediastinal hemorrhage after trauma may result from blunt or penetrating injuries. Tamponade should be suspected if hypotension, cyanosis, dyspnea, and venous congestion occur.

31. **(B)** Dissecting thoracic aneurysm should be suspected in Marfan's syndrome, pregnancy, bicuspid aortic valves, and coarctation. The onset of pain is sudden and severe and radiates to the back. Pulse discrepancy is frequently seen. The hypertension should be treated initially before any surgery is contemplated. The mortality rate of immediate (within 24 hours) surgical resection of the ascending aorta (type A) is 20%; however, if surgery is delayed, the mortality is 50% at 2 weeks and 90% at 3 months.

32. **(E)** The eleventh and twelfth ribs are free anteriorly and like other ribs articulate with costal cartilage anteriorly. However, the anterior margins of these ribs are free (float) and do not form part of the costal margins. The pleural reflection posteriorly intersects the twelfth rib. Ribs that articulate with the sternum are called true (ribs 1–6 or 7); the remainder are called false ribs.

33. **(D)** In ARDS, poor alveolar gas exchange and interstitial edema are evident in the presence of normal or lowered PCWP. The changes are caused by damage to capillary and alveolar epithelial cells consequent to the release of proinflammatory cytokines, which, in turn, arise from stimulated lymphocytes and macrophages. Other clinical features suggestive of ARDS are diffuse ("fluffy") pulmonary infiltrates and refractory hypoxemia (PaO_2/FiO_2 <200).

34. **(C)** ARDS is caused by pulmonary or systemic insult. It is characterized by bilateral pulmonary infiltrates, hypoxemia, noncompliant lungs, and a normal or low PCWP, and steroids have no proved value in the management of ARDS, and their use may be deleterious in the presence of sepsis. PEEP, if required, should be used cautiously with the lowest FiO_2 that maintains the PO_2 above 60 mm Hg. Excessive fluid overload should be avoided. Ventilation should be with lower tidal volumes and decreasing peak airway pressures. Management strategies in ARDS are aimed largely at supportive care, maintaining tissue oxygenation and preventing further lung injury secondary to mechanical ventilation. Smaller tidal volumes are used (5–7 mL/kg) to prevent volutrauma as well as to decrease the peak inspiratory pressures.

35. **(E)** Culture for mycobacterium usually requires 6 weeks before a diagnosis can be made. The clinical and x-ray features are suggestive of tuberculosis. The sedimentation rate is increased in the presence of active disease. The incidence of tuberculosis in the United States has increased in recent years. In many cases of primary infection, resolution occurs without symptoms. The pulmonary focus remains dormant (Ghon) and may become activated, causing caseation of the lung, formation of a thick-walled fibrous cavity, tuberculous bronchitis, bronchiectasis, hemoptysis, and cavitation. Sputum examined for acid-fast bacilli may be inadequate, because saprophytic organisms may be detected. The Kveim test is used in the differential diagnosis to exclude sarcoid.

36. **(D)** In the early stages of HIV infection, skin testing for tuberculin is intact; however, false-positive results occur because of infection by nontuberculous mycobacteria and are common because of the immune disorder. Most patients with tuberculosis, who are compliant, can be treated on an outpatient basis.

37. **(B)** Bronchiectasis is caused by a congenital or acquired dilation of the segmental, subsegmental, or branches of the bronchi. Patients with B lymphocyte disorders are more likely to develop lower respiratory tract infection and bronchiectasis than those with impaired T-cell immunity. Treatment is aimed at obtaining maximal drainage. Resection may be indicated when the disease is localized and persistent symptoms and complications occur.

38. **(A)** Cystic fibrosis is an autosomal-recessive disorder of the exocrine glands and occurs in neonates who survive an episode of intestinal obstruction due to mucoviscidosis. Cystic fibrosis accounts for more than one-half of the cases of bronchiectasis seen today. Other causes include acute and chronic lung infections, humoral immunodeficiency, and localized bronchial obstruction (e.g., carcinoma). The basal segments of the lung, lingula, and right middle lobes are involved most frequently.

39. **(C)** Bronchogenic cysts are located in the mediastinum but are seen most frequently behind the carina. They have a thin wall, are lined by bronchial epithelium, and contain mucus. Bronchogenic cysts are usually asymptomatic, but symptoms may occur because of compression, with cough, wheezing, and possibly dysphagia. Bronchogenic cysts may become infected and rupture into surrounding organs. Cysts constitute 20% of mediastinal mass lesions. The most common mediastinal cyst is the pericardial cyst, which is found most often at the right costophrenic angle.

40. **(D)** Bronchopulmonary sequestration can be differentiated from a bronchogenic cyst; in that it is composed of nonfunctioning lung tissue that is disconnected from the remaining lung; it has a separate blood supply. Glomus tumors are rare tumors that arise in the middle ear or jugular bulb. Patients complain of tinnitus and hearing loss.

41. **(D)** There are three major openings of structures that penetrate the diaphragm at differing thoracic vertebra levels. The IVC enters at T8 (to the right of the midline), the esophagus at T10 (to the left of the midline), and the aorta at T12 in the midline.

42. **(A)** Funnel chest (Fig. 3–9) is the most important congenital chest wall deformity. It is usually present at birth, and there is marked asymmetry. The heart is displaced to the left. There is often a familial history, and associated congenital heart disease may frequently be encountered. Correction is recommended in asymptomatic patients with prominent deformity to avoid permanent cardiopulmonary changes. In flail chest, paradoxical respiration occurs as the chest wall deformity is sucked inward during inspiration. It occurs after extensive rib trauma where individual ribs are separated in two different sites.

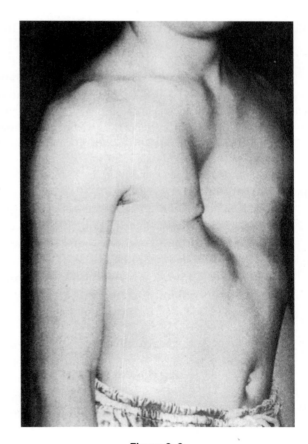

Figure 3–9.
Funnel chest is the most important congenital chest wall deformity. *(Reproduced, with permission, from Doherty GM: Current Surgical Diagnosis and Treatment, 12th ed. 1283. McGraw-Hill, 2006.)*

43. **(A)** Any object that compromises the blood supply to the tracheal mucosa or cartilage can cause stenosis. When the mean intramural pressure exceeds 20–30 mm Hg, damage may be anticipated. Riedel struma is a rare fibrosing thyroid condition, which must be differentiated from carcinoma and may cause severe tracheal stenosis. Achalasia is a neuromuscular defect at the lower end of the esophagus causing dysphagia, because of nonmechanical esophageal obstruction.

44. **(A)** On the left side, the pleural reflection deviates to the left, anteriorly between the fourth and sixth costal cartilages, to accommodate the cardiac notch. Although the right and left pleural reflections approach each other in the midline, there is no direct communication between the two sides.

45. **(D)** Frequently, a fracture cannot be seen on the chest x-ray; however, the patient should be treated for fracture, although none is seen on the x-ray. Pneumothorax may occur if more than one rib is involved, but a chest tube is indicated only if it is of substantial size or increasing in amount. Hemothorax usually occurs because of a tear in the intercostal or other intrathoracic vessels.

46. **(D)** A thoracoabdominal incision is still used occasionally where access to both the upper abdomen and posterior thoracic structures is required. The main reasons for less frequent use of this incision are poor healing of the divided costal margin, postoperative pain, and an increased risk of infection in both the thoracic and abdominal compartments.

47. **(B)** Sternal injuries usually involve the body or manubriosternal junction in a transverse direction and frequently cause displacement. Sternal injuries occur most commonly as a result of injury by steering wheel impact in car accidents. It is important to exclude cardiac and major vessel injury in such injuries.

48. **(B)** Most lesions of the trachea, except infiltrating adenoid cystic carcinoma, that cause tracheal stenosis should be resected when possible.

In general, up to 50% of the trachea may be resected. Unequivocal postintubation stenosis is treated by surgical repair. Congenital tracheal stenosis should be treated by surgery if symptoms necessitate it. Dilatation can result in rupture of the trachea.

49. **(B)** Patients with hyperparathyroidism develop demineralization, and 1.5% shows osteitis fibrosa cystica. The presence of subperiosteal resorption of bone of the phalanges and lamina dura of the teeth are fairly diagnostic radiological findings of hyperparathyroidism. Chondromas account for 20% of benign tumors of the rib and occur at the costochondral junction. Osteochondromas arise from the cortex and usually occur in men. Eosinophilic granuloma results in a destructive lesion apparent on x-ray.

50. **(D)** Antibiotics and vigorous attempts to obtain bronchial drainage will treat the abscess adequately in the majority of cases. Lung abscesses commonly are associated with aspiration pneumonia, where the abscess is found posteriorly. In the presence of an unexplained lung abscess, bronchoscopy is essential to exclude a foreign body or tumor that could cause bronchial obstruction.

51. **(B)** Branchial cleft cysts (Fig. 3–9) arise from the second and third branchial clefts. Branchial cysts may become evident after an URTI and present as a mass anterior to the sternocleidomastoid muscle. Intraoperatively, they can be traced to pass between the and external carotid artery to the piriform sinus or tonsillar fossa.

52. **(C)** Cystic hygromas are relatively rare tumors. Most are encountered in the posterior triangle of the neck, but occasionally they are found in the mediastinum, axilla, or groin. They are often noted at birth and represent persistence of primary lymphatic buds. They extend into the surrounding tissues but are not associated with malignancy. Transillumination is a useful sign to diagnose this lesion.

53. **(D)** Females are affected by myasthenia gravis twice as commonly as males. It is an autoimmune disease that produces antibodies to

acetylcholine receptors. The external ocular and other cranial muscles are often involved at an early stage. There is a deficiency in acetylcholine receptors, and thymectomy is often helpful.

54. **(D)** Squamous carcinoma of the lip comprises 15–20% of all malignant tumors of the oral cavity. In approximately 30%, there is a clear association with heavy exposure to the sun. The incidence increases in those areas where there is more southerly latitude, the air is dry, and the altitude is higher.

55. **(C)** If the lesion is treated early, patients will achieve a cure in most cases. The upper lip is involved in 10% of patients.

56. **(C)** Hyperkeratosis of the lip is a premalignant lesion and usually occurs in people exposed excessively to the sun. The mucosa undergoes metaplasia to keratosquamous epithelium. The lip becomes pale, thin, and fragile, with cracks and fissures, and is covered with a white base.

57. **(D)** Ameloblastoma is a benign tumor and usually occurs at the junction of the body and ramus of the mandible. Although it is a benign tumor, it recurs if inadequately excised. It is relatively radioresistant. Histologically, odontogenic epithelium is seen in connective tissue stroma with extensive areas of cystic degeneration.

58. **(B)** The lingual nerve swings forward deep to the mylohyoid muscle and crosses twice over the submandibular (Wharton's) duct. The mandibular branch of the facial nerve (not listed in the answer choices) may accidentally be injured below the angle of the mandible (Fig. 3–10). Injury to this branch causes serious facial deformity.

59. **(C)** Squamous cell carcinoma of the tongue frequently (40–60%) metastasizes to the lymph glands. Carcinoma of the tongue usually commences at the tip or side. The 5-year survival rate for carcinoma of the tongue is 40%, but it improves to 55% if lymph nodes are not involved.

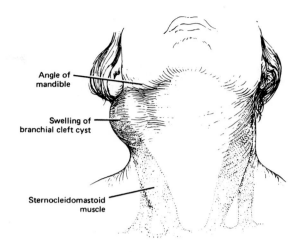

Figure 3–10.
Branchial cyst. (Reproduced, with permission, from Lindner, HH: Clinical Anatomy. Appleton & Lange, 1989.)

60. **(B)** Carcinoma of the posterior third of the tongue is often detected late and carries a worse prognosis. Posterior-third tongue tumors are also called lymphoepitheliomas. These lesions can be poorly differentiated.

61. **(A)** Tumors of the hard palate usually arise from the minor salivary glands. Cancers of the lip, tongue, esophagus, and larynx are often squamous cell carcinoma.

62. **(A)** Poorly differentiated squamous cell carcinoma of the floor of the mouth tends to be more invasive than better-differentiated tumors. Poorer prognosis can be expected when invasion is larger than 9 mm, perineural invasion is noted, and lymph node metastasis is evident.

63. **(C)** Nasopharyngeal carcinoma is prevalent in China. It has been associated with high levels of Epstein-Barr virus titers. The most common sign is a neck mass, even when the primary lesion is microscopic. The first cranial nerve to be affected is the abducent (VI) and indicates cranial extension.

64. **(A)** Any object that compromises the blood supply to the tracheal mucosa or cartilage can cause stenosis. When the mean intramural

pressure exceeds 20–30 mm Hg over a prolonged period, damage occurs.

65. **(A)** Verrucous carcinoma is a low-grade malignancy and is seen more frequently in the southern part of the United States. It is found most commonly on the gingival-buccal junction in tobacco chewers. It is grayish white and exophytic. Radiation is associated with possible metastases. If not excised, the lesion tends to invade locally.

66. **(D)** Juvenile nasopharyngeal hemangiofibromas are rare nonmalignant tumors containing both fibrous and vascular tissue. They occur exclusively among boys.

67. **(C)** If the neck nodes are removed, some patients have surgically curable primary disease. In some series, as many as 20% remain free of disease for more than 5 years without any manifestation of a primary tumor. It is essential to search extensively for a primary source before labeling the lesion as a possible branchial cleft carcinoma, which is extremely rare.

68. **(D)** More than 80% of neck gland tumors arise from structures above the clavicle. The piriform fossa is lateral to the aryepiglottic folds and is a major site where a primary cancer may remain hidden from early detection. Twenty percent of neck gland tumors are primary and 80% represent metastatic disease.

69. **(D)** The response is transient, lasting only 2–3 months. The results of this type of therapy, combined with those of artery occlusion, radiotherapy, or other modes of chemotherapy, require further evaluation.

70. **(B)** The classic block dissection includes sternocleidomastoid muscle, the external and internal jugular veins, the spinal accessory nerve, the submandibular gland, and the lymphatic tissue of the lateral compartment of the neck. Procedures that preserve muscle, nerve, or vessels are called modified neck dissection.

71. **(B)** The chorda tympani (branch of the facial nerve) join the lingual nerve in the infratemporal fossa to supply the anterior two-thirds of the tongue with taste fibers (cell stations in the geniculate ganglion of the facial nerve). It also contains the secretory parasympathetic fibers to the submandibular and sublingual glands.

72. **(D)** The thymus gland is removed in certain cases of myasthenia gravis. It is located in the anterior mediastinum and can be approached by a cervical or mediastinal approach. It arises from the third and fourth branchial arches. Pneumococcal infections are particularly likely to develop after splenectomy performed in children.

73. **(A)** The most common organisms isolated in acute pharyngitis are streptococci, virus, *Neisseria gonorrhoeae*, and mycoplasma.

74. **(C)** Odynophagia is a sensation of sharp retrosternal pain on swallowing. It is usually caused by severe erosive conditions such as *Candida*, herpes virus, and corrosive injury following caustic ingestion.

75. **(B)** The most common source of epistaxis is Kisselbach's vascular plexus on the anterior nasal septum. Predisposing factors include foreign bodies, forceful nose-blowing, nose-picking, rhinitis, and deviated septum.

76. **(D)** Carotid body tumor is the most common type of paraganglioma in the head and neck region, followed by the glomus jugular tumor. Carotid body tumor grows slowly, rarely metastasizes, and may secrete catecholamines. The tumor usually is supplied by the external carotid artery, and dissection to remove it off the carotid bifurcation may be difficult and cause bleeding. Malignancy occurs in 6% of patients.

77. **(E)** Bell's palsy (of the facial nerve) has been attributed to an inflammatory condition of the facial nerve at the site where it exits through the stylomastoid foramen. Its cause remains unclear, and recent studies indicate a possible association with reactivation of herpes simplex virus in some cases. Facial paresis usually comes on abruptly.

78. (B) Prospective nonrandomized evaluations of treatment duration of acute otitis media reveal no difference in outcome if given over 5-day, 7-day, or 10-day duration. However, 10-day treatment is indicated for children with history of acute otitis media within the preceding month.

79. (A) Neuroleptic anesthesia is the use of agents that suppress psychomotor activity. Droperidol produces marked sedation and tranquilization. The onset of action is 3–10 minutes after injection, but the full effect may not be noted until 30 minutes after injection. The sedative action lasts 2–4 hours. It potentiates the action of central nervous system (CNS)-depressant drugs, can cause hypotension, and causes mild α-adrenergic blockade.

80. (C) The most common complication of thyroid and parathyroid surgery is iatrogenic injury to the recurrent laryngeal nerve, which can result in temporary (up to 7.1%) or permanent (up to 3.6%) paralysis of the vocal cord.

81. (B) Laryngomalacia is characterized by inspiratory stridor and is caused by redundant epiglottis and aryepiglottic folds in young children. The condition usually resolves without surgical intervention.

82. (B) Jet irrigation (e.g., *Water Pik*) should be avoided to remove cerumen impaction. Detergent ear drops (such as 3% hydrogen peroxide) may be used. Aqueous irrigation should be avoided if organic material is present, because further swelling will be induced.

83. (A) The presence of a nasogastric tube causes swelling and irritation of the nasal mucosa. This, in turn, may partly occlude drainage of the sinus into the meatus.

84. (B) Foreign bodies in the ear canal are more frequently encountered in children than adults. In general, foreign bodies in the ear are removed under microscopic control to avoid further injury.

85. (D) Rapid testing for streptococci with latex agglutination (LA) antigen test is much less sensitive than with solid-phase enzyme-linked immunoassay (ELISA).

86. (B) Pharyngeal (branchial arch) remnants account for many cysts or fistulas in the lateral neck. The associated tract can be found in various locations. Thyroglossal duct cysts associated with the decent of the thyroid gland are usually midline, extending as high as the base of tongue.

87. (A) Epistaxis in children and young adults usually arises from the anterior nasal septum (Kiesselbach's plexus). In elderly persons, however, spontaneous rupture of a sclerotic blood vessel in the posterior nasal septum is usually the cause of bleeding, especially in combination with hypertension.

88. (A) Tinnitus is the perception of abnormal noise in the ear or head. It is usually attributed to a sensory loss; pulsatile tinnitus occurs with conductive hearing loss and is due to carotid pulsations becoming more apparent.

89. (E) Surgical drainage of otitis media (myringotomy) is performed in either chronic infections or severe infections. Complications of otitis media include mastoiditis and meningitis.

90. (E) These may be difficult to excise because of the focal nerve involvement by the hemangioma.

91. (D) Blowout fractures of the orbit exhibit epistaxis; subcutaneous emphysema and periorbital ecchymosis are also frequently encountered. Treatment of most severe injuries is by surgical repair, often by a lower lid blepharoplasty incision. Enopthalmous, lateral diplopia and blindness do not generally occur.

92. (E) Tympanostomy tube placement is performed through the external auditory canal with microscopic guidance. The tympanic membrane is directly visualized after clearing wax and debris from external auditory canal. Otorrhea is the most common sequela, requiring tube removal in 13.5% of long-term tubes and 0.9% of short-term tubes.

93. **(C)** The external laryngeal nerve supplies the cricothyroid muscle, which assists in tensing the cords.

94. **(A)** Scrofula is tuberculosis lymphadenitis. It may occur in immunocompromised hosts as well as in patients from underdeveloped countries. A chest x-ray must be obtained and a purified protein derivative (PPD) skin test must be carried out. The response rate to antituberculous drugs is good, but excision of the residual lesion may be required.

95. **(D)** Mucor is an opportunistic mold that causes mucormycosis. At least 50% of reported cases are associated with uncontrolled diabetes, and many of the remaining patients are immunosuppressed. It appears as black crusting in the nose and sinuses and spreads rapidly to involve the cerebrum. Biopsy reveals nonseptate hyphae, which confirms the diagnosis. Treatment is directed toward control for diabetic ketoacidosis and use of amphotericin B.

96. **(B)** Dermoid cysts arise along line of fusion of embryonic parts. In the floor of the mouth, the swelling forces the tongue upward. Alternatively, the swelling may occur below the mylohyoid muscle, where it gives the impression of a double chin. It is not a premalignant lesion. It has an epithelial lining and may contain secretions, sloughed-off cells, and hair.

97. **(D)** In Peutz-Jegher syndrome, pigmented melanin spots are found in the buccal and perineal region. The lesions are flat and greenish black in the buccal region and remain after puberty. Pigmentation is found inside the mouth, nostrils, palms, and feet. Usually at about 20–30 years of age, hamartomatous polyps are found in the small intestine, but other parts of the alimentary tract may also be involved. Adenocarcinoma develops in 23% of patients.

98. **(D)** Benign mixed tumor (pleomorphic adenoma) requires appropriate excision (superficial parotidectomy). If the tumor is shelled out,

recurrence is likely. Approximately 80% of tumors of the salivary glands occur in the parotid gland.

99. **(B)** The trigeminal nerve exits from the foramen ovale to enter the infratemporal fossa. The motor mandibular division of cranial nerve V also exits through the same opening.

100. **(A)** If the thyroid gland is absent from the neck, it may be in the lingual position at the foramen cecum. Excision of this lesion from the tongue will require thyroid hormone replacement.

101. **(B)** Nasopharyngeal cancer is most closely associated with Epstein-Barr virus. This virus is also associated with infective mononucleosis and Burkitt's lymphoma.

102. **(E)** If the tumor should extend upward into the sphenoid bone, the cavernous sinus may be involved.

103. **(B)** The tip of the tongue drains into the submental lymph nodes, whereas, the side of the tongue drains into the submandibular lymph nodes.

104. **(G)** Dermoid cysts form along lines of fusion of embryological dermatomes of the skin. In the neck, they are commonly above the thyroid cartilage and may be classified as one of four varieties, central or lateral in the midline and above or below the mylohyoid muscle.

105. **(G)** The thyroid develops from the foramen cecum in the tongue and descends to its definitive position in the neck. Failure of the tract to close may result in a thyroglossal duct cyst.

106. **(A)** An elevated ionic calcium and elevated blood levels of intact PTH clinches the diagnosis of hyperparathyroid. Primary hyperparathyroidism can result in bone demineralization and renal calculi if neglected. Hyperparathyroidism may be manifestation of the multiple endocrine neoplasia syndrome. Pancreatic islet cell tumors, vi2 gastinomas and insulinomas, and pituitary tumors are part of the multiple endocrine neoplasia MEAN 1 syndrome.

Myoglobin in the urine is present in patients with rhabodmyolysis and is not associated with elevated serum calcium, and is after associated with hyperkalemia.

107. **(B)** An ectopic thyroid gland can be located anywhere from the base of the tongue to the mediastinum. It often results in the failure of descent resulting in either a linginal thyroid or ectopic thyroid in the midline of the neck. The so called lateral aberrant thyroid is usually a metastasis from papillary carcinoma of the thyroid.

Angioneurotic edema is an acute allergic reaction, which causes a sudden swelling of the whole tongue with airway obstruction.

108. **(E)** Hyperthyroidism could be diffuse primary hyperthyroidisms, Graves' disease, or a toxic nodular goiter. Graves' disease is an autoimmune hyperthyroidism. The treatment consists of medical management with use of antithyroid drugs such as methimazole, or ablation of the gland with radioactive I_{131}, or surgically with subtotal thyroidectomy. Failure of medical management requires oblation procedures either with I_{131} or surgery.

Lugols iodine is used in preparation to surgery. Steroids are not used in the treatment of hyperthyroidism. It may be used in the management of thyroid storm, a life threatening condition.

109. **(B)** Definitive treatment of hyperparathyroidism is parathyroidectomy. When serum calcium is above 14 mgm/dL the patient is in hypercalcemic crisis. Immediate treatment of this condition requires hydration with normal saline and use of diuretics to bring down the serum calcium level.

A positive parathyroid scan will help to locate an adenoma of the parathyroid preoperatively.

CHAPTER 4

Cardiac and Thoracic

Marshall O. Kramer and E. A. Bonfils-Roberts

Questions

DIRECTIONS (Questions 1 through 30): Each of the numbered items in this section is followed by five answers. Select the ONE lettered answer that is BEST in each case.

1. A 14-year-old boy is seen by a pediatric cardiologist because of increasing shortness of breath. Studies reveal increased pulmonary vascular resistance, left axis deviation on Electrocardiogram (ECG), and mitral regurgitation murmur. What is the most likely diagnosis?

   (A) Ostium primum defect
   (B) Tetralogy of Fallot
   (C) Right aortic arch
   (D) Ostium secundum defect
   (E) Atrioventricular canal

2. A cyanotic female neonate is born with transposition of the great arteries. Metabolic acidosis and hypoxemia are present and are life threatening. Which of the following is the best initial treatment?

   (A) Urgent Mustard operation
   (B) Prostaglandin E1
   (C) Atrial septotomy
   (D) Pulmonary artery banding
   (E) Prostaglandin E1 and atrial septotomy

3. A 65-year-old man undergoes cardiac surgery for triple vessel coronary artery disease. What can he anticipate?

   (A) 95% chance his grafts will occlude after 12 months.
   (B) 5% chance of living for 5 years.
   (C) If the internal mammary artery is used as a conduit, patency is increased.
   (D) Mortality if 10–20% in most centers.
   (E) Functional improvement with the saphenous vein graft is better than internal memory artery.

4. Three months after aortic valve replacement with a mechanical prosthesis, a 60-year-old man describes malaise, and increasing shortness of breath. Examination reveals pulsus paradoxus. ECG shows low voltage precordially. What test is most useful for making the diagnosis?

   (A) Stress thallium exam
   (B) Computer Tomography (CT) examination of chest
   (C) Coronary angiography
   (D) Echocardiography
   (E) Serum creatinine phosphokinase (CPK)

5. In the patient described above urine output decreases to 20 cc/h. Studies reveal paradoxical septal motion. What is the next course of therapy?

   (A) Expectant medical therapy
   (B) Redo aortic valve surgery
   (C) Left chest tube
   (D) Ontra-aortic balloon
   (E) Pericardial window

6. A 58-year-old man is in cardiogenic shock in the emergency department after sustaining an acute myocardial infarction (MI). An intra-aortic balloon pump (IABP) is inserted. Which statement is TRUE about IABP?

   (A) The balloon increases coronary perfusion during diastole.
   (B) The balloon increases coronary perfusion during systole.
   (C) The balloon increases peripheral resistance.
   (D) The balloon is inflated in systole and diastole.
   (E) The pump must be removed after 24 hours.

7. A 66-year-old female has had two MIs in the past. She is admitted to the emergency department in congestive heart failure. After admission and appropriate therapy her Holter monitor shows frequent PVCs and her ejection fraction is found to be 35%. Appropriate treatment would include which of the following?

   (A) Single chamber pacemaker
   (B) Cardioversion
   (C) Dual chamber pacemaker
   (D) Internal cardiac defibrillator (ICD)
   (E) Greenfield filter

8. During a routine examination of a 30-year-old female actuary seeking life insurance, she is found to have a ventricular septal defect (VSD). She undergoes subsequent studies including ECG, chest x-ray, echocardiography, and Doppler ultrasound. What is the major determinant of operability in VSD?

   (A) Age of patient
   (B) Pulmonary vascular resistance
   (C) Size of the VSD
   (D) Location of the VSD
   (E) Presence of cyanosis

9. At the age of 3 years, a child with a VSD becomes progressively short of breath and requires urgent surgery. What is the most common type of VSD (Fig. 4–1)?

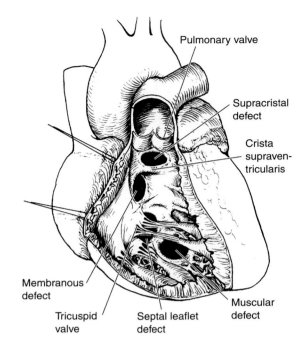

Figure 4–1.
Anatomical locations of various ventricular septal defects. The wall of the right ventricle has been excised to expose the ventricular septum. *(Reproduced, with permission, from Doherty GM: Current Surgical Diagnosis and Treatment, 12th ed. 433. McGraw-Hill, 2006.)*

   (A) Defect anterior to the crista supraventricular
   (B) Membranous septal defect
   (C) Posterior septal defect
   (D) Low muscular defect
   (E) Right-to-left shunt

10. A 1-year-old girl is found to have a posterior membranous VSD. Peripheral resistance of the pulmonary system is 40% that of the systemic. How should you proceed?

   (A) Observe the child, because most VSDs close spontaneously.
   (B) Band the pulmonary artery and fix the defect at age 6.
   (C) Repair electively at age 14.
   (D) Repair electively between ages 4 and 6 years.
   (E) Repair immediately as an emergency.

11. At birth, the 6 weeks premature infant is noted to have progressive dyspnea. There is a continuous murmur in the pulmonic area

(second left intercostal space), and cyanosis is absent. ECG findings are normal. An x-ray of the heart shows cardiomegaly, and the pulse is bounding. Patent ductus arteriosus (PDA) is diagnosed. What does treatment include?

(A) Immediate surgical correction
(B) Administration of indomethacin
(C) Administration of cortisone
(D) Renal dialysis
(E) Endotracheal intubation in all cases

12. During a routine preschool physical examination, the physician notes that a 3-year-old girl has a machinery-type murmur on auscultation of the chest. The pulse is bounding and palpable in the femoral and radial region of both sides of her body. There were no symptoms, and she has excellent exercise performance. Persistent PDA is confirmed on subsequent examination. The parents should be advised that the girl requires which of the following:

(A) Surgical correction and closure of the PDA
(B) Indomethacin
(C) Coronary angiography
(D) No treatment unless symptoms occur
(E) CT scan of the heart

13. At the age of 34 years, a female long-distance runner notes increasing dyspnea after running more than 10 mi. On inspection and palpation, a prominent right ventricular heave is noted. There is a loud systolic murmur in the left third interspace. The ECG shows right-axis deviation with right bundle branch block. An x-ray of the chest shows a small aortic knob. What sign or test will most likely reveal the cause of the congenital heart abnormality thought to be atrial septal defect?

(A) Beading (scalloping) of the ribs on x-ray
(B) Decreased carotid pulse
(C) Left ventricular hypertrophy on ECG
(D) Elevated sedimentation rate
(E) Increased oxygen saturation gradient between the superior vena cava and the right ventricle

14. The only son of a physiology instructor dies suddenly at the age of 12 years following worsening symptoms of tetralogy of Fallot. What would an autopsy reveal?

(A) Dextroposition of the appendix
(B) Brachiocephalic vein draining into the right renal vein
(C) Inferior vena cava (IVC) draining to the superior mesenteric vein
(D) Atrial Septal Defect (ASD)
(E) Decreased vascularity of the lung field.

15. After suffering a streptococcal throat infection, a 12-year-old immigrant boy develops cardiac symptoms that are attributed to rheumatic fever. Years later, at the age of 34 he is admitted to the hospital with pulmonary edema. Further examination reveals a diastolic murmur at the apex and mitral stenosis is diagnosed. Before surgical evaluation, which of the following findings can be attributed to mitral stenosis?

(A) Large left ventricle
(B) Indentation of the middle third of the esophagus by an enlarged left atrium
(C) Notching of the ribs
(D) Bounding, full pulse
(E) Angina pectoris

16. A 23-year-old ballet dancer is concerned about the recent sudden death of a young famous Russian dancer on a New York stage. The patient seeks advice about his own risk for developing cardiac disease. His father died suddenly from ischemic heart disease at the age of 40. What is the most important risk factor that would further indicate the possibility of coronary artery heart disease?

(A) Diabetes mellitus
(B) Personality type
(C) Elevated high-density lipoprotein
(D) Elevation of total cholesterol/ high-density lipoprotein ratio
(E) Obesity

17. In evaluating the risk factors involved in advising elective cholecystectomy in a 52-year-old man with heart disease, which of the following conditions should alert the surgeon to avoid an elective procedure?

    (A) MI 9 months earlier
    (B) Persistent nonspecific changes on ECG
    (C) Increased frequency and severity of attacks of angina
    (D) Elevated alkaline phosphatase levels
    (E) Hypertension controlled with diuretics

18. After his first heart attack 3 years ago, a 63-year-old painter complained of central chest pains that radiated to the left arm after exercise. The pain was alleviated by nitroglycerin. Recently, he fell on a steel object and severed the median nerve and flexor tendons at the wrist. The skin was sutured but he is now scheduled to have a second operation that will require anesthesia. What is the best method to diagnose angina pectoris?

    (A) Cholesterol/high-density lipid ratio
    (B) Isoenzymes
    (C) Stress electrocardiography
    (D) Echocardiography
    (E) Chest x-ray

19. Eight days after undergoing a hysterectomy, a 64-year-old woman complains of chest pain. After 12 hours, the internist orders tests to exclude MI. Which test will most likely support this diagnosis?

    (A) Serum glutamic oxaloacetic transaminase (SGOT) elevation
    (B) Increased sedimentation rate
    (C) ^{99m}Tc pyrophosphate scintigraphy showing a "hot spot"
    (D) Thallium 201 (^{201}Tl) scintigraphy showing a ("hot spot")
    (E) Dimethyliminodiacetic acid (HIDA) scan

20. After undergoing repair of a left indirect inguinal hernia, a 72-year-old obese man is admitted to the emergency department with severe retrosternal pain of 1-hours duration. The pain radiates to the medial aspect of the left hand. The ECG shows Q waves and an elevated ST-segment. A diagnosis of acute MI is established 1 hour after admission. Immediate management should include which of the following?

    (A) Thrombolytic therapy with tissue plasminogen activator (tPA)
    (B) Vitamin K
    (C) Ampicillin, 2 mg tid PO
    (D) Hydrochlorthiazide, 50 mg/d
    (E) Sodium, nitroprusside 0.5 mg/kg/min

21. Following recovery from an acute MI, a 44-year-old embryology lecturer is discharged from the hospital with what instructions?

    (A) Angiogram every 3 months to evaluate the degree of atherosclerosis
    (B) Nitroglycerin three times a day
    (C) Digoxin
    (D) 325 mg of aspirin on alternate days
    (E) Pacemaker insertion

22. A 63-year-old woman fell while crossing the street after her Thursday afternoon bridge game. Attempts at resuscitation for cardiac arrest by the emergency medical service (EMS) team were unsuccessful. The woman had previously been diagnosed as having aortic stenosis and left ventricular hypertrophy. In addition to these factors, which of the following predisposes to sudden cardiac death?

    (A) Split first heart sound
    (B) Hypokalemia
    (C) Soft murmur at left of sternum that varies with inspiration
    (D) Failure of the central venous pressure (CVP) to rise more than 1 cm H_2O with 30-second pressure on the liver (hepato-jugular reflux)
    (E) CVP of -1 cm H_2O

23. Three days after a patient underwent hip replacement for a fracture of the neck of the femur, the resident is called to examine the patient and notes hypotension (85/60 mm Hg) and a pulse rate of 104 beats per minute (bpm). Fluids are administered, but there is no

improvement. The ECG shows peaked T waves and ST-elevation. Bedside monitoring reveals a cardiac index (CI) of 1.7 L/min/m² (normal >2.2), stroke work index of 16 g/m² (normal >30), and a pulmonary artery wedge pressure (PAWP) of 22 mm Hg (normal <15). Urgent treatment should involve which of the following?

(A) Rapid hypertonic saline solution administration

(B) Adrenaline

(C) Inotropic agents and, if necessary, intra-aortic balloon counterpulsation

(D) Indomethacin

(E) Atropine

24. A 58-year-old neurologist is admitted to the emergency department with persistent hypotension and shock following an acute MI. He is placed on an IABP. Which following statement is true about IABP?

(A) The balloon is inflated during systole.

(B) The balloon is inflated during diastole and systole.

(C) The pump must be removed after 10 minutes.

(D) The balloon usually is inserted via the femoral artery.

(E) Use of an IABP worsens diastolic coronary blood flow.

25. While lying on the examining table before colonoscopy, a 68-year-old electrician notes palpitations. The colonoscopy was scheduled as a routine procedure following removal of a benign polyp 1 year earlier. He had rheumatic fever in infancy. His atrial rate on ECG is 450 bpm, and his ventricular rate is 160 bpm. His pulse rate is 88 bpm. The left atrium is enlarged. Similar findings were noted 1 year ago, but he declined to take any medication. Treatment should entail which of the following?

(A) Continue with colonoscopy

(B) Continue with colonoscopy after administration of parenteral antibiotics

(C) Immediate administration of antibiotics and follow-up colonoscopy at a later date

(D) Immediate administration of anticoagulation and digoxin and follow-up colonoscopy at a later date

(E) Immediate electrocardioversion with a current of 300–400 J

26. During routine clinical examination of a 23-year-old seeking consultation to remove a mole on her left cheek, she develops tachycardia with a pulse rate of 186 bpm. Her pulse is regular and is otherwise asymptomatic. An ECG reveals supraventricular tachycardia. What should the treatment be?

(A) Alternate pressure on the right and left carotid sinus

(B) Bilateral simultaneous pressure over right and left carotid sinus

(C) Deep eyeball pressure

(D) Morphine sulfate, 4–8 mg IV, given cautiously

(E) Electrical cardioversion

27. After experiencing progressive chest pain for 2 months, a surgical-supply store owner undergoes a CT scan that reveals a space-occupying lesion of the wall of the left atrium, which was confirmed to be a myxoma. There is no evidence of disease elsewhere. What would the next line of treatment be?

(A) Excision of a myxoma performed with a bypass procedure

(B) Excision of a myxoma performed without a bypass procedure

(C) Insertion of a pacemaker

(D) Chemotherapy

(E) Radiotherapy

28. During examination of a 49-year-old male schoolteacher who presents with a swelling in the neck, palpation by a bounding pulse. Which test would be most likely to establish a possible cause of the underlying condition?

(A) Funduscopic eye examination

(B) Liver–spleen scan

(C) Thyroid function studies

(D) X-ray of the chest and cervical spine

(E) Carotid sinus pressure

29. Following a car accident, a 52-year-old lawyer complains of pain in the left abdomen and back. After arrival of the EMS team, her pulse rate is 84 bpm, but of small volume. She states that she has some cardiac condition but is uncertain of its nature. Which is the most likely cause of the small pulse volume?

    (A) Aortic stenosis
    (B) Syphilis
    (C) Hyperthyroidism
    (D) Carcinoid syndrome
    (E) Aortic incompetence

30. Stenosis of which of the following vessels is associated with the highest patency rates following angioplasty or stenting?

    (A) Medial circumflex artery
    (B) Iliac artery
    (C) Superficial femoral artery
    (D) Popliteal artery
    (E) Tibial arteries

DIRECTIONS (Questions 31 through 42): Each set of matching questions in this section consists of a list of lettered options followed by several numbered items. For each numbered item, select the appropriate lettered option. Each lettered option may be selected once.

Question 31

    (A) History of angina and prior MI
    (B) Left ventricular ejection fraction of over 50%
    (C) Aortic stenosis
    (D) Signs of left ventricular failure
    (E) Lowered jugular venous distension
    (F) Minimal decrease in hematocrit
    (G) Presence of groin hernia
    (H) Decreased bowel motility

31. A 83-year-old retired navy general shows improvement in claudication following aortoiliac bypass surgery. What is the factor that would cause the greatest concern over the possibility of developing cardiac complications? SELECT ONE.

Questions 32 through 37

    (A) A double aortic arch
    (B) Tetralogy of Fallot
    (C) PDA
    (D) Coarctation of the aorta
    (E) Tricuspid atresia
    (F) Umbilical caput medusa
    (G) Neurofibromatosis (von Recklinghausen's disease)
    (H) Noncyanotic ASD
    (I) Spider nevi
    (J) Femoral AV fistula
    (K) Beading (notching) of the ribs

32. Cerebrovascular accident occurs most often in which? SELECT ONE.

33. Dyspnea and dysphagia occur with what? SELECT ONE.

34. Differential pressure in right arm and right leg indicates what? SELECT ONE.

35. A child was born with congenital heart disease. The mother had rubella during pregnancy. The child has what? SELECT ONE.

36. Notching of ribs occurs in what? SELECT ONE.

37. Hypoplasia of the right ventricle occurs in what? SELECT ONE.

Questions 38 and 39

A 62-year-old black physician complains of headache, nocturia, and dysuria of 3 weeks duration. Rectal examination reveals a palpable mass in the prostate, and a biopsy confirms the presence of prostatic carcinoma. He is advised to undergo prostatectomy. His blood pressure is 160/105 mm Hg.

    (A) Verapamil
    (B) Propanalol (inderal)
    (C) Deep eyeball pressure
    (D) Hydrochlorthiazide diuretic
    (E) Calcium phosphate
    (F) Digoxin

(G) Cardiac catheterization

(H) Repeat blood pressure assessment in the supine position

(I) Antihistamine

38. The next step in management is which? SELECT ONE.

39. The patient's blood pressure remains elevated when assessment is repeated on several occasions. Investigations fail to reveal an underlying cause of hypertension. Before surgery, he should receive what? SELECT ONE.

Questions 40 and 41

While undergoing a physical examination for life insurance purposes, a 46-year-old executive is noted to have a harsh systolic murmur in the left third and fourth parasternal area. Further evaluation, including echocardiography, reveals pulmonary stenosis.

(A) Right ventricular/pulmonary artery gradient of 20 mm Hg

(B) Right ventricular/pulmonary artery gradient of 65 mm Hg

(C) Left ventricular hypertrophy

(D) Right ventricular hypoplasia

(E) Absence of symptoms

(F) Hyperbaric oxygen

(G) Surgical correction

(H) Outflow tract (tunnel) to divert blood from the aorta to the right ventricle

(I) Percutaneous balloon valvuloplasty

40. The indication for surgery in pulmonary stenosis is what? SELECT ONE.

41. The appropriate treatment for significant pulmonary stenosis involves which? SELECT TWO.

Question 42

On the day of admission for elective cataract surgery, an 84-year-old retired bus driver is noted to have a blood pressure of 255/120 mm Hg.

(A) Undergo cataract surgery after oral diuretic therapy

(B) Undergo cataract surgery without general anesthesia

(C) Be given a discharge order and referred to the cardiology clinic

(D) Undergo electrocardioversion

(E) Be given sodium nitroprusside intravenously

(F) Undergo a CT scan of the head

(G) Undergo central venous pressure monitoring

(H) Undergo arterial blood gas (ABG) measurement

42. Blood pressure assessment is repeated on two occasions, and the same measurements are obtained. What should he do? SELECT ONE.

DIRECTIONS (Questions 43 through 54): Each of the numbered items or incomplete statements in this section is followed by five answers. Select the ONE lettered answer that is BEST in each case.

43. A 61-year-old man with a long history of heavy smoking shows on computed axial tomography (CAT) scanning a right upper lobe tumor and enlarged paratracheal nodes. The tumor has been diagnosed as malignant by bronchoscopy. Your next move should be:

(A) Esophagoscopy to rule out invasion of the esophagus.

(B) Proceed with lobectomy and paratracheal node dissection.

(C) Begin radiation of the tumor and paratracheal area.

(D) Perform a mediastinoscopy for staging.

(E) Wait 3 months and repeat CAT scan to evaluate further disease progression.

44. A young man is shot at the level of the right sternoclavicular joint. His blood pressure is 80/60 mm Hg, pulse 120 bpm, and a chest x-ray shows a right hydropneumothorax. The first step should be:

    (A) Insert a chest tube and observe for drainage.
    (B) Perform an immediate right thoracotomy.
    (C) Perform an angiogram to rule out great vessels injury.
    (D) Perform median sternotomy with extension along with right anterior boarder of the sternocleidomastoid muscle.
    (E) Perform a CAT scan with contrast, to evaluate extent of injury.

45. A patient with a long history of smoking, diabetes, and hypertension develops a carcinoma of the right lung. Along the staging process he presents enlarged right mediastinal (paratracheal) nodes that, upon biopsy, are found to contain cancer cells. He is at stage:

    (A) IA N0 M0
    (B) IA N1 M1
    (C) IA N1 M0
    (D) IIIA
    (E) IV

46. During a car crash a young man suffers bilateral multiple fracture ribs. He is alert and presents shortness of breath. His blood pressure is 100/60 mm Hg and chest is unstable. Treatment for this is:

    (A) Prolonged intubation and ventilatory support until rib fractures heal along with aggressive bronchial toilette.
    (B) Once the patient is stable, open rib fracture reduction and stabilization with plates.
    (C) Fracture stabiliztion, with towel clips on ribs and attached to weights (external fixation).
    (D) Avoid intubation, control pain, and perform aggressive bronchial toilette.
    (E) Temporary extracorporeal circulation to allow fractures to heal.

47. Immediately following a bout of pneumonia, a young woman develops a large pleural effusion. A chest tube is inserted and 600 mL of thin pus is obtained. A CAT scan shows incomplete drainage and multiple intrapleural loculations. Management of this empyema requires:

    (A) Insertion of multiple chest tubes under CAT guidance to drain either most or all loculations.
    (B) Treat the patient with antibiotics and continue single chest tube drainage.
    (C) Treat patient with antibiotics and continue single chest tube drainage waiting for a thick peel to develop and then proceed with open total lung decortication.
    (D) Proceed with thoracoscopy and intrapleural toilette. Break the loculations and place drains.
    (E) A thorough open total lung decortication immediately.

48. A 40-year-old woman treated for many years for gastroesophageal reflux develops dysphagia and weight loss. Previous esophagoscopy has revealed cellular atypia. An esophagoscopy is about to be performed. What is it most likely to reveal?

    (A) Leiomyoma arising from the long esophageal muscular layer
    (B) Squamous cell carcinoma arising from esophageal mucosal lining
    (C) Adenocarcinoma originated from islands of Barrett's esophagus
    (D) Adenocarcinoma extending from the stomach
    (E) A large ulcer at the gastroesophageal junction

49. A young woman has suffered severe achalasia of the lower most esophagus. Attempted dilations have failed. The best treatment is:

    (A) Left thoracotomy and extensive myotomy
    (B) Resection of the gastoesophageal junction and reanastomosis

(C) Left thorcotomy, myotomy, and stomach wrap (fundoplication)

(D) Laparoscopic myotomy and partial fundoplication

(E) Transthoracic esophagogastrostomy (side-to-side) anastomosis to avoid disrupting the gastroesophageal sphincter

50. Shortly after an esophagoscopy, the patient develops shortness of breath, chest pain, and fever. A contrast study shows extravasation of contrast into the left chest cavity. You should:

(A) Perform a cervical esophagostomy, gastrostomy, insert a chest tube and begin high dose antibiotic therapy

(B) Insert a nasogastric tube and begin high dose antibiotic therapy

(C) Perform immediate left thoracotomy and repair the esophageal tear

(D) Depoly an endoscopic intraesophageal stent to "plug the hole"

(E) Stop all ingestion of food, insert a chest tube and begin high dose antibioic therapy

51. An 80-year-old woman walks into the emergency room complaining of vomiting and severe retrosternal pain. This has happened many times in the past. A nasogastric tube is inserted and there is immediate clinical improvement. On chest x-ray the tube is found looped in the chest. This patient has:

(A) A large diveticulum of the mid-esophagus

(B) The tube perforated the esophagus

(C) Achalasia

(D) A short esophasus

(E) A gastric volvulus

52. The best treatment of this 80-year-old woman with vomiting retrosternal pain and a looped nasogastric tube in her left chest is:

(A) Remove the tube because the patient is now well and discharged.

(B) Evaluate the esophageal myotomy to treat achalasia.

(C) Immediate left thoracotomy to treat perforation.

(D) Consider surgical reduction of volvulus and diaphragmatic repair.

(E) Do not consider any surgical repair because the patient is too old.

53. While landing at the end of flight a young woman develops shortness of breath and right-sided pressure chest pain. She is tall and thin. The pain, although less in intensity, occurs during her menstrual periods. She has not previously consulted a doctor. A chest film is likely to show?

(A) Left pleural effusion

(B) Pneumothorax

(C) Dilated stomach

(D) Widening of the mediastinum

(E) Cardiomegaly

54. And the treatment is:

(A) Insertion of a chest tube

(B) Immediate cardiology consult

(C) Thoracentesis

(D) Insertion of a nasogastric tube

(E) A CAT scan

DIRECTIONS (Questions 55 through 58): Each set of matching questions in this section consists of a list of lettered options followed by several numbered items. For each numbered item, select the appropriate lettered option. Each lettered option may be selected once.

(A) Transvalvular gradient of 50 mm or more

(B) History of congestive heart failure

(C) Transient ischemic attacks (TIA)

(D) Angina

(E) Aortic insufficiency

(F) Aortic dissection

(G) Ventricular fibrillation

(H) Mitral insufficiency

(I) Acute MI

55. A 50-year-old man has a systolic heart murmur best heard in the second interspace on the right side. He is increasingly short of breath. Which of the above clinical settings would determine the decision to operate? SELECT ONE.

56. A 68-year-old female with aortic stenosis needs a valve replacement. Which of the above might result in a poor result for this patient? SELECT ONE.

57. A 55-year-old man with a diastolic murmur heard in the second interspace on the right that radiates toward the apex of the heart. The cardiac index is normal at rest but decreases with exercise. The most likely diagnosis is? SELECT ONE.

58. A 45-year-old tall, thin, male has acute onset of chest pain radiating into the back. In the emergency room his right radial pulse is bounding but his femoral pluses are absent. The most likely diagnosis is? SELECT ONE.

Answers and Explanations

1. **(A)** Ostium primum. Typically ostium primum in an adolescent would be diagnosed by increasing symptoms, increased pulmonary resistance, left axis on ECG, and a mitral regurgitation murmur due to a cleft mitral valve. Ostium secundum would cause increased pulmonary resistance later in life, not at age 14. AV canal is seen most commonly in Down syndrome. Right aortic arch and tetralogy of Fallot do not have this symptom complex.

2. **(E)** Prostaglandin E1 and Aterial septotomy. Prostaglandin E1 is used to keep the ductus arteriousus open in transposition. Desaturated "systemic" blood can pass through the pulmonary circulation to be oxygenated. The aterial septotomy creates an ASD, which aids in saturated blood being pumped peripherally, decreasing the cyanosis. The mustard operation is not commonly done as the arterial switch operation is most common in this era, and in this acutely ill neonate definitive operation would not be the best initial treatment. Pulmonary artery banding does not apply.

3. **(C)** Internal thoracic artery. The internal thoracic artery is the conduit of choice especially for grafting the left anterior descending (LAD) artery. Arterial and venous grafts 95% of the time do *not* occlude after 12. Seventy-five percent of patients under coronary artery bypass graft (CABG) survive 5 years. Mortality is 2% or lower in most centers.

4. **(D)** Echocardiography. This patient has a pericardial effusion. Echocardiography is the most useful in making the diagnosis. CAT scan of the chest can be used but is not the best exam. The other choices do not apply.

5. **(E)** Pericardial window. The patient developed decreased cardiac output (decreasing urine output,)and cardiac tamponade. Emergent pericardial window is the treatment of choice. Medical therapy will result in the patient's death. The other choices do not apply.

6. **(A)** IABP increases coronary perfusion during distole. The IABP inflates during diastole and propels blood into the coronary circulation. IABP decreases peripheral resistance and decreases afterload on the heart. The IABP can stay in the patient for longer than 24 hours.

7. **(D)** ICD. In a patient with history of MI, congestive heart failure, and decreased ejection fraction coupled with frequent premature ventricular beats studies have shown that this subset of patient benefits from internal cardiac defibrillators, as the most frequent cause of death in these patients is sudden cardiac death from ventricular fibrillation. Single and dual chamber pacemakers are used for bradyarrythmias. The other choices do not apply.

8. **(B)** Increase in pulmonary vascular resistance causes an increased cardiac output. Small shunts (with a pulmonary/systemic flow ratio >1.5) do not require surgery but must be treated with prophylactic antibiotics. Larger shunts should be repaired, because the mortality rate exceeds 50% when severe pulmonary pressure (>85 mm Hg) occurs. Closure of the VSD in the presence of cyanosis with established reversal of the direction

of flow (right to left) would be detrimental, carrying a very high mortality.

9. **(B)** VSD is the most common cardiac congenital abnormality and results from failure of fusion of the uppermost part of the interventricular septum with the aortic septum. Membranous septal defects account for 90% of VSDs. There is usually a left-to-right shunt and cyanosis does not occur until pulmonary hypertension is severe enough to reverse flow across the VSD. Surgery is indicated in large shunts only when symptoms occur and pulmonary hypertension is evident. Forty percent will close spontaneously in childhood.

10. **(D)** Increase in pulmonary resistance would require more urgent intervention. Because nearly half the cases of VSD in childhood will close spontaneously, elective surgery is deferred to late childhood. Banding procedures are used less frequently today because of the high mortality rate. If symptoms increase in severity and pulmonary pressure is high, more urgent intervention is indicated. If the pulmonary systolic pressure is over 85 mm Hg and the left-to-right shunt is small, surgical mortality exceeds 50%.

11. **(B)** Management of compromised respiratory status in the premature infant with PDA includes fluid restriction, adequate oxygenation, attempted closure by medication with indomethacin, and surgical ligation (undertaken when indomethacin is contraindicated). Good results can be anticipated in the absence of other serious complications.

12. **(A)** In full-term infants born with persistent PDA, the anomaly must be closed or excised between 6 months and 3 years of age to avoid cardiac complications, including endocarditis. In PDA, persistence of the communication between the pulmonary trunk and aorta increases pulmonary blood flow, left atrial flow, left ventricular flow, and ascending aorta flow. PDA accounts for 15% of all congenital cardiac abnormalities. Cyanosis does not occur initially, because oxygenated blood is shunted from the aorta to the pulmonary trunk. The murmur is continuous (sounds like machinery) and has harsh features. Its intensity is maximum over the left second intercostal space but radiates to the chest wall and the neck.

13. **(E)** Cardiac catheterization is the definitive test for confirming the diagnosis of ASD. It quantifies the size of the shunt and confirms the increase in oxygen saturation between the right ventricle and the superior vena cava. Beading of the ribs is seen in coarctation, and a decreased carotid pulse is found in aortic stenosis. An elevated sedimentation rate occurs in the presence of infection such as bacterial endocarditis.

14. **(E)** There is decreased vascularity of the lungs seen on chest x-ray. Tetralogy of Fallot includes VSD, right ventricular outflow obstruction, dextroposition of the aorta, and right ventricular hypertrophy. Tetralogy of Fallot accounts for over one-half the cases of congenital cyanotic heart disease.

15. **(B)** Dilation of the left atrium is the obvious complication following long-standing mitral stenosis. Echocardiography is the simplest and most precise method of showing enlargement of the left atrium. Frequently, there is a latency period of 15–20 years before symptoms become evident. Important complications of mitral stenosis include exertional dyspnea caused by an increase in left atrial pressure and backup of blood with possible pulmonary edema, decreased cardiac output, atrial fibrillation, emboli (15%), and pressure in the intermediate third of the esophagus as seen on an esophogram after barium swallow. The pulse in mitral or aortic stenosis is reduced.

16. **(D)** Elevation of total cholesterol/high-density lipoprotein is a useful predictor of coronary artery disease (CAD). Other known main risk factors include genetic predisposition, high cholesterol level, arterial hypertension, and cigarette smoking. Obesity, diabetes mellitus, and personality type are of probable importance as independent risk factors. The presence of elevated high-density lipoprotein is a favorable factor.

17. **(C)** Changes in the nature of angina should alert the physician to the possible progression of the underlying cardiac status. The pain may become more severe and more frequent, may last longer, and may occur with a lesser degree of exertion. Nocturnal pain should likewise signal concern. In the face of unstable angina, 30% of patients are likely to develop MI within a 3-month period.

18. **(C)** In about one-quarter of patients with angina pectoris, the ECG findings will be normal. Exercise electrocardiography will reveal ST-segment depression and possibly precipitate symptoms if angina pectoris is present. There is a risk of myocardial death in patients tested, and patients with symptoms after minimal exertion and/or unstable angina are at particular risk with this procedure. If hypotension, ventricular arrhythmia, and supraventricular arrhythmia occur or if the ECG shows a fall in segment ST of over 3 mm, the test should be discontinued. In these cases, ^{201}Tl scintigraphy would be used to detect cardiac ischemia or infarction. Echocardiography during supine exercise may be a helpful test in selected circumstances.

19. **(C)** ^{99m}Tc pyrophosphate scintigraphy showing a "hot spot." Following injection of ^{99m}Tc pyrophosphate, scintigraphy may show a hot spot in the infarcted area. The hot spot is developed as the radiotracer forms a complex with calcium in necrotic tissue. The test should be requested within the first 18 hours following the onset of acute MI. It is not sensitive enough to detect small infarctions. Following ^{201}Tl scintigraphy, a "cold spot" occurs because of hypoperfusion. The test is performed where exercise or dipyridamole (Persantine) injection can be given. SGOT levels are elevated in liver disease. The HIDA scan is used to exclude gallbladder disease. Cardiac enzyme levels and ECG findings are useful to establish a diagnosis of MI.

20. **(A)** Thrombolytic therapy intravenously with streptokinase, urokinase, or tPA is indicated in most patients with MI presenting early for treatment. This therapy, however, is effective only if initiated within 6 hours after the onset of pain in patients with acute MI. These drugs are fibrinogenolytic, and aspirin and heparin are frequently included in the anticoagulant protocol. Reperfusion rates of 60% can be anticipated; reocclusion rates of 15% usually occur. Vitamin K is not indicated, because it would increase the coagulability of blood. If a diuretic, such as hydrochlorothiazide, 25–50 mg/d is indicated to treat milder hypertension, hypokalemia must be avoided.

21. **(D)** Studies have shown that in men over the age of 50, taking 1 tablet of aspirin (325 mg) on alternate days reduces the incidence of subsequent CAD complications. Nitroglycerin is prescribed if angina pectoris develops, and digoxin would be indicated if congestive heart faliure (CHF) is evident. Progression of atherosclerosis should be minimized by appropriate diet and exercise. The intake of excess of cholesterol and saturated fats in the diet causes changes in the vascular endothelium and smooth muscle proliferation, with subintimal fat and fibrous tissue accumulation leading to occlusion of the coronary arteries, their branches, and other arteries.

22. **(B)** Sudden cardiac death is defined as an unexpected death occurring within 1 hour after the beginning of symptoms in a patient who was previously hemodynamically stable. In asymptomatic patients presenting initially with cardiac disease, 20% will die within the first hour of symptoms. Electrolyte imbalance, hypoxia, and conduction system defect are additional factors that increase the risk of sudden death syndrome. Split first heart sound accentuated on inspiration occurs in normal individuals. In CHF, the CVP changes more than 1 cm when pressure is applied below the right costal margin to the liver (hepatojugular reflex) for a 30-second period.

New York Classification of Functional Changes in Heart Disease

Class	Limitation of Physical Activity
I	None
II	Slight
III	Marked
IV	Complete (even at rest)

23. **(C)** The patient described has cardiogenic shock due to postoperative MI. The mortality rate for patients who develop MI is increased to more than 60% if hypotensive cardiogenic shock also supervenes. Pathology studies of patients dying after such episodes reveal that more than 40% of the heart will have infarcted. Inotropic drugs such as dobutamine are used. If a rapid response is not obtained, intra-aortic balloon tamponade is provided to unload the left ventricle during systole and increase diastolic coronary arterial flow. Hypertonic solutions in graded amounts would be given only if hypovolemia is evident. Atropine and adrenaline would be contraindicated.

24. **(D)** The balloon usually is inserted via the femoral artery. The balloon is inflated during diastole and deflated during systole. It is important that the balloon be adequately deflated during systole to avoid damage to the left ventricle. The pump can be used for a few days if required.

25. **(D)** The major complications occurring in atrial fibrillation are cardiac failure, coronary ischemia, and emboli. Emboli may lead to stroke. Urgent cardioversion is required in patients with auricular fibrillation if heart failure, hypotension, or angina are also present. Immediate cardioversion is indicated in ventricular tachycardia or ventricular fibrillation. If treatment with lidocaine is ineffective, electrocardioversion with 100–200 J for ventricular tachycardia or 300–400 J for ventricular fibrillation is urgently indicated.

26. **(A)** Alternate pressure over the carotid sinus for 20 seconds will end an attack of paroxysmal tachycardia in nearly one-half of cases. The procedure is contraindicated in patients who have had a cerebral TIA or those who have a carotid bruit. Bilateral simultaneous pressure on the carotid sinus carries an additional risk of stroke and must be avoided. The common carotid artery usually divides at the level of the upper border of the thyroid cartilage or hyoid bone (C3). The carotid sinus may be located either on the proximal internal carotid artery or distal common carotid bifurcation.

Eyeball pressure may be effective but carries the risk of retina detachment. If initial measures are unsuccessful, the arrhythmia is treated with intravenous administration of verapamil or a similar drug. Electrocardioversion is indicated in severe cases, particularly if there are adverse symptoms caused by the tachycardia.

27. **(A)** Myxomas constitute more than 50% of all primary cardiac tumors. They are usually polypoid and attached to the septum. Sarcomas constitute 20–25% of primary cardiac tumors. Cardiac metastases are seen in patients with metastatic disease.

28. **(C)** The pulse is bounding when the pulse pressure is magnified because of a wide difference between the systolic and diastolic pressure. It may be due to aortic incompetence, PDA, or noncardiac causes that result in increase in cardiac output and decreased peripheral resistance (e.g., hyperthyroidism, peripheral AV fistula, or anemia).

29. **(A)** A small pulse occurs when the cardiac output is decreased and/or the peripheral resistance is increased. The pulse is reduced in aortic stenosis, heart failure, pulmonary hypertension, pulmonary incompetence, mitral stenosis, and pericardial effusion. The typical cardiac lesion in syphilis is aortic incompetence, which results in a forceful bounding pulse with a wide pulse pressure. Other noncardiac conditions that result in an *increased* pulse pressure include hyperthyroidism, carcinoid syndrome, and aortic incompetence.

30. **(B)** Angioplasty and stenting of the iliac vessels has a patency rate of 75% at 5 years; PTA and stenting of all other vessels has a much lower patency than bypass procedures. The FDA has only approved illiac artery stenting.

31. **(D)** The single most serious prognostic sign for adverse changes after vascular surgery is the presence of CHF. Every effort must be made to correct pulmonary congestion and improve left ventricular function before undertaking elective procedures. MI occurring within 3 months before operation carries a high mortality rate

that will be reduced by delaying surgery for 3–6 months when possible.

32. **(B)** Cerebrovascular accident is the most important cause of death during the first year of life in patients with tetralogy of Fallot. Over 65% of patients with the tetralogy have cyanosis before 1 year of age. These patients have more severe polycythemia and are particularly liable to develop cyanotic spells of unconsciousness, cerebral thrombosis, hemiplegia, and death. Brain abscess may develop subsequent to infarction and bacteria's entering the systemic circulation via a right-to-left shunt.

33. **(A)** A double aortic arch implies that there are two arches of the aorta; one passes posterior to the esophagus and the other anterior to the trachea. The right side is more common than the left side, and usually one of the arches is smaller than the other. Respiratory difficulty with a labored type of respiration (often precipitated by feeding) usually occurs within the first few months of life. Dysphagia occurs less frequently. Treatment is required only if symptoms are troublesome.

34. **(D)** Coarctation of the aorta is a relatively common anomaly and accounts for approximately 15% of all congenital anomalies. The most common site of coarctation is immediately distal (within 3–4 cm) to the origin of the left subclavian artery. Normally, pressure in the lower extremity is higher than that in the upper extremity, but in coarctation of the aorta, the femoral pulses are absent or markedly reduced. Magnetic resonance imaging (MRI) (cine) of chest shows coarctation (Fig. 4–2).

35. **(C)** In the fetus, the sixth left aortic arch diverts blood in the pulmonary artery away from the undeveloped lungs. After birth, the channel closes and becomes the ligamentum arteriosum. In rubella, a PDA may be associated with mental retardation and cataracts. Most cases of PDA occur without a clear-cut cause.

36. **(D)** In the presence of coarctation of the aorta, left ventricular enlargement, hypertrophy, and failure to develop occur. As the child grows,

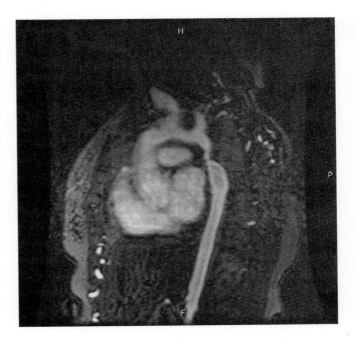

Figure 4–2.
MRI (cine) shows coarctation of the aorta distal to the left subclavian artery origin.

collaterals develop between the subclavian artery and the aorta via the intercostal and internal thoracic vessels. In children older than 8 years of age, the intercostal arteries cause typical notching on the inferior margin of the ribs.

37. **(E)** Tricuspid atresia accounts for 5% of cyanotic heart disease. Blood to the lungs is maintained by a PDA.

38. **(H)** Repeat blood pressure assessment in the supine position. Hypertension can be defined as a diastolic pressure above 90 mm Hg or systolic pressure above 160 mm Hg. Anxiety in an office setting may provide a false high reading of blood pressure. The pressure usually decreases when the individual remains seated and still for a short while. Essential hypertension implies that there is no clear associated cause to explain the hypertension. Approximately 10–15% of white adults and 20–30% of black adults in the United States suffer from hypertension.

39. **(D)** Diuretics and angiotensinogen-converting enzyme (ACE) inhibitors are more likely to be effective in elderly black men presenting with hypertension. ACE inhibitors inhibit

the renin–angiotensin–aldosterone system, sympathetic nervous system activity, and bradykinin degradation and cause an increase in prostaglandin (vasodilator) synthesis. P-Blockers (e.g., propanalol) and calcium channel blockers (e.g., verapamil, nifedipine) are the first line of drugs chosen for young white men presenting with hypertension.

40. **(B)** The presence of mild stenosis (valve gradient/right ventricular pulmonary artery <30 mm Hg) in asymptomatic patients does not require surgical correction; such patients can anticipate a normal life expectancy. Moderate to severe stenosis (right ventricular/pulmonary artery gradient of 50–80 mm Hg) requires surgical correction.

41. **(G, I)** Percutaneous balloon valvuloplasty is now used in many centers as an initial approach to correct pulmonary stenosis. Right ventricular hypertrophy accounts for the parasternal heave noted on examination. Left ventricular hypertrophy does not occur consequent to pulmonary stenosis. Pulmonary stenosis was once considered rare but now accounts for 10% of cases of congenital heart disease.

42. **(E)** Sodium nitroprusside, 0.5–10 mg/kg/min IV, is given to patients (such as the one here) presenting as an urgent hypertensive emergency (e.g., symptomatic hypertension with systolic blood pressure >200 mm Hg, or asymptomatic with systolic pressure >240 mm Hg). Sodium nitroprusside lowers blood pressure by causing arteriolar and venous dilation. Untreated hypertension may lead to cardiovascular, cerebrovascular, and renal disease. Other complications of hypertension include pulmonary edema, aortic dissection, progressive atherosclerosis, accelerated (malignant) hypertension, and, in pregnant patients, eclampsia.

43. **(D)** Next move should be sampling of mediatinal nodes to stage this carcinoma of the lung. If the nodes are positive, the patient is *not* a surgical candidate. He needs chemo-radiotherapy. Radiation to the mediastinal nodes should not begin without pathologic confirmation of nodal metastasis. Waiting constitutes malpractice.

44. **(D)** This patient has probably suffered a penetrating injury to the vessels of the thoracic outlet and/or superior mediastinum. Immediate operation is needed. This incision gives excellent exposure on the right and also gives access to both chest cavities.

45. **(D)** Positive ipsilateral parathracheal nodes defines stage IIIA.

46. **(D)** In the past, prolonged intubation (internal fixation) was performed with enthusiasm because the pulmonary failure was thought to be secondary to chest wall instability. Today is known that pulmonary failure and breathing problems are due to lung contusion and pain, respectively. Avoiding intubation, controlling pain, and performing aggressive bronchial toilette yield better results.

47. **(D)** During the early period of the fibrinopurulent stage of empyema, thoracoscopy is the standard of care.

48. **(C)** Adenocarcinoma, originated from islands of Barrett's esophagus, is today the most common cancer of the esophagus in the United States.

49. **(D)** Today, the standard of care for classic achalasia is laparoscopic myotomy and partial fundoplication.

50. **(C)** Perforation of the esophagus is associated with serious complications and death. Earliest repair is mandatory. Antibiotics would also be given. The other choices allow an on-going leak.

51. **(E)** The esophagus is not perforated because of the patient's dramatic improvement. Achalasia is usually accompanied by chronic dysphagia. Short esophagus does not present with severe retrosternal pain. The nasogastric tube is looped inside the intrathoracic, volvulated stomach and the patient has improved because of decompression.

52. **(D)** Recurrent volvulus of the stomach into the chest is a serious condition that can lead to incarceration and gangrene. Every attempt should be made to repair this diaphragmatic hernia.

53. **(B)** The presentation itself should alert the clinician to the possibility of a pneumothorax (Fig 4–3). This condition is seen quite frequently with patients that are thin and tall. This lady presents with a catamenial pneumothorax syndrome.

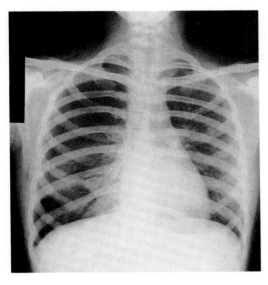

Figure 4–3.
Spontaneous pneumothorax on right side. *(Reproduced, with permission, from Doherty GM: Current Surgical Diagnosis and Treatment, 12th ed. 349. McGraw-Hill, 2006.)*

54. **(A)** This is the first documented pneumothorax on this patient. The treatment of choice is insertion of a chest tube. If the air leak persists for more than 3 days or if she develops a recurrence after discharge, a thoracoscopy, resection of bullae and pleurodesis becomes the treatment of choice.

55. **(A)** The decision to operate in patients with aortic stenosis is based on transvalvular gradient. 50-mm gradient is termed critical aortic stenosis and the valve should be replaced in a symptomatic patient.

56. **(B)** Congestive heart failure. In patients with aortic stenosis, risk factors include a history of agina, stroke or TIAs, and a history of congestive heart failure, which indicates a compromised left ventricle. Of the three, congestive heart failure is the factor which is the greatest risk factor for patients undergoing surgery.

57. **(E)** Aortic insufficiency. This is the murmur of a patient with aortic insufficiency. Typically, these patients will be well compensated at rest but will have decreased cardiac output with exercise. These patients should be operated on.

58. **(F)** Aortic dissection. This describes a patient with Marfan syndrome, who are typically at risk for aortic dissection. With dissection you may preserve right radial pulse but lose femoral pulses.

CHAPTER 5

Stomach, Duodenum, and Esophagus

Soula Privolous and Max Goldberg

Questions

DIRECTIONS (Questions 1 through 97): Each of the numbered items in this section is followed by five answers or by completions of the statement. Select the ONE lettered answer or completion that is BEST in each case.

1. A 45-year-old man complains of burning epigastric pain that wakes him up at night. The pain is relieved by eating or using over-the-counter antacids and H_2 blockers. Diagnosis is best confirmed by which of the following?

   (A) Urea breath test
   (B) Serum gastrin levels
   (C) Barium meal examination
   (D) Upper endoscopy
   (E) Upper endoscopy and biopsy

2. A 64-year-old woman with arthritis is a chronic NSAID user. She develops severe epigastric pain and undergoes an upper endoscopy. She is told that she has an ulcer adjacent to the pylorus. Which of the following is TRUE about the pylorus?

   (A) It cannot be palpated at laparaotomy.
   (B) It is not covered completely by omentum.
   (C) It is a distinct anatomic entity that can be distinguished during laparotomy.
   (D) It is a true physiologic sphincter.
   (E) It is a site where cancer is rarely found.

3. A 30-year-old executive learns that he has a duodenal ulcer. His gastroenterologist prescribes and outlines medical therapy. The patient worries that if medical therapy fails he may need surgery. Which of the following is the best indication for elective surgical therapy for duodenal ulcer disease?

   (A) An episode of melena
   (B) Repeated episodes of pain
   (C) Pyloric outlet obstruction due to scar formation from an ulcer
   (D) Frequent recurrences of ulcer disease
   (E) Referral of pain to the back, suggestive of pancreatic penetration

4. A 44-year-old dentist was admitted to the hospital with a 1-day history of hematemesis caused by a recurrent duodenal ulcer. He has shown considerable improvement following operative treatment by a truncal vagotomy and pyloroplasty, 10 years prior to this incident. Which is TRUE of truncal vagotomy?

   (A) It is performed exclusively via the thorax.
   (B) It can be performed in the neck.
   (C) If complete, it will result in increased acid secretion.
   (D) It requires a gastric drainage procedure
   (E) It has been abandoned as a method to treat ulcer disease.

5. A 42-year-old executive has refractory chronic duodenal ulcer disease. His physican has suggested several surgical options. The patient has chosen a parietal (highly selective) vagotomy instead of a truncal vagotomy and antrectomy because?

(A) It results in a lower incidence of ulcer recurrence.

(B) It benefits patients with antral ulcers the most.

(C) It reduces acid secretion to a greater extent.

(D) The complication rate is lower.

(E) It includes removal of the ulcer.

6. A 63-year-old woman is admitted to the hospital with severe abdominal pain of 3-hour duration. Abdominal examination reveals board-like rigidity, guarding, and rebound tenderness. Her blood pressure is 90/50 mm Hg, pluse 110 bpm (beats per minute), and respiratory rate is 30 breaths per minute. After a thorough history and physical, and initiation of fluid resuscitation, what diagnostic study should be performed?

(A) Supine abdominal x-rays

(B) Upright chest x-ray

(C) Gastrograffin swallow

(D) Computerized axial tomography (CAT) scan of the abdomen

(E) Abdominal sonogram

7. A frail elderly patient is found to have an anterior perforation of a duodenal ulcer. He has a recent history of nonsteroidal anti-inflammatory drug (NSAID) use and no previous history of peptic ulcer disease. A large amount of bilious fluid is found in the abdomen. What should be the next step?

(A) Lavage of the peritoneal cavity alone

(B) Lavage and omental patch closure of the ulcer

(C) Total gastrectomy

(D) Lavage, vagotomy, and gastroenterostomy

(E) Laser of the ulcer

8. Three months after recovery from an operation to treat peptic ulcer disease, a patient complains that she has difficulty eating a large meal. A 99m Tc-labeled chicken scintigraphy test confirms a marked delay in gastric emptying. A delay in gastric emptying may be due to which of the following?

(A) Zollinger-Ellison syndrome (ZES)

(B) Steatorrhea

(C) Massive small-bowel resection

(D) Previous vagotomy

(E) Hiatal hernia

9. A 64-year-old supermarket manager had an elective operation for duodenal ulcer disease. He has not returned to work because he has diarrhea with more than 20 bowel movements per day. Medication has been ineffective. The exact details of his operation cannot be ascertained. What operation was most likely performed?

(A) Antrectomy and Billroth I anastomosis

(B) Gastric surgery combined with choleystectomy

(C) Truncal vagotomy

(D) Highly selective vagotomy

(E) Selective vagotomy

10. A 40-year-old man has had recurrent symptoms suggestive of peptic ulcer disease for 4 years. Endoscopy reveals an ulcer located on the greater curvature of the stomach. A mucosal biopsy reveals *Helicobacter. pylori*. What is TRUE about *H. pylori*?

(A) Active organisms can be discerned by serology.

(B) It is protective against gastric carcinoma.

(C) It is associated with chronic gastritis.

(D) It causes gastric ulcer but not duodenal ulcer.

(E) It can be detected by the urea breath test in <60% of cases.

11. A 35-year-old CEO underwent an antrectomy and vagotomy for a bleeding ulcer. Although usually careful with his diet, he ate a large

meal during a business lunch. Within 1 hour, he felt lightheaded and developed abdominal cramping and diarrhea. His symptoms may be attributed to:

(A) Anemia

(B) Jejunogastric intussusception

(C) Dumping syndrome

(D) Afferent loop syndrome

(E) Alkaline reflux gastritis

12. A 63-year-old man has an upper gastrointestinal (UGI) study as part of his workup for abdominal pain. The only abnormal finding was in the antrum, where the mucosa prolapsed into the duodenum. There were no abnormal findings on endoscopy. What should he do?

(A) Sleep with his head elevated.

(B) Be placed on an H_2 antagonist.

(C) Undergo surgical resection of the antrum.

(D) Be observed and treated for pain accordingly.

(E) Have laser treatment of the antral mucosa.

13. A 63-year-old man underwent gastric resection for severe peptic ulcer disease. He had complete relief of his symptoms but developed "dumping syndrome." This patient is most likely to complain of which of the following?

(A) Gastric intussusception

(B) Repeated vomiting

(C) Severe diarrhea

(D) Severe vasomotor symptoms after eating

(E) Intestinal obstruction

14. A 65-year-old man was admitted to the hospital for severe bilious vomiting following gastric surgery. This occurs in which circumstance?

(A) Following ingestion of gaseous fluids

(B) Spontaneously

(C) Following ingestion of fatty foods

(D) Following ingestion of bulky meals

(E) In the evening

15. A 64-year-old man has had intermittent abdominal pain as a result of duodenal ulcer disease for the past 6 years. Symptoms recurred 6 weeks before admission. He is most likely to belong to which group?

(A) A and secretor (blood group antigen in body fluid)

(B) B and Lewis antigen

(C) AB

(D) O and nonsecretor

(E) O and secretor

16. A 64-year-old man was evaluated for moderate protein deficiency. He underwent a gastrectomy 20 years earlier. He is more likely to show which of the following?

(A) Porphyria

(B) Hemosiderosis

(C) Aplastic anemia

(D) Hemolytic anemia

(E) Iron deficiency anemia

17. A 68-year-old woman has been diagnosed with a benign ulcer on the greater curvature of her stomach, 5 cm proximal to the antrum. After 3 months of standard medical therapy, she continues to have guaiac positive stool, anemia, and abdominal pain with failure of the ulcer to heal. Biopsies of the gastric ulcer have not identified a malignancy. The next step in management is which of the following?

(A) Treatment of the anemia and repeat all studies in 6 weeks

(B) Endoscopy and bipolar electrocautery or laser photocoagulation of the gastric ulcer

(C) Admission of the patient for total parenteral nutrition (TPN), treatment of anemia, and endoscopic therapy

(D) Surgical intervention, including partial gastric resection

(E) Surgical intervention, including total gastrectomy

18. Investigations of a 43-year-old woman with pluriglandular syndrome were scheduled to determine if a gastrinoma (ZES) was present. The serum gastrin level was slightly elevated. Further assessment to establish the diagnosis can be made by repeating the serum gastrin level after stimulation with which of the following?

   (A) Phosphate
   (B) Potassium
   (C) Calcium
   (D) Chloride
   (E) Magnesium

19. Over the past 6 months, a 60-year-old woman with long standing duodenal ulcer disease has been complaining of anorexia, nausea, weight loss and repeated vomiting. She recognizes undigested food in the vomitus. Examination and workup reveal dehydration, hypokalemia, and hypochloremic alkalosis. What is the most likely diagnosis?

   (A) Carcinoma of the fundus
   (B) Penetrating ulcer
   (C) Pyloric obstruction due to cicatricial stenosis of the lumen of the duodenum
   (D) ZES (Zollinger Ellison Syndrome)
   (E) Anorexia nervosa

20. A 50-year-old woman presents with duodenal ulcer disease and high basal acid secretory outputs. Secretin stimulated serum gastrin levels are in excess of 1000 pg/mL. She has a long history of ulcer disease that has not responded to intense medical therapy. What is the most likely diagnosis?

   (A) Hyperparathyroidism
   (B) Pernicious anemia
   (C) Renal failure
   (D) ZES
   (E) Multiple endocrine neoplasia

21. A 44-year-old man underwent partial resection of the stomach. Following the operation, there was a reduction in serum gastrin levels. The site of resection of the stomach that removed the normal source of gastrin is which of the following (Fig. 5–1)?

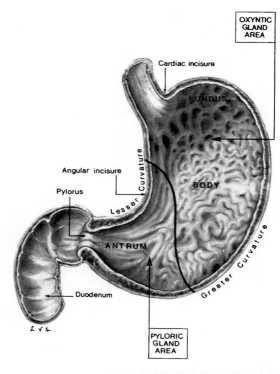

Figure 5–1.
Site of gastrin release. *(Reproduced, with permission, from Doherty GM: Current Surgical Diagnosis and Treatment, 12th ed. 509. McGraw-Hill, 2006.)*

   (A) Gastroduodenal junction
   (B) Lower esophagus
   (C) Antrum
   (D) Body of the stomach
   (E) Fundus of the stomach

22. A 50-year-old man presents with vague gastric complaints. Findings on physical examination are unremarkable. The serum albumin level is markedly reduced (1.8 g/100 mL). A barium study of the stomach shows massive gastric folds within the proximal stomach. These findings are confirmed by endoscopy. What is the correct diagnosis?

   (A) Hypertrophic pyloric stenosis
   (B) Gallstone ileus
   (C) Mallory-Weiss tear
   (D) Hypertrophic gastritis
   (E) Crohn's disease

23. A 2-cm ulcer on the greater curvature of the stomach is diagnosed in a 70-year-old woman by a barium study. Gastric analysis to maximal acid stimulation shows achlorhydria. What is the next step in management?

    (A) Antacids, H_2 blockers, and repeat barium study in 6 to 8 weeks

    (B) Proton pump inhibitor (PPI) (e.g., omeprazole) and repeat barium study in 6 to 8 weeks

    (C) Prostoglandin E (misoprostol) and repeat barium study in 6 to 8 weeks

    (D) Immediate elective surgery

    (E) Upper endoscopy with multiple biopsies (at least 8 or 9) for the ulcer

24. A 55-year-old school bus driver was diagnosed 3 months ago with an antral ulcer. He was treated for *H. pylori* and continues to take a PPI. Repeat endoscopy demonstrates that the ulcer has not healed. What is the next treatment option?

    (A) Treatment with H_2 blockers

    (B) Vagotomy alone without additional surgery

    (C) Endoscopy and laser treatment of the ulcer

    (D) Distal gastrectomy with gastroduodenal anastomosis (Billroth I)

    (E) Elevating the head of the bed when asleep

25. A 70-year-old woman complains of abdominal discomfort, anorexia, and a 10-lb weight loss. Endoscopy reveals a polypoid lesion in the antrum. The lesion is biopsied and the patient is informed that she has early gastric cancer (EGC). Why?

    (A) Because it involves only the mucosa and does not invade the muscular wall of the stomach

    (B) Because it is demonstrable on a barium study

    (C) Because it has a 5 year survival rate of 5%

    (D) Because surgery always cures it

    (E) Because it does not require tumor free margins when resected

26. A 62-year-old man presents with guaiac positive stool. He is asymptomatic. Workup reveals a 2-cm ulcerated carcinoma on the antral lesser curvature. Tumor markers are negative. A CAT scan is negative for metastatic disease and lymphadenopathy liver function tests are normal. What is the correct treatment for this patient?

    (A) Chemotherapy only

    (B) Radiation therapy only

    (C) Combination chemotherapy and radiation therapy without resection

    (D) Total gastrectomy

    (E) Distal gastrectomy with en bloc removal of lymph nodes

27. A 55-year-old man complains of anorexia, weight loss, and fatique. A UGI study demonstrates an ulcerated lesion at the incisura. Where is the incisura?

    (A) Cardia

    (B) Fundus

    (C) Greater curvature

    (D) Lesser curvature

    (E) Gastrocolic ligament

28. A 36-year-old man presents with weight loss and a large palpable tumor in the upper abdomen. Endoscopy reveals an intact gastric mucosa without signs of carcinoma. Multiple biopsies show normal gastric mucosa. A UGI study shows a mass in the stomach. At surgery, a 3-kg mass is removed. It is necessary to remove the left side of the transverse colon. What is the most likely diagnosis?

    (A) Gastric cancer

    (B) Gastrointestinal stromal tumor (GIST)

    (C) Choledochoduodenal fistula

    (D) Eosinophilic gastroenteritis

    (E) Linitis plastica

29. A 74-year-old man presents with anorexia and self-limited hematemesis. During endoscopy a mass is discovered and a biopsy is done. A hematopathologis diagnoses non-Hodgkin's lymphoma. What is the recommended therapy?

(A) Chemotherapy alone
(B) Immunotherapy
(C) Radiation and chemotherapy
(D) Surgery, radiation, and chemotherapy
(E) Surgery alone

30. A 63-year-old woman is admitted to the hospital with a UGI bleed that subsides spontaneously within a short time after admission. A barium study shows a gastric ulceration that is described by the radiologist as having a "doughnut sign." What is the most likely diagnosis?

(A) Lipoma
(B) Gastric ulcer
(C) Ectopic pancreas
(D) GIST
(E) Carcinoma

31. A 50-year-old woman is diagnosed with multiple hyperplastic polyps in the stomach during endoscopy and biopsy. How are these best treated?

(A) Total gastrectomy
(B) Partial gastrectomy
(C) Staged endoscopic removal after brushing for cytologic examination
(D) Ablation by laser
(E) No treatment other than repeated endoscopy and multiple brush biopsies

32. During a surveillance upper endoscopy, a 35-year-old woman who was successfully treated for multiple familial polyposis of the colon, is found to have several polyps in the antrum. Biopsies show adenomatous polyps. What is the best therapy?

(A) Observation and repeated endoscopy at frequent intervals
(B) Antrectomy

(C) Endoscopic polypectomies with repeat endoscopy to monitor subsequent polyp development
(D) Endoscopic laser ablation of the polyps
(E) Total gastrectomy to remove all existing polyps and to prevent the formation of potential future polyps

33. A 64-year-old woman presents with severe upper abdominal pain and retching of 1-day duration. Attempts to pass a nasogastric tube are unsuccessful. X-rays show an air-fluid level in the left side of the chest in the posterior mediastinum. An incarcerated paraesophageal hernia and gastric volvulus is diagnosed. What is the next step in management?

(A) Insertion of a weighted bougie to untwist the volvulus
(B) Elevation of the head of the bed
(C) Placing the patient in the Trendelenburg position with the head of the bed lowered
(D) Laparotomy and vagotomy
(E) Surgery, reduction of the gastric volvulus, and repair of the hernia

34. A 78-year-old woman undergoes an uncomplicated minor surgical procedure under local anesthesia. At the completion of the operation, she suddenly develops pallor, sweating, bradycardia, hypotension, abdominal pain, and gastic distension. What is the next stem in management?

(A) Rapid infusion of 3 L of Ringer's lactate
(B) Digoxin
(C) Insertion of a nasogastric tube
(D) Morphine
(E) Neostigmine

35. A 35-year-old teacher has a family history of gastric cancer. She has an upper endoscopy performed for epigastric symptoms. The endoscopy is negative. The patient ask her endoscopist if there are any conditions that predispose to gastric carcinoma. He provides her with the following answer.

(A) Environmental metaplastic atrophic gastritis (EMAG)

(B) Autoimmune metaplastic atrophic gastritis (AMEG)

(C) Menetrier's disease

(D) Duodenal ulcer

(E) Hiatal hernia

36. A 48-year-old man undergoes surgery for a chronic duodenal ucler. The procedure is a truncal vagotomy and which of the following?

(A) Gastroenterostomy

(B) Removal of the duodenum

(C) Closure of the esophageal hiatus

(D) Incidental appendectomy

(E) No further procedure

37. A healthy 75-year-old man bleeds from a duodenal ucler. Medical management and endoscopic measures fail to stop the bleeding. What is the next step in management?

(A) Continued transfusion of 8 U of blood

(B) Administration of norepinephrine

(C) Oversewing of the bleeding point

(D) Oversewing of the bleeding point, vagotomy. and pyloroplasty

(E) Hepatic artery ligation

38. A 60-year-old woman undergoes vagotomy and pyloroplasty for duodenal ulcer disease. Gallstones are noted at the time of the original operation. Eight days following surgery, she develops abdominal pain and right upper quadrant tenderness. To determine if the gallbladder is the cause of her symptoms, she should undergo which study?

(A) Supine x-ray

(B) Hepatobiliary scan (HIDA)

(C) Ultrasound

(D) Erect x-ray

(E) Cholangiogram

39. A recent immigrant to the United States has had persistent epigastric discomfort. He delays seeking treatment because he could not afford to pay a doctor. He finally went to the emergency department and was referred to an endoscopist. A submucosal mass was seen and it was thought to be a GIST. The most common site of a GIST is which of the following?

(A) Esophagus

(B) Stomach

(C) Jejunum

(D) Ileum

(E) Colon

40. A 60-year-old woman complains of early satiety and undergoes an upper endoscopy. A small mass is seen in the antrum with sparing of the mucosa. GIST is suspected. A CAT scan of the chest, abdomen, and pelvis is performed. What does she require next?

(A) Fulguration of the tumor

(B) Distal gastrectomy

(C) Laser therapy followed by radiation therapy

(D) Chemotherapy alone

(E) Total gastrectomy

41. A 67-year-old woman complains of paresthesias in the limbs. Examination shows loss of vibratory sense, positional sense, and sense of light touch in the lower limbs. She is found to have pernicious anemia. Endoscopy reveals an ulcer in the body of the stomach. What does she most likely have?

(A) Excess of vitamin B_{12}

(B) Deficiency of vitamin K

(C) Cancer of the stomach

(D) Gastric sarcoma

(E) Esophageal varices

42. A 79-year-old retired opera singer presents with dysphagia, which has become progressively worse during the last 5 years. He states that he is sometimes aware of a lump on the left side of his neck and that he hears gurgling sounds during swallowing. He sometimes regurgitates food during eating. What is the likely diagnosis?

(A) Carcinoma of the esophagus
(B) Foreign body in the esophagus
(C) Plummer-Vinson (Kelly-Patteson) syndrome
(D) Zenker's (pharyngoesophageal) diverticulum
(E) Scleroderma

43. A symptomatic patient has a barium swallow that reveals a 3-cm Zenker's diverticulum. The next step in management is?

(A) H$_2$ blockers
(B) Anticholinergic drugs
(C) Elemental diet
(D) Bougienage
(E) Surgery (cricopharyngeal myotomy and diverticulectomy)

44. A 30-year-old psychiatric patient has a barium swallow after removal of a foreign body to rule out a small perforation of the esophagus. No perforation is seen, but an epiphrenic diverticulum is visualized. An epiphrenic diverticulum may be associated with which of the following?

(A) Duodenal ulcer
(B) Gastric ulcer
(C) Cancer of the tongue
(D) Cancer of the lung
(E) Hiatal hernia

45. A 64-year-old man develops increasing dysphagia over many months. A barium swallow is performed. What is the most likely cause of his clinical presentation?

(A) Carcinoma of the esophagus
(B) Achalasia

(C) Sliding hiatal hernia
(D) Paraesophageal hernia
(E) Esophageal diverticulum

46. A 63-year-old woman from Norway is visiting the United States. She presents with dysphagia. On endoscopy, an esophageal web is identified and the diagnosis of Plummer-Vinson syndrome is established. What would be the next step in management?

(A) Esophagostomy
(B) Dilatation of the web and iron therapy
(C) Esophagectomy
(D) Gastric bypass of the esophagus
(E) Cortisone

47. A 53-year-old moderately obese woman presents with heartburn aggravated mainly by eating and lying down in the horizontal position. Her symptoms are suggestive of gastroesophangeal reflux disease (GERD). Which of the following statements is TRUE?

(A) It is best diagnosed by an anteroposterior (AP) and lateral film of the chest.
(B) It may be alleviated by certain drugs, especially theophylline, diazepam, and calcium channel blockers.
(C) It is not relieved by cessation of smoking.
(D) If it is associated with dysphagia, it suggest a stricture or motility disorder.
(E) It should be immediately treated with surgery.

48. A 64-year-old man has symptoms of reflux esophagitis for 20 years. The barium study shown (Fig. 5–2) demonstrates a sliding hiatal hernia. Whis is TRUE in sliding hiatal hernia?

(A) A hernia sac is absent.
(B) The cardia is displaced into the posterior mediatstinum.
(C) Reflux esophagitis always occur.
(D) A stricture does not develop.
(E) Surgery should always be avoided.

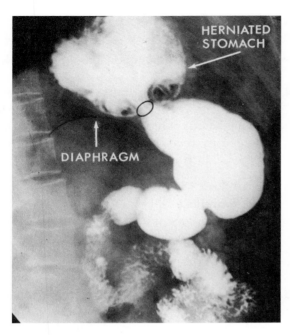

Figure 5–2.
Large sliding hiatal hernia. Diaphragmatic hiatis is encircled. *(Reproduced, with permission, from Doherty GM: Current Surgical Diagnosis and Treatment, 12th ed. 467. McGraw-Hill, 2006.)*

49. A 45-year-old man presents with a long history of heartburn, especially at night. He uses three pillows to sleep and has medicated himself with a variety of antacids over the past 15 years. Recently he has been complaining of dysphagia that he localized to the precordial area. Which is the most likely diagnosis?

    (A) Adenocarcinoma of the esophagus
    (B) Angina pectoris
    (C) Benign peptic stricture of the esophagus
    (D) Achalasia of the esophagus
    (E) Lower esophageal ring (Schatzki's ring)

50. A 54-year-old man presents with dysphagia, heartburn, belching, and epigastric pain. A barium swallow shows a sliding hiatal hernia and a stricture situated higher than usual in the mid-esophagus. Endoscopic findings suggest Barrett's esophagus (ectopic gastric epithelium lining the esophagus). Marked esophagitis with linear ulcerations are seen during endoscopy. A biopsy shows columnar epithelium at the affected area and normal squamous epithelium above, confirming the diagnosis. What statement is TRUE regarding this condition?

    (A) Adenocarcinoma is less common in Barrett's esophagus
    (B) Most patients do not have associated gastroesophageal reflux
    (C) The presence of ectopic gastric lining protects against aspiration during sleep and prevents recurrent pneumonitis.
    (D) The present treatment is aimed at preventing esophagitis.
    (E) When strictures form, they are always malignant.

51. A 75-year-old woman presents with a paraesophageal hiatal "rolling" hernia. Diagnosis is made by radiologic studies (Fig. 5–3). What can this patient be told about paraesophageal hernias?

    (A) They constitute about 50% of all esophageal hiatal hernias and are more common in women over the age of 60.
    (B) They cause the gastroesophageal (GE) junction to become displaced from its normal position below the diaphragm to above the diaphragm.
    (C) They prevent herniation of the stomach and intestine above the diaphragm.
    (D) They may result in volvulus and stangulation of the stomach or bleeding.
    (E) They are treated medially with attention to diet, position during sleep, antacids, and omeprazole [H+/K+ adenosine triphosphate (ATP-ase) pump inhibitors]

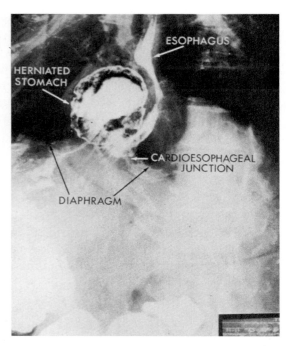

Figure 5–3.
Paraesophageal hernia. *(Reproduced, with permission, from Doherty GM: Current Surgical Diagnosis and Treatment, 12th ed. 468. McGraw-Hill, 2006.)*

52. A 52-year-old gastroenterologist suffers from intermittent dysphagia attributed to the presence of a lower esophageal stricture. The doctor's condition is characterized by which of the following?

    (A) A full thickness scar in the upper esophagus
    (B) Symptoms of mild-to-moderate dysphagia
    (C) A low incidence in men
    (D) The absence of a sliding hiatal hernia in most case
    (E) The need for antireflux surgery at an early stage

53. A 54-year-old clerk complains of having had dysphagia for 15 years. The clinical diagnosis of achalasia is confirmed by a barium study. What is TRUE in this condition?

    (A) The most common symptom is dysphagia.
    (B) In the early stages, dysphagia is more pronounced for solids than liquids.

(C) The incidence of sarcoma is increased.
(D) Recurrent pulmonary infections are rare.
(E) Endoscopic dilatation should be avoided.

54. A 69-year-old man is admitted to the emergency department with an acute UGI hemorrhage following a bout of repeated vomiting. Fiberoptic gastroscopy reveals three linear mucosal tears at the GE junction. What is the diagnosis?

    (A) Reflux esophagitis with ulceration
    (B) Barrett's esophagus
    (C) Carcinoma of the esophagus
    (D) Mallory-Weiss tear
    (E) Scleroderma

55. A 60-year-old man presents with excruciating chest pain. The pain follows an episode of violent vomiting that occurred after a heavy meal. Subcutaneous emphysema was noted in the neck. X-rays shows air in the mediastinum and neck, and a fluid level in the left pleural cavity. What is the most likely diagnosis?

    (A) Perforated duodenal ulcer
    (B) Spontaneous rupture of the esophagus
    (C) Spontaneous pneumothorax
    (D) Inferior wall myocardial infarction
    (E) Dissecting aortic aneurysm

56. A patient is diagnosed with Boerhaave's syndrome. Management involves which of the following?

    (A) Administration of intravenous antibiotics and TPN
    (B) Administration of intravenous antibiotics and TPN, and insertion of a chest tube and a nasogastric tube
    (C) Administration of intravenous antibiotics and TPN, and insertion of a nasogastric tube
    (D) Resuscitation and emergency surgery either by laparotomy or thoracotomy
    (E) Resuscitation, administration of intravenous antibiotics, replacement of fluids and electrolytes; elective surgical intervention when the general status of the patient improves

57. A chest CAT scan is done to further delineate an abnormality seen on a chest x-ray. The superior mediastinum at the level of T4 is evaluated. Which structure is remote from the esophagus?

    (A) Trachea
    (B) Recurrent laryngeal nerves
    (C) Aorta
    (D) Azygous vein
    (E) Brachiocephalic vein

58. A 69-year-old man is informed that the cause of his dysphagis is a benign lesion. The barium swallow is shown in (Fig. 5–4). What should he be told regarding benign tumors and cysts of the eosphagus?

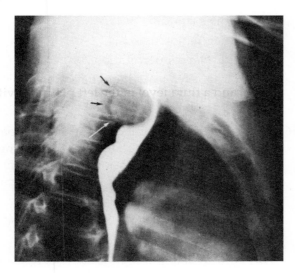

Figure 5–4.
Leiomyoma of esophagus. Note smooth rounded density causing extrinsic compression of esophageal lumen. *(Reproduced, with permission, from Doherty GM: Current Surgical Diagnosis and Treatment, 12th ed. 469. McGraw-Hill, 2006.)*

    (A) They occur more commonly than malignant tumors.
    (B) They are symptomatic at an early age.
    (C) Diagnosis is best confirmed on chest x-ray.
    (D) Leiomyoma is the most common benign tumor encountered in the esophagus.
    (E) Malignant transformation of a benign leiomyoma into a malignant leiomyosarcoma is common.

59. A 45-year-old pilot has retrosternal burning, especially when he eats and lies down to go to sleep. He has self-medicated himself with over the counter heartburn medications. Upper endoscopy reveals an erythematous and inflammed distal esophagus. In severe reflux esophagitis, the resting pressure of the LES is decreased. This may be physiologically increased by which of the following?

    (A) Pregnancy
    (B) Glucagon
    (C) Gastrin
    (D) Secretin
    (E) Glucagon

60. A 46-year-old man has a long history of heartburn (GERD). His barium study shows an irregular, ulcerated area in the lower third of his esophagus. There is marked mucosal disruption and overhanging edges. What is the most likely diagnosis?

    (A) Sliding hiatal hernia with GERD
    (B) Paraesophageal hernia
    (C) Benign esophageal stricture
    (D) Squamous carcinoma of the esophagus
    (E) Adenocarcinoma arising in a Barrett's esophagus

61. A 46-year-old man present with dysphagia of recent onset. His esophogram shows a lesion in the lower third of his esophagus. Biopsy of the lesion shows adenocarcinoma. His general medical condition is excellent, and his metastatic workup is negative. What should his management involve?

    (A) Chemotherapy
    (B) Radiation therapy
    (C) Insertion of a stent to improve swallowing
    (D) Surgical resection of the esophagus
    (E) Combination of chemotherapy and radiation therapy

62. A 25-year-old man arrives in the emergency department in respiratory distress following a motor vehicle collision. A chest x-ray shows abdominal viscera in the left thorax. What is the most likely diagnosis?

    (A) Traumatic rupture of the diaphragm
    (B) Sliding esophageal hernia
    (C) Short esophagus with intrathoracic stomach
    (D) Rupture of the esophagus
    (E) Bochdalek hernia

63. A 32-year-old man undergoes a laparotomy for multiple organ injury resulting from trauma. He is discharged after 2 weeks in the hospital, only to be readmitted 3 days later because of abdominal pain and sepsis. The CAT scan shows an accumulation of fluid in the subhepatic space (Fig. 5–5). This space is likely to be directly related to an injury involving which structure?

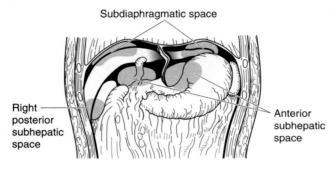

Figure 5–5.
Subhepatic space; anterior view. *(Reproduced, with permission, from Doherty GM: Current Surgical Diagnosis and Treatment, 12th ed. 498. McGraw-Hill, 2006.)*

    (A) Inferior pole of the right kidney
    (B) Stomach
    (C) Uncinate process of the pancreas
    (D) Aortic bifurcation
    (E) Right psoas muscle

64. A 38-year-old man attempts suicide by ingesting drain cleaner fluid. His family brings him to the local emergency department. Which of the following is TRUE?

    (A) Copious neutralizing (acid) solutions should be given.
    (B) Emetics should be administered.
    (C) Stricture formation is inevitable.
    (D) Fluids and solid foods can usually be started several days after the injury.
    (E) Esophagoscopy should be performed to visualize the distal extent of the injury.

65. A patient is admitted to the hospital after ingesting lye. The following day he complains of chest pain. His pulse is 120 bpm. On physical examination he is found to have subcutaneous crepitus on palpation. His chest x-ray shows widening of the mediastinum and a pleural effusion. What has occurred?

    (A) Aortic rupture
    (B) Coagulation necrosis
    (C) Esophageal perforation
    (D) Oropharyngeal inflammation
    (E) Spontaneous pneumothroax

66. Following an emergency operation for hepatic and splenic trauma, the surgeon inserts a finger into the foramen of Winslow in an attempt to stop the bleeding. Which is TRUE of the hepatic artery?

    (A) It is called the common hepatic artery at this level.
    (B) It is medial to the common bile duct and anterior to the portal vein.
    (C) It is posterior to the portal vein.
    (D) It is posterior to the inferior vena cava.
    (E) It forms the superior margin of the epiploic foramen.

67. A 44-year-old patient develops a mass on the anterior abdominal wall. He notes that the mass has gradually increased in size over the last 3 months. On examination, the lesion is a 5 × 8 cm mass in the left iliac fossa and hypogastrium. Which test will establish whether the tumor is arising from the abdominal wall or the abdominal cavity?

    (A) Needle biopsy
    (B) Ability to elicit a cough impulse

(C) Transillumination

(D) Examination of the mass with the patient in a prone position

(E) Examination of the mass with the patient instructed to attempt sitting up

68. A 26-year-old man is diagnosed with adenocarcinoma of the stomach. He wants to know what could have caused him to develop this condition. He does an internet search. Which of the following is a risk factor for developing gastric cancer?

(A) Exposure to ionizing radiation

(B) Blood group B

(C) A diet high in fiber

(D) *H. pylori* infection

(E) North American descent

69. A 44-year-old woman is scheduled for gastric surgery. She has no comorbid disease. The anesthesiologist has difficulty inserting the orotracheal tube. In between intubation attempts he uses an ambu-bag to oxygenate the patient. The patient's abdomen gets distended and tympany is noted in the left upper quadrant. Suddenly the patient becomes hypotensive. Which of the following can cause a vosogvagal response during anesthesia?

(A) The gastric remnant following a distal gastrectomy

(B) Corrosive gastritis

(C) Pernicious anemia

(D) Gastric volvulus

(E) Acute gastric dilatation

70. A 42-year-old taxi driver is diagnosed with a gastric tumor. He delays definitive therapy because he is afraid of losing his job. He finally has surgery and the mass is invading the transverse colon. Which of the following has the best long term survival despite local invasion?

(A) Adenocarcinoma

(B) Lymphosarcoma

(C) Linitis plastica

(D) Chordoma

(E) GIST

71. A 46-year-old man remains disease free following a total colectomy for familial adenomatous polyposis 24 years ago. He now presents with obstructive jaundice of 1 month's duration and guaiac positive stool. He does not have calculus disease. What is his diagnosis?

(A) Adenomatous gastric polyps

(B) Leiomyosarcoma

(C) Lymphosarcoma

(D) Linitis plastica

(E) Ampullary carcinoma

72. A 40-year-old woman complains of heartburn located in the epigastic and retrosternal areas. She also has symptoms of regurgitation. Endoscopy shows erythema of the esophagus consistent with reflux esophagitis. The patient has tried conservative measures, including PPls with no improvement in symptoms. Which of the following is TRUE?

(A) Manometry does not add any additional information.

(B) The 24-hour pH test is no longer used.

(C) If endoscopy has been done, an esophagogram is unnecessary.

(D) Nissen fundoplication is the surgical treatment of choice.

(E) Toupet fundoplication is 360 nic nerve.

73. A 50-year-old man is involved in a major motor vehicle collision and suffers multiple trauma. He is admitted to the intensive care unit. After 2 days of hospital admission he bleeds massively from the stomach. What is the probable cause?

(A) Gastric ulcer

(B) Duodenal ulcer

(C) Hiatal hernia

(D) Mallory-Weiss tear

(E) Erosive gastritis

74. A 65-year-old lawyer has an elective colon resection. On postoperative day number five, the patient develops fever, leukocytosis, and increasing abdominal pain and distension. An anastomotic leak is suspected. During the preparation for a CAT scan, fresh blood and coffee grounds are seen in the nasogastric tube. Acute stress gastritis is best diagnosed by?

    (A) CAT scan
    (B) UGI series
    (C) Angiogram
    (D) Capsule endoscopy
    (E) Upper endoscopy

75. A previously healthy florist presents to the emergency department after vomiting blood in his flower shop. While waiting to be seen he has another episode of hematemesis. What is the most likely cause of his bleeding?

    (A) Peptic ulcer disease (stomach or duodenum)
    (B) Hiatal hernia
    (C) Mallory-Weiss tear
    (D) Gastric carcinoma
    (E) Esophagitis

76. A 22-year-old student is involved in a motorcyle accident. He sustains multiple injuries including an intracranial hemorrage and a pelvic fracture. Despite ulcer prophylaxis he develops a UGI bleed. Which of the following is effective in protecting the gastric mucosa but has not proven useful in the management of erosive gastritis because of side effects (diarrhea)?

    (A) H₂ blockers
    (B) Intrinsic factor
    (C) Cortisone
    (D) Adrenaline
    (E) Protaglandin E (misoprostol)

77. A 33-year-old man is admitted to the hospital for evaluation and treatment of a gastrojejunal ulcer. At age 25, he was treated surgically with an omental (Graham) patch for a perforated duodenal ulcer. At age 30, he was treated with a truncal vagotomy and antrectomy for a chronic duodenal ulcer. He now has a stomal (gastrojejunal) ulcer that is refractory to medical therapy. Which of the following should be checked?

    (A) Intrinsic factor
    (B) Gastrin level
    (C) Adrenaline
    (D) Corstisol
    (E) Potassium

78. A 73-year-old woman is admitted to the hospital with a mild UGI hemorrhage that stopped spontaneously. She did not require transfusion. She had ingested large amounts of aspirin in the past 4 months to relieve the pain caused by severe rheumatoid arthritis. Endoscopy confirms the presence of a duodenal ulcer. A biopsy is done. What is the next step in the management of a duodenal ulcer associated with a positive biopsy for *H. pylori*?

    (A) H₂ blockers
    (B) Bipolar electrocautery of the ulcer
    (C) Triple therapy
    (D) Photocoagulation
    (E) Elective surgery

79. A 52-year-old artist develops epigstric pain that is relieved by antacids. She also complains that her stool has changed color and is black and tarry. What is the most important cause of the entity presenting above other than *H. pylori*?

    (A) Submucosal islet cells
    (B) Hyperglycemia
    (C) Diet
    (D) Acid secretion
    (E) Acute erosive gastritis

80. An 80-year-old grandfather gets admitted to the hospital for a UGI bleed. He undergoes upper endoscopy and bleeding ulcer is visualized. Attempts at endoscopic cauterization and epinephrine injection are unsuccessful at stopping the bleeding. A previous attempt at angioembolization was also unsuccessful. What is the next definitive step in therapy?

    (A) Elective surgery
    (B) High-dose antibiotics

(C) Blood transfusion

(D) Repeated attempts at bipolar electocanter

(E) Emergency surgery

81. An elderly patient delayed seeking medical attention for his early satiety and weight loss because he attributed these changes to aging. When he underwent upper endoscopy a large mass was seen in the stomach. Which statement is TRUE regarding gastric carcinoma?

(A) During resection, it is safe to leave cancer at the cut edges.

(B) The incidence is increased in patients with gastric ulcer disease.

(C) Draining lymph nodes should not be removed.

(D) It is caused by diverticulitis.

(E) It is associated with hyperchlorhydria.

82. An alert nursing home patient is unable to swallow because of a neurologic disease and has lost a significant amount of weight. What treatment should be offered?

(A) Central hyperalimentation

(B) Intralipids

(C) Percutaneous endoscopic gastrostomy (PEG)

(D) Nasogastric feeding

(E) Cervical esophagostomy

83. A 32-year-old waitress is interested in learning about gastric bypass surgery. She consults her primary care physician to see if she is a candidate. Her doctor refers her to an obesity center because?

(A) She has not lost enough weight after her pregnancies.

(B) She is hypertensive and overweight.

(C) Her weight is 50 lb greater than her ideal body weight.

(D) She has a body mass index (BMI) greater than 35 kg/mg.

(E) She is tired of diet and exercise.

84. A morbidly obese patient is told that he qualifies for bariatric surgery. He is given several options. He chooses to undergo a gastric bypass procedure (GBP). Which of the following is TRUE?

(A) Malabsorptive jejunoitial bypass is a more effective operation with less complications.

(B) Vertical banded gastroplasty is technically easier and more effective than gastric bypass surgery.

(C) Patients lose up to two-thirds of their excess weight.

(D) Gastrojejunal leakage rate is in excess of 20%.

(E) The gastric pouch capacity should be 100cc.

85. A 50-year-old gynecologist complains of dysphagia, regurgitation, and weight loss. She also states that she feels as if food is stuck at the level of the xiphoid. An upright chest x-ray shows a dilated esophagus with an air-fluid level. Which of the following is FALSE?

(A) A barium swallow will show a "bird's beak" deformity

(B) Manometry will demonstrate that the LES fails to relax during swallowing.

(C) Upper endoscopy should be avoided because of the risk of complications.

(D) Medical treatment includes nitrates and calcium channel blockers.

(E) Intersphincteric injection of botulinum toxin can be therapeutic.

86. A patient has been diagnosed with achalasia. He refused surgery initially, preferring to try nonoperative therapy. He tried life style modification, calcium channel blockers, botulin toxin injection, and endoscopic pneumatic dilatation. None of the treatments alleviated his symptoms. What are his surgical options?

    (A) Esophagectomy
    (B) Surgical esophagomyotomy proximal to the LES
    (C) Modified Heller myotomy and partial fundoplication
    (D) Repeat pneumatic dilation using pressures of loops
    (E) Nissen fundoplication

87. A 50-year-old man presents to the emergency department with chest pain. The patient is evaluated for an myocardioinfarction. The workup is negative. On further questioning, his symptoms include dysphagia (with both liquids and solids). Which of the following is TRUE?

    (A) A barium swallow will always show a corkscrew esophagus.
    (B) Manometry shows simultaneous high-amplitude contractions.
    (C) Initial evaluation should exclude coronary artery disease.
    (D) A pulsion diverticulum may be present.
    (E) Patients refractory to medical management may respond to long esophagomyotomy.

88. A 60-year-old man with a long history of GERD has worsening symptoms. He has an upper endoscopy that shows esophagitis. A biopsy is taken that shows intestinal metaplasia. Which of the following is TRUE?

    (A) Barrett's esophagus is more common in women.
    (B) 50% of patients with GERD have Barrett's esophagus.
    (C) High-grade dysplasia is an indication for prophylactic esophagectomy.

    (D) Cells typically found in the esophagus are columnar develop adenocarcinoma.
    (E) 100% of patients with Barrett's esophagus develop adenocarcinoma.

89. A 60-year-old man has been having vague symptoms of upper abdominal discomfort, early satiety, and fatigue. He is referred to a gastroenterologist, who performs an upper endoscopy. Although a discrete mass is not visualized, the stomach looks abnormal. It does not distend easily with insufflation. A biopsy shows signet ring cells. Which of the folowing is TRUE?

    (A) Signet ring cells are typically found in intestinal type gastric adenocarcinoma.
    (B) Signet ring cell cancer is the most common type of gastric cancer.
    (C) "Leather bottle stomach" is a term used to describe a nondistensible stomach infiltrated by cancer.
    (D) The gross appearance of the stomach always shows classic findings of linitus plastica.
    (E) Linitus plastica has an excellent prognosis.

90. A patient presents to the emergency department with obstructive jaundice. A percutaneous transhepatic cholangiogram and biliary drainage is performed. Shortly afterward, the patient develops a UGI bleed. What is the most likely cause?

    (A) The patient has developed stress gastritis.
    (B) The patient has ingested NSAIDs after the procedure.
    (C) The patient has developed hemobilia.
    (D) The patient is bleeding from esophageal varices.
    (E) The catheter has migrated from the biliary tree into the stomach.

91. A 56-year-old woman with Sjörgen's syndrome complains of fatigue and melena. She is pale and anemic. Endoscopy reveals ectatic vessels radiating from the pylorus. Which of the following is TRUE?

(A) These findings are very common.

(B) This condition occccurs exclusively in patients with autoimmune diseases.

(C) The only treatment for this condition is surgery.

(D) It occurs more often in men.

(E) Ectatic vessels are frequently found in the colon.

92. A known HIV positive patient complains of severe odynophagia. He avoids eating and drinking because of the intense pain, and he has lost a significant amount of weight. Which of the following is TRUE?

(A) Esophagectomy is the treatment of choice.

(B) Cancer is the only condition that can explain these findings.

(C) UGI series is not useful.

(D) Candida is the most common cause of infectious esophagitis.

(E) Esophageal candidiasis is almost certain if the patient has oral thrush.

93. A 54-year-old man presents with a massive UGI bleed. After resuscitation, endoscopy is performed. No esophageal varices, gastritis, or gastric ulcers are seen. After copious irrigation, a pinpoint lesion is seen near the GE junction. What can be said about this lesion?

(A) It is a carcinoid.

(B) It is related to alcohol use.

(C) It is exclusively a mucosal lesion.

(D) Surgery if first-line therapy.

(E) Bleeding is from a submucosal vessel.

94. A 60-year-old diabetic woman had a partial gastrectomy 15 years ago for peptic ulcer disease. He now complains of nausea, vomiting, early satiety, and weight loss. She has palpable upper abdominal mass. She reluctantly agrees to have an upper endoscopy because she is fearful of being told that she has cancer. She is happy to hear that she does not have a maligancy and agrees to ingest meat tenderizer and have a repeat endoscopy. Which of the following is TRUE?

(A) She has a GIST.

(B) She is in denial.

(C) She has a cancer at the gastrojejunal anastomosis.

(D) A barium study is nondiagnostic.

(E) She has a phytobezoar.

95. A 65-year-old man has a chest x-ray done for an insurance physical. A posterior mediastinal mass is seen. After a complete evaluation, he is diagnosed with an esophageal duplication cyst. Which of the following is TRUE regarding these congenital cysts?

(A) Communication with the true lumen is uncommon.

(B) Malignant degeneration is common.

(C) Most cysts are symptomatic.

(D) All cysts should be removed.

(E) Thoracoscopic excision is contraindicated.

96. A patient has compressive symptoms of the esophagus. He has a barium esophagram that shows posterior extrinsic compression of the esophagus. Which of the following is true?

(A) Vascular rings are acquired atherosclerotic lesions.

(B) Both the trachea and esophagus can be affected by vascular rings.

(C) The two most common types of complete vascular rings are double aortic arch and left aortic arch.

(D) There is no role for Echo and Doppler.

(E) Surgery involves division of the esophagus.

97. A 70-year-old man has surgery for an abdominal aortic aneurysm. About 1 month later the patient presents with a massive UGI bleed. Which of the following statements is TRUE?

(A) He should be given PPLs and observed in the intensive care unit.

(B) Most aortoenteric fistulas are primary.

(C) Most aortoenteric fistulas occur between the aorta and duodenum.

(D) It is not improtant to separate the aorta from the eosphagus after aortic surgery.

(E) This condition is always fatal.

Answers and Explanations

1. **(E)** Duodenal ulcer is best diagnosed by upper endoscopy and biopsy. Findings of gastritis and the presence of *H.pylori* are indications to prescribe appropriate therapy. This typically includes a PPI and two antibiotics (one regimen includes amoxicillin and clarithromycin). Although the urea breath test is the most sensitive and specific test used to detect *H. pylori*, it is not readily available in all settings.

2. **(C)** The pylorus is palpable but it is not a true physiologic sphincter. It does not demonstrate reciprocal contraction when the stomach relaxes, nor does it relax when the stomach contracts. The pylorus is normally in tonic contraction It is partially covered by omentum and cancer is commonly found there.

3. **(C)** Surgical intervention for peptic ulcer disease is uncommon. It is indicated by four clinical situations—intractable pain, hemorrhage, perforation, and obstruction. Noncompliance with medication is often the cause of recurrence. Patients with gastic decompression need a nasogastric tube and fluid and electrolyte correction prior to surgery.

4. **(D)** If vagotomy alone is performed, gastric stasis occurs in more than 40% of cases. Branches of the vagus nerve innervate the pylorus. A drainage procedure is necessary; a pyloroplasty or a gastroenterostomy should be performed and both of these require a laparotomy. Truncal vagotomy can also be done through a thoracic approach. Transection of the vagus nerve in the neck results in paralysis of the recurrent laryngeal nerve.

5. **(D)** In highly selective vagotomy (Fig. 5–6), the nerve supply to the pylorus is left intact

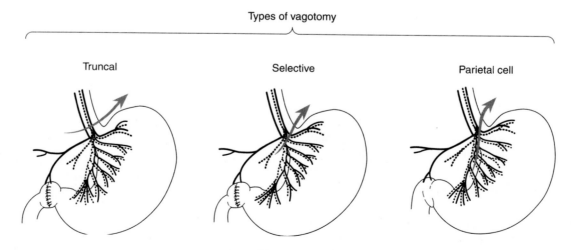

Types of vagotomy

Truncal   Selective   Parietal cell

Figure 5–6.
Various types of vagotomy currently popular for treating duodenal ulcer disease. *(Reproduced, with permission, from Doherty GM: Current Surgical Diagnosis and Treatment, 12th ed. 517. McGraw-Hill, 2006.)*

(and therefore no drainage procedure is necessary). During this operation, the branches of the vagus nerve that supply the parietal cell mass are meticulously divided, leaving the main anterior and posterior nerves of Latarjet intact. The main vagal trunks are also left intact, thus sparing the nerve supply to the liver, gallbladder, pancreas, and intestines. To ensure completeness of the procedure, great care is taken to divide the proximal (criminal) nerve of Grassi. Although the complication rate is lower, the recurrence rate is higher than that of an antrectomy and truncal vagotomy.

6. **(B)** An upright chest x-ray will demonstrate free air below the diaphragm in about 70–75% of patients presenting with a perforated duodenal ulcer. An abdominal sonogram may demonstrate free fluid, but not free air. Although a CAT scan will show both free fluid and free air, it will take longer to perform and may delay the definitive treatment. The combination of an acute abdomen and an upright chest x-ray with free air under the diaphragm provides enough information to take the patient to the operating room for exploration.

7. **(B)** Although surgery is generally recommended for perforation, conservative measures can be considered in select cases. A patient who has a benign clinical presentation or one who is improving, might be considered for treatment with antibiotics and nasogastric decompression.

   Patients who have an acute abdomen and are hemodynamically unstable should not be observed. Board-like rigidity of the abdomen occur as a result of chemical peritonitis. These patients should have fluid and electrolyte repletion, and anitbiotics followed by surgery.

   Choice of the operative procedure should be guided by the information obtained during the history, the presence of comorbid disease, and hemodynamic stability during the operation. A omental (Graham) patch will seal the ulcer, but it will not prevent recurrence.

8. **(D)** Following truncal land selective vagotomy, gastric emptying is delayed. If a vagotomy (truncal or selective) is performed, a drainage procedure is necessary (e.g., pyloroplasty). A disturbance is gastric motility with a delay in gastric emptying may occur with a mechanical gastric outlet obstruction, diabetes, myxedema, hypokalemia, or the administration of anticholinergic or opiate drugs. Rapid gastric emptying may be seen with ZES, retained gastric antrum syndrome, steatorrhea, or massive small-bowel resection where there is impared ability to reduce gastric acid secretion. Failure of switch-off mechanism to inhibit acid secretion also results in increased motility and emptying of the stomach.

9. **(C)** Although a milder type of diarrhea is not uncommon after gastrectomy, fulminant diarrhea may be a problem after vagotomy (it is one of the many complications collectively referred to as *post vagotomy syndromes*). The exact mechanism is not known. It occurs in 1–2% of patients following truncal vagotomy and is less likely to be found after selective or highly selective vagotomy.

10. **(C)** *H. pylori* (previously called *Campylobacter pylori*) is associated with chronic gastritis, duodenal ulcers, gastric ulcers, and gastric cancer. Serology can accurately detect *H. pylori* but remains positive for up to 1 year post treatment. The urea breath test is highly sensitive (96%) and specific (94%). In 2005, Barry Marshall and J. Robbin Warren won the Nobel Prize in medicine for their work on *H. pylori* and its role in gastritis and peptic ulcer disease.

11. **(C)** *Postgastrectomy syndromes* collectively refer to complications that can occur after gastric surgery. This constellation of syndromes includes delayed gastric emptying, recurrent ulcers, diarrhea, anemia, jejunogastric intussusception, afferent loop syndrome, alkaline reflux gastritis, and dumping syndrome. There are two types of dumping syndrome, early and late. Early dumping occurs within 30 minutes and is caused by rapid gastric emptying of a hyperosmolar load into the small bowel. Late (hypoglycemic) dumping occurs 1–3 hours after eating. Symptoms are mostly vasomotor. They are related to the excessive release of insulin in response to the rapid rise in postprandial glucose.

12. **(D)** Prolapse of gastric mucosa into the duodenum may be difficult to distinguish from a polyp in the antrum. It may be detected in a patient who is asymptomatic. Surgical correction should be reserved for patients with obstructive symptoms (e.g., vomiting). Sleeping with they head elevated, H_2 antagonist, and laser treatment have no role.

13. **(D)** Dumping syndrome is a symptom complex ocurring after gastric surgery. It is characterized by fatigue, abdominal distension, pain, and vasomotor symptoms caused by the rapid entry of food into the small intestine. Tachycardia, sweating, and feeling lightheaded after eating are symptoms patients may feel. There are two types of dumping syndrome, early and late.

14. **(B)** Bilious vomiting is usually spontaneous and should be differentiated from vomiting that occurs after eating. The most likely cause of this complication is reflex of bile into the stomach. Bile gastritis with intestinalization of the gastric mucosa is a likely cause.

15. **(D)** Group O is the most common blood type in patients with duodenal ulcer disease. In patients who have bled from a duodenal ulcer, this observation is even more striking. Secretors have an excess of blood group antigen that is absent in nonsecretors. The secretor antigen on the red blood cell appears in body fluids also. Nonsecretors are more prone to develop dueodenal ulcers than secretors.

16. **(E)** There is a varying degree of impairment in carbohydrate, fat, protein, and mineral absorption after gastrectomy. These changes are most severe after a subtotal gastrectomy and gastrojejunostomy (Billroth II) (Fig. 5–7), in most patients these changes are mild. An acid environment is necessary to release ferric ion from food and make it available for absorption in the small intestine.

17. **(D)** In general, vagotomy with a gastric drainage procedure is less satisfactory in the treatment of primary gastric ulcer. Treatment of a gastric ulcer may include partial gastrectomy with a gastroduodenal anastomosis (Billroth I). Vagotomy is

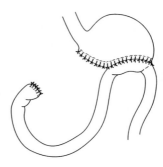

Subtotal gastrectomy
(Billroth II)

Figure 5–7.
Subtotal gastrectomy; Billroth II. *(Reproduced, with permission, from Doherty GM: Current Surgical Diagnosis and Treatment, 12th ed. 517. McGraw-Hill, 2006.)*

not necessary because gastric ulcers are usually not associated with acid hypersecretion. A gastric ulcer that fails to heal despite medical therapy should be excised.

18. **(C)** In ZES gastrin levels may be only mildly elevated but can be increased with provocation with intravenous calcium or secretin. Most patients with gastrinoma have serum gastrin levels that exceed 500 pg/mL. When the range is lower than 200–500 pg/mL, a stimulation test is performed to confirm the diagnosis. A rise of 200 pg/mL after 15 minutes, or a doubling of the fasting level is diagnostic. ZES can occur sporadically or as part of multiple endocrine neoplasia (MEN) I.

19. **(C)** Chronic duodenal ulcer, with recurrent episode of healing and repair, may lead to pyloric obstruction due to scarring and stenosis of the duodenum. Painless vomiting of undigested food may occur once or twice a day. Surgical intervention should be carried out after correction of fluid and electrolyte imbalances. Preoperative antibiotics should be used due to bacterial overgrowth secondary to gastric statis.

20. **(D)** ZES is characterized by duodenal ulcer disease, high basal acid secretory output, and a pancreatic tumor. Stimulated serum gastrin levels may be in excess of 1000 pg/mL or as

high as 10,000 pg/mL. ZES is due to a true pancreatic tumor in adults, but may be secondary to hyperplasia in children. Growth of the tumor is usually slow and survival is often prolonged. If an isolated tumor is found on CAT scan, surgical resection is indicated. About two-thirds of these tumors are malignant. About one-forth of patients have MEN I syndrome tumors of parathyroid pituitary and pancreas.

21. **(C)** Gastrin is produced in the antrum, duodenum, and small intestine. It is not present in the fundus of the stomach. When the distal stomach is removed gastrin levels decrease significantly. Gastrin stimulates parietal cells to secrete acid and it stimulates chief cells to secrete pepsinogen.

22. **(D)** Hypertrophic gastritis is characterized by massive loss of plasma protein through the affected gastric mucosa. Most cases can be managed medically by maintenance of adequate nutrition. An increased incidence of gastric cancer has been reported in some series.

23. **(E)** The distinction between a benign and malignant ulcer can be difficult. The presence of achlorhydria rules out peptic ulceration. Endoscopy is indicated so that biopsy can be performed.

24. **(D)** A gastric ulcer that does not respond to medical therapy requires surgical intervention. An appropriate operation for an antral ulcer is an antrectomy with a gastroduodenal anastomosis (Billroth I). Vagotomy is not nearly as effective in preventing recurrences in gastric ulcers. It is important to realize that the management of gastric and duodenal ulcers is not identical because the etiologies are different. Duodenal ulcers are associated with acid hypersecretion while gastric ulcers are associated with impaired mucosal defense mechanisms. Both are associated with *H. pylori* (duodenal ulcers 90% and gastric ulcers 75%). A gastric ulcer is much more likely to harbor a malignancy as compared to a duodenal ulcer. A gastric ulcer should always be biopsied. If a gastric ulcer fails to heal after appropriate medical management, it should be excised.

25. **(A)** EGC is found only in the mucosa and submucosa. Regional lymph nodes may or may not be involved. EGC can be missed on a UGI series (low sensitivity). Treatment is gastric resection with care to ensure that the resection margins and the anastomosis are tumor free. Selected cases may be treated by endoscopic mucosal resection. In the United States, EGC is found in only 15% of patients diagnosed with gastric cancer. In Japan the incidence is up to 40%. Up to 14% of patients will have synchronous cancers. Five-year survival is 85–90%.

26. **(E)** The treatment of an antral gastric cancer is distal subtotal gastrectomy with lymph node dissection (provided there is no metastatic disease). Surgical resection is the only potential curative therapy. Proximal margins should be 5–6 cm. Total gastrectomy does not improve 5-year survival. Postoperative chemoradiation may increase 5-year survival (limited studies).

27. **(D)** The incisura is located at the distal portion of the lesser curvature. It is the point at which the body of the stomach ends and the antrum begins.

28. **(B)** GISTs were previously called leiomyosarcomas. They are rare (4% of all gastrointestinal tumors). They can cause confusion because the overlying mucosa may remain intact. They grow slowly, invade locally, and are not responsive to radiation or chemotherapy. Eosinophilic gastroenterisit is an infiltrative lesion that usually involves the gastric antrum. It is of unknown origin and differs from Menetrier's disease, where the mucosal folds of the proximal stomach are intially involved.

29. **(C)** The stomach is the most common site of involvement in extranodal non-Hodgkin's lymphoma (NHL). Lymphoma is the second most common malignancy of the stomach. Surgery was previously the treatment of choice for gastric lymphoma. More recent studies show that nonoperative treatment with chemotherapy and radiation therapy results in similar 5-year survival and is currently first-line therapy. Surgery is used mainly to treat complications of gastric

lymphoma (e.g., perforation, bleeding). Mucosa associated lymphoid tissue (MALT) lymphoma is a type of NHL. It is associated with *H. pylori*. Treatment with a PPl and antibiotics will cure up to 75% of low-grade MALTomas.

30. **(D)** A GIST (previously called leiomyoma or leiomyosarcoma) can occur in any part of the stomach. Most commonly they are found in the submucosa and grow towards the lumen. Ulceration may occur and give rise to the characteristic "doughnut sign" on barium studies. Hematemesis and/or melena may sometimes be massive. Local resection is curative.

31. **(C)** Hyperplastic polyps are unlikely to harbor carcinoma. Multiplicity of hyperplastic polyps does not seem to predispose to the development of cancer. Adenomatous polyps occur more commonly in the antrum. Hyperplastic polyps are distributed more evenly throughout the stomach. For this reason, antral polyps should be removed first. (Adenomatous polyps may have a focus of cancer within them.)

32. **(C)** Adenomatous polyps of the stomach resemble colon polyps. Coexisting carcinoma may be present in up to 20% of cases. The incidence of carcinoma is increased if lesions are larger than 2 cm. Both hyperplastic and adenomatous polyps are more common in long-term follow-up of patients treated successfully for familial polyposis. All adenomatous polyps should be removed.

33. **(E)** Gastric volvulus is often associated with a large paraesophageal hiatal hernia. The twist causes a cut-off at the cardia above and at the pylorus below leading to distension and ischemia, which may progress to gangrene. Organoaxial volvulus is more common and rotation occurs along the axis between the cardia and the pylorus. In the less common type of gastric volvulus, rotation occurs through an axis that is at the right angle to the organoaxial axis described.

34. **(C)** Acute gastric distension can lead to a vasovagal reaction. Treatment consists of nasogastric decompression for 24–48 hours to allow normal gastric tone to return. Appropriate parenteral fluids should also be administered.

35. **(B)** Autoimmune metaplastic atrophic gastritis is associated with hypochlorhydria parietal cell antibodies, and high gastrin levels. There is an increased risk for developing gastric carcinoid tumors or adenocarcinomas. Other premalignant conditions include adnomatous polyps, gastric ulcer, previous gastric resection (>15 years), chronic atrophic gastritis, and histologic changes showing intestinal metaplasia and dysplasia.

36. **(A)** In 1948, Dragstedt introduced a gastric drainage procedure to overcome stasis that occurred in over 30–40% of cases following vagotomy. Pyloroplasty, gastrojejunostomy, and antrectomy are the three recognized drainage procedures performed in conjunction with vagotomy. The decision on which one to perform is based on the overall condition of the patient and the severity of the ulcer, amongst other things. A drainage procedure is not necessary with a highly selective vagotomy because the innervation to the pylorus is left intact.

37. **(D)** In general, surgery for peptic ulcer bleeding is indicated at an earlier stage in an older patient because vessels are atherosclerotic and less likely to stop bleeding spontaneously. In addition, diminished perfusion of the heart, brain, and kidneys is less well tolerated in elderly patients. At surgery, the gastroduodenal artery is oversewn, and a vagotomy and drainage procedure is performed.

38. **(B)** The scan will fail to visualize the gallbladder if acute cholecystitis is present. In a patient with cholelithiasis, the incidence of cholecystitis and associated biliary complications is increased following truncal vagotomy. A sonogram will show gallstones but may not distinguish acute cholecystitis.

39. **(B)** GIST is the most common sarcoma of the gastrointestinal tract. It is most commonly found in the stomach (60–70%). Other sites include small intestine (25%), rectum (5%), esophagus (2%), and other less frequent locations. It may be

difficult to distinguish between malignant and benign GISTs. Factors that are correlated with improved prognosis include gastric location, low mitotic index <2 cm diameter, and absence of tumor rupture and spoilage during resection.

40. **(B)** If the mass is deemed resectable, the goal of surgery is resection with grossly negative margins. Precautions should be taken to prevent rupture of the mass. Radiation and chemotherapy have traditionally been ineffective. Clinical trials with the drug imatinib mesylate (Gleevec) are promising.

41. **(C)** Patients with pernicious anemia have achlorhydria and an increased risk (about 5%) of developing gastric carcinoma. There is a deficiency in vitamin B_{12} that leads to megaloblastic anemia and neurologic involvement (subacute degeneration of the dorsal and lateral spinal columns).

42. **(D)** A Zenker's (pharyngoesophageal) diverticulum is a mucosal outpouching through the triangular bare area between the cricopharyngeus muscle and the inferior constrictor muscle of the pharynx (Killian's triangle). Most present on the left side of the neck.

43. **(E)** The current surgical treatment for a symptomatic pharyngoesophageal diverticulum is myotomy. If the diverticulum is >2 cm, it should be resected. Small asymptomatic diverticulae require no treatment. Failure of relaxation of the cricopharyngeus muscle is thought to result in the development of the diverticulum.

44. **(E)** An epiphrenic (supradiaphragmatic) diverticulum is a pulsion diverticulum and is associated without any obvious lesions (35%) or with hiatal hernia (30%), diffuse esophageal spasm (DES) (20%), achalasia (10%), and miscellaneous causes (5%). It is located with 10 cm of the cardia. An epiphrenic diverticulum is commonly asymptomatic and should not be treated surgically unless symptoms are clearly related to it. Parabronchial lymphadenopathy can cause traction diverticulae (which are located at a higher level).

45. **(A)** The appearance of unexplained dysphagia in adults requires urgent evaluation. Esophageal carcinoma is particularly prevalent in certain parts of Africa and Asia, but the incidence is increasing in Western countries. In achalasia there is initially a greater tolerance for solids over liquids. In carcinoma, dysphagia for solids is noted initally, and later there is difficulty in swallowing liquids as well. Esophagoscopy is required in the workup of dysphagia. It is imperative to rule out an underlying carcinoma.

46. **(B)** In addition to the presence of an upper esophageal web leading to dysphagia, the Plummer-Vinson syndrome is characterized by atrophic oral mucosa, spoon-shaped brittle nails (koilonychia), and iron deficiency anemia. Endoscopy reveals a fibrous web just below the cricopharyngeus muscle. There is an increased risk of developing cancer of the esophagus.

47. **(D)** Nonoperative therapy is the initial treatment of GERD. The treatment is weight loss, avoidance of fatty meals, smoking cessation, abstinence from alcohol, positional awareness, avoidance of lying supine, and avoidance of certain foods (e.g., chocolate) and drugs (e.g., theophylline, anticholinergic agents, α-adrenergic antagonists). Dysphagia requires special attention to rule out a stricture, cancer, or a motility disorder. Poor results are more likely when previous surgery has failed and in patients with scleroderma.

48. **(B)** The cardia is displaced into the posterior mediastinum. The term sliding hernia (Fig. 5–8) indicates that a part of the peritoneum slips or slides with the hernia into the posterior mediastinum. The wall of the sac is formed medially by the stomach and laterally by the peritoneum. Reflux esophagitis is more likely to occur with this type of hernia. The sliding hiatal hernia may be entirely symptomatic or lead to reflux esophagitis and possibly esophageal stricture.

49. **(C)** Benign peptic strictures of the esophagus are submucosal fibrotic rings that narrow the lumen and obstruct the passage of food. They present with dysphagia. They tend to be

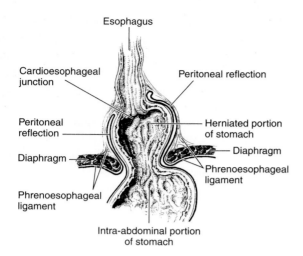

Figure 5–8.
Sliding esophageal hiatal hernia; correlate with x-ray in
Fig. 5–2. *(Reproduced, with permission, from Doherty
GM: Current Surgical Diagnosis and Treatment, 12th ed.
467. McGraw-Hill, 2006.)*

between 1 and 4 cm in length. GERD is the
most common cause. Other associated motility
disorders often occur. Heartburn may improve
because of the obstruction to refluxed bile.

50. **(D)** The present treatment is aimed at preventing esophagitis. Barrett's esophagus is regarded
as a premalignant condition and is characterized by columnar metaplastic of the normal
squamous epithelial lining of the esophagus.
The cancer risk is increased 20–50-fold. About
one-third of patients present with malignancy,
and many cases of adenocarcinoma of the
esophagus arise from Barrett's mucosa. There is
an increased risk for the development of squamous carcinoma. It is found in 8–10% of
patients with long standing reflux.

51. **(D)** This is a type 4 hiatal hernia (Fig. 5–9). In
the classic case of a paraesophageal "rolling"
hernia, the GE junction remains below the
hiatus, allowing the stomach and sometimes
other viscera to migrate upward into the chest
alongside the esophagus. Paraesophageal hernias are prone to obstruction, bleeding, and
volvulus (either mesoaxial or organoxial rotation). Chronic symptoms include pain and
postprandial fullness, with heartburn in 90% of
cases. Gastric ulcers develop in as many as 30%
of cases and they may cause acute or chronic

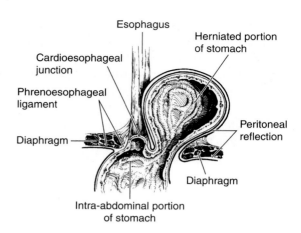

Figure 5–9.
Paraesophageal hernia; correlate with x-ray in Fig. 5–3.
*(Reproduced, with permission, from Doherty GM:
Current Surgical Diagnosis and Treatment, 12th ed. 468.
McGraw-Hill, 2006.)*

(MISSING BOTTOM LINE) indicated and
effective to relieve symptoms and to prevent
complications, which may be catastropic.

52. **(B)** Schantzki's ring is a thin, circumferential
scar in the lower esophagus, more common in
men (65) or greater. It is acquired and probably
results from repeated trauma to the mucosa
with chronic inflammation and fibrosis.
Endoscopic dilation is the usual treatment. It is
usually successful but antireflux surgery is
occasionally necessary for severe GERD, especially if it is worsened by dilatation. Associated
hiatal hernia is very common.

53. **(A)** Dysphagia in esophageal achalasia is
described as paradoxical in that it is more pro-
nounced for liquids than solids. There are
numerous reports of an increased incidence of
carcinoma in achalasia, ranging from 3% to
10%. In 1975, Belsey reported a 10% incidence
in 81 patients in whom symptoms tended to
occur at a younger age. Recurrent lung infections from aspiration of esophageal contents
are a troublesome complication. The treatment
is surgical myotomy or endoscopic dilatation.

54. **(D)** A Mallory-Weiss tear is characterized by
acute and sometimes massive UGI hemorrhage.
It accounts for up to 10% of UGI bleeds. It is due
to arterial bleeding following repeated vomiting
(which causes mucosal tears at the GE junction).

The cause is the same as that for spontaneous rupture of the esophagus (i.e., an increase in intra-abdominal pressure against a closed glottis). Causes other than vomiting such as paroxysmal coughing or retching, may sometimes lead to this condition. Upper endoscopy confirms the diagnosis. Surgery may occasionally be necessary to stop the bleeding.

55. **(B)** Spontaneous rupture of the esophagus, or Boerhaave's syndrome, is most common in men between 35 and 55 years of age. The usual presentation is severe pain in the precordium, lower thorax, or epigastrium. Clasically it follows an episode of violent vomiting. A chest film show hydropneumothorax usually on the left side, but it may be on the right side or bilateral. Free air below the diaphragm is not a usual finding. The tear is usually located above the diaphragm and is longitudinal on the left posterolateral wall. Air passes around the mediastinum, which results in subcutaneous emphysemia.

56. **(D)** Spontaneous rupture of the esophagus is an acute emergency. It requires efforts to establish a rapid diagnosis followed by an emergency operation. Rapid resuscitation and antibiotics should be instituted prior to surgery. Shock is not a contraindication to surgery because it is unlikely that the patient's condition will improve until surgery has been performed. The surgical approach is usually thoracic, but the abdominal approach may also be used.

57. **(E)** The esophagus is a posterior mediastinal structure in much of its course. The thymus gland is located in the anterior mediastinum. The recurrent laryngeal nerve runs between the trachea and the esophagus. The aorta loops backward over the left side of the esophagus. At this level the thoracic duct is on the left side of the esophagus. The brachiocephalic vein is the most anterior structure in the superior mediastinum.

58. **(D)** Leiomyoma is the most common benign tumor encountered in the esophagus. Malignant transformation is thought to be rare. Less than 10% of alimentary tract leiomyomas are found in the esophagus. They are composed of spindle cells and grow slowly and may progressively cause obstructive symptoms. Leiomyomas are not referred to as a benign GIST. Other benign lesions are congenital or acquired cysts, adenomatous polyps, papillomas, lipomas, neurofibromas, and hemangiomas.

59. **(C)** The gastroesophageal zone of elevated pressure is 3–4 cm long and has a resting pressure of 15-cm H_2O. Pregnancy, obesity, and gastric dilatation, all result in increased intra-abdominal pressure and can result in reflux. Alkalinization of the stomach, gastrin, epinephrine, cholinergic agents (bethanecol), and α-adrenergic agents (metoclopromide) increase the resting pressure of the LES. Anticholinergic agents (atropine), glucagon, and secretin decrease the resting pressure, and is released by the vagus nerve and it stimulates the production of acid in the stomach.

60. **(E)** The history of GERD coupled with these findings is highly suggestive of an adenocarcinoma arising in a Barrett's esophagus. Squamous carcinoma is more likely to occur higher up in the middle third of the esophagus. Endoscopy and biopsy prove the diagnosis. The patient should be treated surgically by esophagectomy if carcinoma is confirmed. Inoperable upper esophageal squamous cell carcinomas can be treated with chemoradiation (survival outcomes are similar to surgery with less morbidity).

61. **(D)** Surgical resection of the esophagus remains the recommended treatment for patients with carcinoma of the lower esophagus, provided that there is no metastitic disease and the patient's overall medical condition is compatible with a major operation. This offers the best palliation and the only hope for cure. The 5-year survival rates vary between 15 and 25%. Radiation and chemotherapy, in combination with surgery in selected patients, may improve these statistics. There are four types of esophagectomy—transthoracic, en bloc, transhiatal, and video-assisted. Regardless of what type of operation is performed, complete macroscopic and microscopic removal of tumor, is the goal.

62. **(A)** Blunt trauma is the most common cause of diaphragmatic rupture. Associated injuries are common. In blunt trauma, the left diaphragm is ruptured more frequently than the right. The stomach, spleen, colon, and omentum may enter the left pleural cavity. Diaphragmatic injury without herniation of abdominal contents is difficult to diagnose. Patients may present with symptoms many years after the initial trauma. Early surgery is indicted.

63. **(B)** Subhepatic (intrahepatic) space infection usually occurs after surgery or peritonitis in the supracolic compartment. It is an unlikely amplication of biliary pancreatitis. Infections in the subhepatic space may extend to the infracolic compartment via the paracolic gutter (of Morrison). In addition to the stomach, the subhepatic space may be involved with infection secondary to injury or diseases of the the gallbladder, the first part of the duodenum, the anterior portions of the pancreas, or the liver. The uncinate lobe of the pancreas is the part of the head located posteriorly to the superior mesentric artery vein.

64. **(D)** Oral fluids and solid foods can usually be started several days after the injury. Feeding at this stage is encouraged if the patient continues to show favorable improvement. If the caustic injury is superficial, stricture formation is unlikely to occur. Endoscopy to the proximal extend of the injury is recommended unless perforation is suspected. No attempt should be made to pass the endoscope beyond the proximal protion of the inflammatory segment. Emetics should not be administered because the esophagus will be reexposed to the agent when the patient vomits.

65. **(C)** Esophageal perforation has occurred. Caustic alkali ingestion results in liquefactive necrosis while acid ingestion causes caogulation necrosis. The esoophagus is more often involved than the stomach during alkaline ingestion (and conversely, the stomach is more often involved than the esophagus during acid ingestion). Features on x-ray suggesting esophageal perforation include pneumothorax, pneumomediastinum, and pleural effusion.

Ewald tubes or nasogastric tubes should be avoided because of the risk of perforation.

66. **(B)** The hepatic artery is medial to the common bile duct and anterior to the portal vein. The inferior vena cava passes posterior to the (epiploic) foramen of Winslow, where it lies behind the portal vein. The foramen represents the only natural communication between the lesser and greater peritoneal bursa (sac).

67. **(E)** This test is a useful method of determining if a mass is due to an abdominal wall lesion or an intra-abdominal lesion. Attempts by the patient to sit up will make the anterior abdominal wall muscles taut and thus reduce the palpability definition of an intra-abdominal mass. An abdominal wall mass will still be palpable after this maneuver. This is called Fothergill's sign.

68. **(D)** *H. Pylori* infection, smoking, and a high salt intake are all risk factors for gastric cancer. A diet high in fruits, vegetables, and fiber may lower the risk for gastric cancer. The incidence of gastric cancer is low in North America. Gastric cancer is one of the most common cancers in Japanese men.

69. **(E)** Acute gastric dilatation may result in a vasovagal response. This response is characterized by typical signs and symptoms of marked gastric and abdominal distension. These are clearly demonstrable in an awake patient. Unfortunately, this condition may occur after anesthesia is administered and thus go unrecognized. Vomiting, aspiration, hypoxia, or bleeding from erosive stress gastritis may occur. Gastritis, gastric volvulus, and pernicious anemia do not cause a vasovagal response.

70. **(E)** GISTs are the most common mesenchymal tumors of the gastrointestinal tract. They may be benign, malignant, or intermediate grade. They demonstrate a mutation of the c-kit oncogene. Distant metastases occur late. Prolonged survival follows resection, including adjacent organs if necessary (e.g., colon, pancreas). Hemorrhage can result if the tumor erodes through the gastric mucosa. Malnutrition results from compromise of the capacity of the stomach.

71. **(E)** Patients with familial adenomatous polyposis are at risk for developing carcinoma in adenomatous polyps arising in the stomach and duodenum. Ampullary and bile duct cancers will result in jaundice.

72. **(D)** Conservative treatment of GERD includes lifestyle modifications (e.g., smoking cessation, decreased caffeine intake, avoidance of large meals before lying down, elevation of the head of the bed, and avoidance of constrictive clothing). PPI's are very effective if nonoperative management fails, surgical intervention should be considered. Preoperative evaluation includes manometry, 24-hour pH test and esophagogram, in addition to endoscopy. Manometry evaluates the LES resting pressure and effectiveness of peristalsis. The 24-hour pH test is the gold standard for diagnosing and quantifying acid reflux. Esophagogram shows the external anatomy of the esophagus and proximal stomach, as well as demonstrating the presence of a hiatal hernia. Nissen fundoplication is a 360° gastric wrap. It can be performed as an open or laparoscopic procedure. It is the most common operation performed for GERD. Partial fundoplications (e.g., Thal, Dor, Toupet) are done if esophageal motility is poor.

73. **(E)** Critically ill patients who have multiple organ involvement, from trauma or other diseases, are at risk for developing bleeding from erosive gastritis. Risk factors include multiorgan dysfunction, sepsis, trauma, and respiratory failure requiring mechanical ventilation. The pathogenesis of acute stress gastritis is multifactorial. One factor is thought to involve hypoperfusion of the gastric mucosa and ischemia.

74. **(E)** Endoscopic findings range from petechiae to multiple ulcers in the body of the stomach and duodenum. Endoscopy can safely be performed at the bedside in the intensive care unit. Because bleeding may be secondary to shallow mucosal erosions, a CAT scan, UGI series, and angiogram will not be diagnostic. Capsule endoscopy is sometimes used in the diagnosis of occult gastrointestinal bleeding when other methods have not been helpful.

75. **(A)** Peptic ulcer disease is the most common cause of UGI bleeding in patients presenting to the emergency department. Most bleeding ulcers (80%) will stop with conservative measures. A visible vessel seen during endoscopy can have up to a 55% chance of rebleeding. Other causes of bleeding include gastritis, gastric cancer, esophagitis, Mallory-Weiss tear, Dieulafoy's lesion, and esophageal varices, but these occur less commonly than peptic ulcer as a likely cause of bleeding.

76. **(E)** Prostaglandin E (misoprostol) has not been useful in the management of erosive gastritis because diarrhea has been a troublesome side effect. At lower doses it can be used as prophylaxis against NSAID associated gastropathy.

77. **(B)** Gastrinoma (ZES) should always be excluded in patients presenting with severe peptic ulcer disease that fails to respond to therapy. It accounts for 0.1–1% of peptic ulcers. It is usually caused by a gastrinoma (a non β-cell tumor found in the pancreas or duodenum). The diagnosis is based partly on an elevated fasting serum gastrin level (normal 60 pg/mL; in ZES > 150 pg/mL and can be over 1000 pg/mL). Basal acid secretion is increased above 15 mEq/h. Duodenal ulcers are the most common ulcers, but ulcers in unusual locations (e.g., jejunum) may also be seen.

78. **(C)** Since the patient is stable, she does not require any therapeutic endoscopic or surgical procedures. Triple therapy (a PPI and two antibiotics) should be initiated to eradicate the *H. pylori* organism. She should also be educated about the association of aspirin and NSAIDs with peptic ulcer disease.

79. **(D)** Duodenal ulcers are associated with acid hypersecretion and impaired neutralization of aid in the duodenum. The other choices are not associated with duodenal ulcers.

80. **(E)** If all nonoperative measures have failed to control bleeding from an ulcer, the next definitive step is surgery. Although the patient may require continued resuscitation with crystalloids

and blood products, the bleeding will not stop without surgical intervention. Elderly patients have poor toleration for hypotension due to comorbidities, therefore emergency surgery not elective is appropriate.

81. **(B)** There is an increased incidence of gastric cancer in patients with gastric ulcer disease. The overall 5-year survival is 12%, but it can be as high as 35% if the nodes are negative (and 7% if the nodes are involved). It is important that the cut edges are free of tumor othewise the cancer will recur. Proximal lymph nodes should be removed from the stomach. The extent of lymph node dissection remains controversial. Extended D_2 lymph nodes dissections are performed in Japan and demonstrate improved survival. These results have not been replicated in the West.

82. **(C)** Endoscopic gastrostomy by percutaneous means is rapid and safe. It should be considered in patients who are unable to maintain an appropriate caloric intake orally. The procedure is performed under local anesthesia and sedation.

83. **(D)** A patient is a candidate for bariatric surgery if he or she meets certain criteria. A patient whose weight is 100 lb greater than his ideal body weight or whose BMI is greater than 35 mg/kg is morbidly obese. Prior to surgery, a patient must have a thorough evaluation by a multidisciplinary team (e.g., internist, dietician, psychologist, surgeon, and the likes). Patients who are not morbidly obese and simply want to lose weight are not candidates for these procedures. Patients are at risk for multiple complications, including fatal pulmonary embolus.

84. **(C)** There are multiple morbid obesity operations. Jejunoileal bypass has a higher incidence of both early and late complications. Gastric restrictive procedures (e.g., vertical banded gastroplasty) are generally less effective than GBP. GBP patients can be expected to lose up to two-thirds of their weight initially. The gastric pouch capacity should be no larger than 30cc. Anastomotic leak rate should be less than 5%.

85. **(C)** The symptoms and radiologic findings in this patient suggest achalasia. Evaluation includes endoscopy to rule out a stricture or cancer. Barium swallow will show a dilated esophagus, failure of the LES to relax during swallowing, and a lack of peristalsis. Nonoperative management is of limited usefulness but may be considered in high-risk patients who are not candidates for surgery.

86. **(C)** A healthy patient with achalasia who has failed nonoperative management should be considered for surgical intervention. Pneumatic dilatation is first-line therapy. It causes disruption of the muscular layers of the LES. A balloon is placed endoscopically at the level of the LES. Fluoroscopically is used to visualize the balloon as it is inflated to pressures no higher than 10 psi. If pneumatic dilatation fails, or if symptoms return after successful dilation, surgery should be considered. The procedure may be done open or endoscopically. The operation involves a myotomy that divides the circular and longitudinal muscle fibers. It extends from the distal 6 cm of the esophagus, through the LES, and the proximal gastric cardia. A partial fundoplication is usually included to prevent gastroesophageal reflux.

87. **(A)** It is important to rule out coronary artery disease in patients who have DES because the symptoms may be similar. Barium swallow and endoscopy are used to evaluate the esophagus. A corkscrew esophagus is highly suggestive of DES, however, it is not always seen. Manometry is the diagnostic study of choice. Medical management includes nitrates and calcium channel blockers.

88. **(C)** Barrett's esophagus is a metaplastic change found in 10–15% of GERD patients. The normal squamous cells of the esophagus are transformed into columnar cells. It is more commonly seen in men. Patients with Barrett's esophagus (without dysplasia) require lifelong surveillance. Patients with severe dysplasia have a 40–50% chance of developing adenocarcinoma of the esophagus. Prophylactic esophagectomy is recommended.

89. (C) The Lauren classification divides gastric adenoccarcinomas into two histolgic types—an intestinal type and a diffuse type. The intestinal type is more common and usually forms a discrete lesion. The diffuse infiltrating type is less common and a mass may not be seen. In the intestinal type, cells form glandular strictives in the diffuse type, cells are poorly organized and full of mucin (signet ring cells). The diffuse type may extensively infiltrate the muscles of the stomach, thus leading to rigidity. Gross appearance may be unremarkable, but palpation aids in the diagnosis. "Leather bottle stomach" refers to a stomach that is entirely involved with diffuse type cancer. The 5-years survival is poor.

90. (C) Hemobilia may be secondary to instrumentation of the biliary tree, or malignancy, or trauma. It involves bleeding from the biliary tract that transits through the ampulla into the duodenum. Bleeding may be subacute or massive. Endoscopic retrograde cholangiopancreatography (ERCP) or angiogram may be diagnostic. Angioembolization may be therapeutic.

91. (D) "Watermelon stomach" is a term used to describe the appearance of the stomach in a condition called GAVE (gastic antral vascular ectasis) syndrome. Dilated blood vessels radiate from the pylorus to the antrum in a pattern that resembles the stripes of a watermelon. It is an uncommon cause of gastrointestinal bleeding. It has been associated with certain autoimmune diseases, however, it may also be seen in individuals not affected by these conditions. It may also be seen with portal hypertension. It is most commonly seen in elderly women. Endoscopic laser treatment is usually effective.

92. (D) Candida is the most common cause of infectious esophagitis. Predisposing factors include malignancy, AIDS, and antibiotic use. A double contrast esophageal swallow or esophagogastroduodenoscopy (EGD) can be used to make the diagnosis. Not all patients with oral thrush have candida esophagitis; cytomegalovirus (CMV) esophagitis can also occur in these patients. Other infecious causes include tuberculosis (TB) and herpes. Antibiotics can be effective. A superficial spreading carcinoma of the esophagus may have a similar appearance in diagnostic studies.

93. (E) A dieulafoy lesion is an uncommon cause of UGI bleeding (0.3–7%). It can occur anywhere in the gastrointestinal tract, but is most commonly found in the stomach (near the GE junction). It is often difficult to visualize because of its small size. A dilated submucosal artery is the source of the bleeding. First-line management is therapeutic endoscopy. There is no association with NSAIDs or alcohol. These lesions are more common in men.

94. (E) Patients with impaired gastric emptying, such as those who have had previous gastric surgery or those with diabetes, can develop bezoars. Bezoars can be classified as two types—phytobezoars (undigested vegetable matter) and trichobezoars (hair). The diagnosis can be made by EGD or barium study. Nonoperative management is often successful. Patients are told to ingest meat tenderizer (which contains papain) and repeat endoscopy is performed for further fragmentation and removal of the bezoar. If the patient is obstructed and endoscopic therapy is unsuccessful, surgery is indicated. Patients who ingest their hair should be referred for psychiatric evaluation.

95. (A) Duplication cysts are congenital. Communication with the true lumen is uncommon. They are usually asymptomatic. Symptoms and complications can include dysphagia, infection, perforation, and bleeding. Malignant degeneration is rare. Symptomatic cysts can be removed by open thoracotomy or videoassisted thoracoscopic (VATS) techniques.

96. (B) Vascular rings are congenital. They can encircle the trachea and esophagus and cause compressive symptoms. The two most common types are double aortic arch and right aortic arch with left ligamentum arteriosum. Diagnostic studies include chest x-ray, barium study, Echo, CAT scan, MRI, and angiogram. Surgery involves division of the ring.

97. **(C)** An aortoenteric fistula should be suspected in any patient who has had previous aortic surgery and presents with massive UGI bleed. Most aortoenteric fistulas are secondary to this type of surgery. It is important to separate an aortic graft from intestine (e.g., retroperitoneal tissue). Most aortoenteric fistulas occur between the aorta and duodenum. Mortality is high, but timely surgical intervention can be successful. Surgery may involve performing an extraanatomic bypass and removing the aortic graft.

CHAPTER 6

Small and Large Intestines and Appendix

Evelyn Irizarry and Nicholas A. Balsano

Questions

DIRECTIONS (Questions 1 through 90): Each of the numbered items in this section is followed by five answers. Select the ONE lettered answer that is BEST in each case.

Question 1 through 3

A 17-year-old female model presents to the emergency room with a 1-day history of lower abdominal pain. On examination she is most tender in the right lower quadrant (RLQ) and also has pelvic tenderness. White blood cell (WBC) count is 13,000 and temperature is 100.6°F. A provisional diagnosis of uncomplicated appendicitis is made and laparoscopic appendectomy is offered.

1. Regarding laparoscopic appendectomy which of the following is TRUE?

    (A) It can be performed safely with minimal morbidity compared to open technique.
    (B) Length of hospital stay is longer than with open technique.
    (C) Procedure cost is less than with open technique.
    (D) Return to full feeding is less than with open technique.
    (E) Wound complication rate is greater with open technique.

2. Possible advantages of the laparoscopic techniques include all except?

    (A) Post hospital recovery is longer.
    (B) More scar formation.
    (C) Not allow thorough inspection of the peritoneal contents.
    (D) Longer operative time.
    (E) No treatment for nonappendical disease.

3. At open operation a normal appendix is found. What is the most common procedure a surgeon should do if he finds a normal appendix?

    (A) Evaluate the pelvis for tuboovarian abscess pelvic inflammatory disease, malignancy or etopic pregnancy
    (B) Removal of appendix
    (C) Evaluate the terminal ileum and cecum for signs of regional or bacterial enteritis
    (D) Evaluate the upper abdomen for cholecystitis or perforated duodenal ulcer
    (E) Evaluate for Meckel's diverticulum

4. A 25-year-old male develops diarrhea and colicky abdominal pain. Ulcertive colitus is diagnosed on colonoscopy. Which of the following findings is consistent with the diagnosis?

(A) The rectum is not involved.
(B) The disease is confluent, there are no skip areas in the colon and the rectum is involved.
(C) The full thickness of the bowel wall is involved.
(D) Microscopic examination of the mucosa reveals normal cells without evidence of dysplasia.
(E) The incidence of colorectal cancer is equal to that of the general population.

5. A 35-year-old man has known ulcerative colitis. Which of the following is an indication for total proctocolectomy?

(A) Occasional bouts of colic and diarrhea
(B) Sclerosing cholangitis
(C) Toxic megacolon
(D) Arthritides
(E) Iron deficiency anemia

6. Ten years after diagnosis of total proctocolitis this patient undergoes colonscopy and biopsy reveals high-grade dysplasia in 2–10 specimens. What should the physician recommend?

(A) Repeat colonoscopy in 1 year
(B) Increase steroid dosage
(C) Early repeat colonoscopy and biopsy area again
(D) Total proctocolectomy
(E) Resection of the involved segment

7. A 55-year-old man presents with left lower quadrant (LLQ) abdominal pain of 2-day duration, associated with constipation. On physical examination, he has tenderness localized to the LLQ with fullness in that area leukocyte count is 22,000 and temperature is 101.5°F. Which would be the best diagnostic study to evaluate this man?

(A) Diagnostic laparoscopy
(B) Barium enema
(C) Plain abdominal roentgenogram

(D) Computed tomography (CT) of the abdomen/pelvis with orally (PO) and intravenous (IV) contrast
(E) Colonoscopy

8. Complications of diverticulitis include:

(A) Carcinoma of the colon
(B) Extraintestinal manifestations such as arthritis, iritis, and skin rashes
(C) Fistulisation to adjacent organs such as the bladder, with insueing colovesical fistula
(D) Artheriovenous fistulae of the intestine
(E) Sclerosing cholangitis

9. A patients CT scan reveals diverticulitis confined to the sigmoid colon. There is no associated pericolic abscess. What is best course of treatment?

(A) Bowel rest, nasogastric suction, IV fluids, and broad spectrum antibiotics
(B) Urgent surgical resection
(C) Steroids
(D) Diverting colostomy
(E) Ileostomy

10. An elderly nursing home patient is brought to the hospital with recent onset of colicky abdominal pain, distension and obstipation on examination, the abdomen is markedly distended and tympanitic. There is no marked tenderness. Plain abdominal x-ray shows a markedly distended loop located mainly in the right upper quadrant. The likely diagnosis is:

(A) Small-bowel obstruction
(B) Large-bowel obstruction
(C) Gallstone ileus
(D) Mesenteric vascular occlusion
(E) Sigmoid volvulus

11. The standard initial therapy for acute sigmoid volvulus is:

(A) Laparotomy to reduce the volvulus and replace the sigmoid colon to its normal position
(B) IV neostigmine
(C) Colonoscopy

(D) Ileostomy

(E) Rigid sigmoidoscopy

12. Protoscopy reveals nonbleeding grade I hem-orrhoids and maroon stool and clots coming from the proximal colon. Which of the following is TRUE in the management of lower gastrointestinal (GI) bleeding?

(A) Barium enema is a good tool in the early evaluation of massive GI bleeding.

(B) Technetium sulfur colloid has excellent sensitivity in localizing lower GI bleeding.

(C) Technetium sulfur colloid scan is useful because it may be repeated 24 hours later with single injection.

(D) Colonoscopy should be avoided in the evaluation of acute lower GI bleeding.

(E) Sensitivity specificity and accuracy rates vary widely and the exact role of red blood cell (RBC) scanning is controversial.

13. The patient responds to resuscitation with nor-malization of vital signs but continues to bleed. He is taken to the angiography suite for further evaluation. Which of the following is TRUE?

(A) The inferior mesenteric artery should be injected first because most diverticula are in the sigmoid colon.

(B) Vasopressin be selectively infused into a bleeding mesentric vessel with virtually no risk to the patient.

(C) Embolization with gel foam or autolo-gous clots may be used to stop bleeding.

(D) Since angiography is both diagnostic and therapeutic surgery will not be necessary.

(E) A bleeding rate of 0.1 mL/min is necessary for a positive scan.

14. A 60-year-old man undergoes sigmoid colec-tomy for cancer of the midsigmoid. Path spec-imen reveals the following involvement. What is this patient's stage?

(A) T1 No Mo—stage I

(B) T2 N1 Mo—stage II

(C) T3 No Mo—stage III

(D) T1 N1 Mo—stage III

(E) T2 N1 Mo—stage III

15. The same patient is otherwise healthy. Which of the following is TRUE?

(A) She does not need chemotherapy because prognosis is largely related to depth of tumor penetration and she has an early tumor.

(B) Postoperative chemotherapy should be offered even though there is no proven benefit in stage III colon cancer.

(C) Oral chemotherapy (capecitabine) is as effective as IV chemotherapy.

(D) Patient should be offered IV 5 fluorouracil(5 FU) chemotherapy.

(E) Patient should be offered 5 fluorouracil (5 FU) and radiation therapy.

16. A male neonate develops small-bowel obstruc-tion due to malrotation of the midgut segment. An x-ray of the abdomen confirms the pres-ence of small-bowel obstruction (Fig. 6–1). He undergoes an emergency laparotomy, untwist-ing of the malrotated intestines, and partial small-bowel resection for intestinal infarction. Which of the following statements is true of the small intestine (jejunum and ileum)?

(A) It is derived entirely from the midgut.

(B) In the fetus, it enters the physiologic umbilical hernia in the the fifth month.

(C) It remains in the physiologic hernia for 4 months.

(D) It is attached to the urachus.

(E) It drains into the lymph nodes around the iliac arteries.

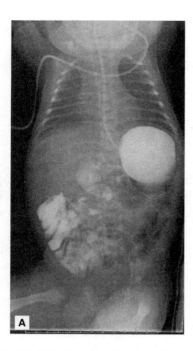

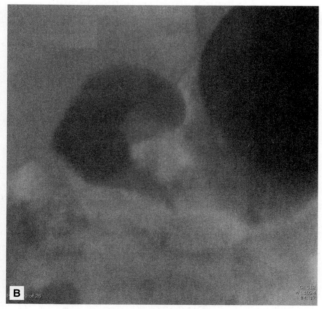

Figure 6–1.
A.Upper GI shows dilation of the bowel secondary to volvulus.
B.Distension of duodenum with beaking of the second portion of the duodenum due to volvulus.

17. A 64-year-old man with mitral stenosis develops mesenteric infarction due to an embolus. At operation and on subsequent pathologic examination, what is noted regarding the small intestine (jejunum and ileum)?

(A) It commences at the right of the midline.
(B) It contains crypts but not villi on histologic examination.
(C) It has a mesentery (parietal) attachment extending 61 cm along the posterior abdominal wall.
(D) It measures approximately 6 m in length.
(E) It is supplied by the inferior mesenteric vessels.

Questions 18 and 19

A 43-year-old woman undergoes investigation for colitis. In her history, it is noted that 20 years earlier she underwent a surgical procedure on the large intestine.

18. The diagnosis is more likely to be Crohn's disease rather than ulcerative colitis because the previous operation was which of the following?

(A) Performed in a young patient
(B) Confined to the colon
(C) Followed by improvement after bypass of the diseased segment
(D) Followed by improvement because steroids were prescribed
(E) Grohn's disease is more premaligent than ulcerative cohitis

19. Is the diagnosis more likely to be ulcerative colitis rather than Crohn's disease because at the previous operation?

(A) All layers of the bowel wall were involved
(B) There was evidence of fistula formation
(C) The serosa appeared normal on inspection, but the colon mucosa was extensively involved
(D) Skip lesions were noted
(E) The preoperative GI series showed a narrowing string like stricture in the ileum (string sign)

Questions 20 and 21

A 64-year-old woman with a known history of cardiac disease is admitted to the hospital with severe abdominal pain. Her blood pressure is 150/95 mm Hg, and her pulse rate is 84 beats per minute (bpm). There are minimal signs of intravascular depletion.

20. The possibility of small-bowel infarction is characterized by which of the following?

    (A) The stack-of-coins sign
    (B) Marked distention of loops of bowel
    (C) Air in the biliary tree
    (D) Air in the bowel wall (intramural)
    (E) Air below the left diaphragm

21. At operation, 2.5 m of distal ileum is found to be gangrenous. There is, however, pulsation in the superior mesenteric artery and its main branches. Small-bowel gangrene in this patient is caused by which of the following?

    (A) Arterial thrombosis
    (B) Embolus
    (C) Nonocclusive ischemic disease
    (D) Von Willebrand's disease
    (E) Idiopathic thrombocytopenic purpura

22. A 48-year-old man undergoes a supine abdominal x-ray for epigastric discomfort. He has been on IV hyperalimentation since an operative procedure performed 5 days previously. Gas is consistently absent from the alimentary tract because he has previously undergone which of the following?

    (A) Appendectomy
    (B) Gastrostomy
    (C) Ligation of the esophagus and cervical esophagostomy
    (D) Lysis of adhesions
    (E) Colostomy for large-bowel obstruction

Questions 23 and 24

A 64-year-old woman is admitted to the hospital with abdominal pain, vomiting, and abdominal distention. Bowel sounds are increased on auscultation, and a plain film shows marked distention of loops of bowel with nonspecific pattern.

23. The most likely diagnosis is which of the following?

    (A) Sigmoid volvulus
    (B) Cecal volvulus
    (C) Jejunal obstruction
    (D) Ileal obstruction
    (E) Pyloric obstruction

24. Management, following rehydration and electrolyte imbalance correction, should initially involve which of the following?

    (A) Nasogastric suction, rehydration, and observation
    (B) Anticholinergic drugs
    (C) Laxatives
    (D) Emergency surgery and bowel resection
    (E) Appendectomy

25. A 42-year-old woman is admitted to the emergency department with severe colicky pain, vomiting, and abdominal distention. She has not passed stools or flatus for 48 hours. X-rays of the abdomen confirm the presence of small-bowel obstruction. What is the most likely cause of small-bowel obstruction in this patient?

    (A) Adenocarcinoma
    (B) Adhesions
    (C) Crohn's disease
    (D) Ulcerative colitis
    (E) Gallstone ileus

26. An 80-year-old woman with a known history of femoral hernia is admitted to the hospital because of strangulation of the hernia. There is a tender swelling in the right femoral region immediately below and lateral to the pubic tubercle. She has had multiple bowel movements without relief of symptoms. What is the most likely diagnosis?

    (A) Lymphadenitis
    (B) Diverticulitis
    (C) Volvulus
    (D) Richter's hernia
    (E) Gastroenteritis

27. A 63-year-old man from Miami presents to the emergency department with abdominal pain due to intestinal obstruction. A diagnosis of small-bowel volvulus is established. Primary small-bowel volvulus is differentiated from secondary small-bowel volvulus. In the latter there is a secondary cause, such as adhesions, that accounts for the volvulus. Which is true of primary small-bowel volvulus?

    (A) It does not lead to gangrene of bowel.
    (B) It is common in the United States.
    (C) It occurs nearly exclusively in women.
    (D) It usually involves the jejunum.
    (E) It may require a limited resection of small intestine.

Questions 28 and 29

A 44-year-old man is stabbed in the abdomen. The injury penetrates the root of the small-bowel mesentery. At laparotomy, resection of 2 cm of ileum is removed.

28. The complication that is more likely to occur after resection of the ileum rather than of an equivalent length of jejunum is the failure to absorb which of the following?

    (A) Iron
    (B) Zinc
    (C) Bile salts
    (D) Medium-chain triglycerides
    (E) Amylase

29. Why is distal resection, as compared to proximal resection, poorly tolerated?

    (A) Transit time in the ileum is slower than that in the jejunum.
    (B) Transit time in the jejunum is slower than that in the ileum.
    (C) The greater bulk of food is absorbed in the ileum.
    (D) Water absorption is mainly in the ileum.
    (E) All minerals are absorbed preferentially in the ileum.

30. A 66-year-old woman is admitted for hyperalimentation due to malnutrition consequent to massive small-bowel resection. What is the most likely condition that leads to the need to perform a massive resection?

    (A) Autoimmune disease
    (B) Mesenteric ischemia
    (C) Mesenteric adenitis
    (D) Cancer
    (E) Pseudomyxoma peritonei

31. A 68-year-old female is known to have had surgery several years previously for a bowel lesion. Her surgeon had told her that she suffers from the blind loop syndrome. In which condition can one anticipate the blind loop syndrome to occur?

    (A) Intestinal bypass
    (B) Vesicocolic fistula
    (C) Duodenal ulcer disease
    (D) Multiple polyposis of the colon
    (E) Anteriovenous fistula of the colon

32. A 33-year-old woman is noted to have a Meckel's diverticulum when she undergoes an emergency appendectomy. The diverticulum is approximately 60 cm from the ileocecal valve and measures 2–3 cm in length. What is the most common complication of Meckel's diverticulum among adults?

    (A) Bleeding
    (B) Perforation
    (C) Intestinal obstruction
    (D) Ulceration
    (E) Carcinoma

33. A 30-year-old male is diagnosed with Peutz-Jeghers syndrome. What findings is consistent with the diagnosis?

(A) Adenomas
(B) Hamartomas
(C) Adenomatous polyps
(D) Villoglandular polyps
(E) Villotubular polyps

34. A 38-year-old male is admitted to hospital with symptoms suggestive of small-bowel obstruction. Examination reveals multiple loops of distended bowel with increased bowel sounds. Treatment with IV fluids and nasogastric suction fails to correct symptoms. Laparotomy is performed. Following surgery, copious volumes of fluid occur through the incision. A diagnosis of intestinal fistula is established.What is TRUE of intestinal fistulas?

(A) They may occur as a complication after an operation to divide adhesions.
(B) They are rare after irradiation.
(C) As a result of Crohn's disease, they almost always close spontaneously.
(D) They should not be treated with a central venous line for fear of sepsis.
(E) They most commonly arise from the distal colon.

35. A 69-year-old female is found to have an enterocutaneous fistula that arises from the proximal small intestine. Which of the following statements is TRUE concerning this fistula?

(A) If internal, it occurs mainly from iatrogenic causes.
(B) It occurs more commonly after an anastomosis than spontaneously.
(C) If internal, it always causes serious complications.
(D) If external, it closes spontaneously in 10% of cases.
(E) If external, it requires immediate closure in most cases.

Questions 36 and 37

36. A 68-year-old retired female plastic surgeon underwent laparotomy through a midline abdominal incision. Intestinal infarction was found and a distal 60% small-bowel resection was performed with ileocecal anastomosis. She was placed on hyperalimentation. Seven days after the operation, she underwent a second operation through the same incision. Wound healing is further impaired by which of the following?

(A) Incision through the same abdominal wall scar
(B) Vitamin A administration
(C) Zinc deficiency
(D) Increased local oxygen tension
(E) Incision through new area of abdominal wall

37. At the second operation an advanced carcinoma of the colon is detected. What factors would cause wound healing to be further impaired?

(A) Doxorubicin is given.
(B) Denervation of bowel or skin incision occur.
(C) Mechanical lavage and oral antibiotics are given before surgery.
(D) Steroids are not given.
(E) Leavage with polyethylene glycol solution.

38. A 79-year-old man has had abdominal pain for 4 days. An operation is performed, and a gangrenous appendix is removed. The stump is inverted. Why does acute appendicitis in elderly patients and in children have a worse prognosis?

(A) The appendix is retrocecal.
(B) The appendix is in the preileal position.
(C) The appendix is in the pelvic position.
(D) The omentum and peritoneal cavity appear to be less efficient in localizing the disease in these age groups.
(E) The appendix is longer in these age groups.

Questions 39 through 41

39. A 12-year-old boy complains of pain in the lower abdomen (mainly on the right side). Symptoms commenced 12 hours before admission. He had noted anorexia during this period. Examination revealed tenderness in the right iliac fossa, which was maximal 1 cm below Mc Burney's point. In appendicitis, where does the pain frequently commence?

    (A) In the right iliac fossa and remains there
    (B) In the back and moves to the right iliac fossa
    (C) In the rectal region and moves to the right iliac fossa
    (D) In the umbilical region and then moves to the right iliac fossa
    (E) In the right flank

40. On examination, patients presenting with appendicitis typically show maximal tenderness over which of the following?

    (A) Inguinal region
    (B) Immediately above the umbilicus
    (C) At a point between the outer one-third and inner two-thirds of a line between the umbilicus and the anterior superior iliac spine
    (D) At a point between the outer two-thirds and inner one-third of a line between the umbilicus and the anterior superior iliac spine
    (E) At the midpoint of a line between the umbilicus and the anterior superior iliac spine

41. What is the mortality rate from acute appendicitis?

    (A) In the general population, it is 4/10,000
    (B) After rupture, appendicitis is 4–5%
    (C) For nonruptured appendicitis, it is 2%
    (D) It is 80% if an abscess has formed
    (E) It has increased in the past 40 years

42. A 29-year-old woman presents to her physician's office with pain in the right iliac fossa. Examination reveals tenderness in this region. Her last menstrual cycle was 2 weeks previously and findings on gynecologic examination and leukocyte count are normal. A provisional diagnosis of acute appendicitis is made. She should be informed that operations to treat this condition reveal acute appendicitis in what percentage of cases?

    (A) A small percentage of cases
    (B) 50–89% of cases
    (C) 90–99% of cases
    (D) More than 99% of cases
    (E) No reliable statistics are available

43. A 28-year-old man is admitted to the emergency department complaining of pain in the umbilical region that moves to the right iliac fossa. Which is a corroborative sign of acute appendicitis?

    (A) Referred pain in the right side with pressure on the left (Rovsing)sign
    (B) Increase of pain with testiculalr elevation
    (C) Relief of pain in lower abdomen with extension of thigh
    (D) Relief of pain in lower abdomen with internal rotation of right thigh
    (E) Hyperanesthesia in the right lower abdomen

44. A 28-old-male from Kosovo, who lives alone, presents with diarrhea. On examination he manifests clear wasting and malnutrition. His hematocrit (HCT) is 28%, serum albumin reduced to 2.8 g%, and the blood analysis shows a macrocytic anemia. The emergency department physician is unable to secure an accurate history of the nature of multiple previous operations he had undergone before his arrival in the United States several months previously. What is the likely diagnosis that explains these features?

    (A) Blind loop syndrome
    (B) Diverticulitis of the sigmoid colon
    (C) Carcinoma of the left colon
    (D) Gastric ulcer
    (E) Carcinoid syndrome

Questions 45 and 46

A 74-year-old patient has a biopsy of the prostate that shows malignancy. He is considering radical prostatectomy or radiation therapy.

45. He is concerned about enterocolitis, which is likely to occur when?

 (A) After local treatment with 15 Gy
 (B) After local treatment with 35 Gy
 (C) After local treatment with 55 Gy
 (D) Less frequently after previous surgery
 (E) Less frequently in the presence of adhesions

46. What complication should be anticipated in this patient?

 (A) Diverticulitis
 (B) Hemorrhoids
 (C) Complete occlusion of superior mesenteric artery
 (D) Complete occlusion of inferior mesenteric artery
 (E) Rectal bleeding

47. A 49-year-old computer technician receives irradiation to the pelvis for cervical cancer. Three months after irradiation, severe rectal proctitis may be shown by the presence of which of the following?

 (A) Ulcers
 (B) Strictures at anal verge
 (C) Mucosa prolapse
 (D) Multiple telangiectasis and polypoid tumor
 (E) Free air under the diaphragm

Questions 48 and 49

A 63-year-old man is admitted to the hospital for abdominal pain and diarrhea of 6-day duration. X-ray of the abdomen shows "thumbprinting" and gaseous distention suggestive of ischemic colitis.

48. What is true of colonic ischemia?

 (A) It occurs in a younger age group (40–60 years of age).
 (B) In most cases, it occurs in patients with cardiac failure.
 (C) It usually causes severe abdominal pain.
 (D) It may have a predisposing associated colonic lesion in 20% of patients.
 (E) It results in the patient's appearing seriously ill.

49. To confirm the diagnosis of ischemic colitis, what test should be requested?

 (A) Selective angiogram of inferior mesenteric artery
 (B) Angiogram of superior and inferior mesenteric arteries
 (C) CT scan of the abdomen
 (D) Barium enema after 2 weeks
 (E) Barium enema as soon as possible

50. A 54-year-old man with diarrhea is found to have ulcerative colitis. Colectomy should be advised in patients with ulcerative colitis who have symptoms that persist for more than which of the following?

 (A) 1 month
 (B) 6 months
 (C) 1–5 years
 (D) 10–20 years
 (E) More than 25 years

51. A 48-year-old woman develops colon cancer. She is known to have a long history of ulcerative colitis. In ulcerative colitis, which of the following is a characteristic of colon cancer?

 (A) Occurs more frequently than in the rest of the population.
 (B) Is more likely to occur when the ulcerative disease is confined to the left colon.
 (C) Occurs equally in the right and left side.
 (D) Has a synchronous carcinoma in 4–5% of cases.
 (E) Has an excellent prognosis because of physician awareness.

52. A 64-year-old train conductor is diagnosed as having carcinoma confined to the descending colon. Before operation, what should be told?

(A) He will most likely require a colostomy.
(B) He should have the cancer excised by cautery.
(C) He should undergo left hemicolectomy.
(D) Radiotherapy is the treatment of choice.
(E) 40% of colorectal cancer involves the colon.

53. A 72-year-old woman is scheduled to undergo right hemicolectomy for cancer of the cecum. In this condition, she can anticipate subsequent recurrence

(A) Of 20–30% if confined to the mucosa
(B) Close to 100% if there is lymph node involvement
(C) Which will not result in small-bowel obstruction
(D) Which will not result in hydronephrosis
(E) Which with microscopic lymph node metastasis would have a lower rate than that with macroscopic spread

54. A pathology specimen indicates that synchronous lesions are present. Which of the following statements are true regarding colon cancer with synchronous lesions?

(A) Cancer occurs in 20% of patients.
(B) Benign lesions occur in 20–30%.
(C) Malignant lesions are usually adjacent to the primary cancer.
(D) Benign lesions are usually adjacent to the primary cancer.
(E) Lesions occur much less frequently than metachronous lesions.

Questions 55 and 56

A 68-year-old dentist undergoes anterior resection (sigmoid resection) for cancer at the rectosigmoid junction. The tests performed before her surgery were colonscopy and biopsy. There were no other lesions detected with sigmoidoscopy or in the pathology specimen.

55. Following operation, she requires which of the following within 2–3 months?

(A) Repeat rectal examination and sigmoidoscopy
(B) Colonoscopy
(C) CT scan of the abdomen
(D) Angiography
(E) Bone scan

56. The patient requests information from her surgeon as to her subsequent prognosis. She is informed that the prognosis for colon and rectal cancer is favorably affected by which of the following?

(A) Minimal serosal extension
(B) Minimal lymph node involvement
(C) Confinement to the mucosa
(D) Right-sided obstructing lesions
(E) Elevated carcinoembryonic antigen (CEA) levels

57. An 83-year-old man is diagnosed on colonoscopy to have cancer of the colon. He refuses surgical intervention and after a 3-month follow-up period is admitted to the emergency department with large-bowel obstruction. Carcinoma of the colon is most likely to obstruct if found in the

(A) Cecum
(B) Ascending colon
(C) Descending colon
(D) Rectum
(E) Transverse colon

58. A 43-year-old man is seen in his physician's office for severe pain in the perineum. Examination reveals exquisite tenderness in the area to the right side of the anal verge due to a perianal abscess. Rectal examination is refused. What should be the next step in management?

(A) Drainage of the abscess in the office under local anesthesia.
(B) Excision of the vertical fold of Morgagni.
(C) Drainage under general anesthesia and immediate colonoscopy.
(D) CT scan of the abdomen.
(E) Insertion of a rectal tube.

59. A 64-year-old man undergoes CEA surveillance for cancer, because his brother and father both had colon cancer. What information should he be provided?

(A) CEA is highly sensitive for diagnosis.
(B) If CEA is elevated preoperatively, it implies unresectable disease.
(C) Increases in CEA after resection may indicate tumor recurrence.
(D) CEA is highly specific for the presence of colon cancer.
(E) CEA is present in normal adult colonic mucosa.

60. A 70-year-old man presents with pallor and breathlessness on exertion. He does not complain of abdominal pain. He has microcytic, hypochromic anemia. What is the most probable cause?

(A) Diverticulosis of the colon
(B) Peptic ulcer disease
(C) Crohn's disease
(D) Ulcerative colitis
(E) Carcinoma of the right colon

61. A 25-year-old man has recurrent, indolent fistula in ano. He also complains of weight loss, recurrent attacks of diarrhea with blood mixed in the stool, and tenesmus. Proctoscopy revealed a healthy, normal-appearing rectum. What is the most likely diagnosis?

(A) Crohn's colitis
(B) Ulcerative colitis
(C) Amoebic colitis
(D) Ischemic colitis
(E) Colitis associated with acquired immunodeficiency syndrome (AIDS)

62. A 65-year-old man presents with chronic constipation and abdominal distention of 5-day duration. He complains of lack of appetite and general malaise. Findings on physical examination are positive for a large distended abdomen with hyperactive bowel sounds. Rectal examination shows minimal stool that is guaiac-positive. Sigmoidoscopy does not reveal any further findings. Abdominal x-rays show a large 10-cm cecum and dilated, fluid-filled transverse and descending colon with very little gas in the rectum. What is the most probable cause of this condition?

(A) Volvulus of the sigmoid colon
(B) Pseudo-obstruction of the colon
(C) Ischemic colitis
(D) Carcinoma of the colon
(E) Diverticulitis of the colon

63. A 27-year-old homosexual male presents with a foreign body in the rectum. During the extraction of the foreign body, a large tear in the sigmoid colon with extensive devitalization and contamination is observed. What is the preferred method of treatment?

(A) Observation
(B) Proctoscopic repair
(C) Laparotomy and closure of sigmoid colon tear
(D) Laparotomy, closure of sigmoid, and proximal colostomy or exteriorization of perforation as a colostomy
(E) Laparotomy, resection of sigmoid colon, and colostomy

64. A 65-year-old woman with a history of chronic constipation is transferred from a nursing home because of abdominal pain and marked abdominal distention. On examination, her abdomen is found to be distended and tender in the LLQ. What is the most likely diagnosis?

(A) Appendicitis
(B) Carcinoma of the colon
(C) Volvulus of the sigmoid colon
(D) Volvulus of the cecum
(E) Small-bowel obstruction

65. A 40-year-old man with a long history of bloody diarrhea presents with increased abdominal pain, vomiting, and fever. On examination, he is found to be dehydrated and shows tachycardia and hypotension. The abdomen is markedly tender with guarding and rigidity. What is the most likely cause?

    (A) Toxic megacolon in ulcerative colitis
    (B) Small-bowel perforation from regional enteritis
    (C) Perforated carcinoma of the sigmoid colon
    (D) Volvulus of the sigmoid colon
    (E) Acute perforated diverticulitis

66. Three days after undergoing an operation for an abdominal aortic aneurysm, a patient has moderate fever, abdominal pain, and rectal bleeding. What is the most helpful investigation?

    (A) Angiography
    (B) Upper GI endoscopy
    (C) Abdominal ultrasound
    (D) Sigmoidoscopy
    (E) Abdominal CT scan

67. A 55-year-old woman presents with pain in the LLQ of the abdomen and fever of 102°F. On examination, she is found to be dehydrated and has tenderness in the LLQ. A CT scan shows a mass in the LLQ involving the sigmoid colon. There is a minimal amount of free fluid and no free air. What should the initial treatment of this patient include?

    (A) IV fluids, penicillin, and steroids
    (B) IV fluids, cefoxitin, and nasogastric drainage
    (C) IV fluids, blood transfusion, and laparotomy
    (D) immediate laparotomy
    (E) bowel preparation followed by laparotomy

Questions 68 and 69

A 72-year-old woman presents with bright red rectal bleeding, not associated with abdominal pain, of 2-day duration. She had previous similar episodes but was never hospitalized. Examination reveals a pale but alert individual with no significant abdominal findings. Findings on rectal examination are positive for bright red rectal bleeding. Her vital signs are stable and her hemoglobin is 9.5 g.

68. What is the most probable cause of her bleeding?

    (A) Diverticulitis of the colon
    (B) Carcinoma of the sigmoid colon
    (C) Meckel's diverticulitis
    (D) Adenomatous polyp of the colon
    (E) Diverticulosis of the colon

69. The patient continues to bleed per rectum and becomes hypotensive to a systolic pressure of 60 mm Hg despite blood transfusion. What is the optimal management plan?

    (A) Emergency colonoscopy and cauterization of bleeding vessels
    (B) Mesenteric angiography and embolization of the bleeder
    (C) Bleeding scan to localize the bleeder
    (D) Laparotomy and right colon resection
    (E) Blood transfusion laparotomy and subtotal colectomy with or without ileoproctostomy

70. A 60-year-old man complains of recurrent attacks of painless rectal bleeding. Colonoscopy reveals normal mucosa between the cecum and the anal verge. What is the most helpful test to determine the cause of bleeding?

    (A) Angiography to look for angiodysplasia
    (B) Technetium scan for Meckel's diverticulum
    (C) Upper GI endoscopy for peptic ulcer
    (D) Small-bowel series for tumor
    (E) Ultrasound for abdominal aortic aneurysm

71. The small intestine is characterized by basal crypts and superficial villi (Fig. 6–2). Where does cell division take place?

    (A) Submucosa
    (B) Crypts
    (C) Villi

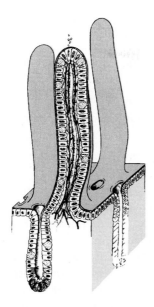

Figure 6–2.
Schematic representation of villi and crypts of Lieberkühn. *(Reproduced, with permission, from Doherty GM: Current Surgical Diagnosis and Treatment, 12th ed. 657. McGraw-Hill, 2006.)*

(D) Small-bowel lumen

(E) Lamina propria

72. A 64-year-old man has a benign lesion of the colon. He is informed that the lesion does not predispose to colon cancer. What is the lesion he has?

(A) Ulcerative colitis

(B) Villous adenoma

(C) Hyperplastic polyp

(D) Adenoma in familial polyposis

(E) Colon mucosa in a patient with colon carcinoma

73. A 25-year-old man complains of rectal bleeding, weight loss, and abdominal pain. He gives a history of similar complaints in his siblings as well as his mother. Findings on physical examination are unremarkable except for guaiac-positive stool. What is the most likely diagnosis?

(A) Peutz–Jegher syndrome

(B) Familial polyposis of the colon

(C) Ulcerative colitis

(D) Carcinoma of the stomach

(E) Crohn's colitis

74. A 55-year-old man has had previous hemicolectomy for a carcinoma of the right colon. At this time, 3 years after the primary resection, a CT scan shows a solitary lesion in the right lobe of the liver. What is the next step in management?

(A) Laser cauterization

(B) Radiotherapy

(C) Hepatic artery catheterization and local chemotherapy

(D) Symptomatic treatment with analgesics, because the colon disease is now stage IV

(E) Exploratory laparotomy and resection of the tumor

75. Following an appendectomy, a 28-year-old man is placed on ceftizoxime sodium (Cefizox). This antibiotic is unlikely to be effective against which of the following?

(A) *Pseudomonas*

(B) *Staphylococcus aureus*

(C) *Neisseria gonorrhoeae*

(D) *Bacteroides fragilis*

(E) *Haemophilus influenza*

76. A 68-year-old man presents with crampy abdominal pain and distention with vomiting. Findings on physical examination are positive for healed abdominal scars. X-rays reveal multiple gas fluid levels. The WBC count is 12,000. What is the most likely diagnosis?

(A) Small-bowel intestinal obstruction due to adhesions

(B) Hernia

(C) Appendicitis

(D) Inflammatory bowel disease

(E) Gallstones and ascites

77. A 55-year-old woman presents with vague RLQ abdominal pain. A palpable mass is noted on abdominal examination. The mass is painless, well defined, mobile, and nonpulsatile. What is the most likely diagnosis?

    (A) A mesenteric cyst
    (B) Appendix mass
    (C) Perforated tubo-ovarian abscess
    (D) Cholecystitis
    (E) Meckel's diverticulum

78. A 74-year-old woman complains of vomiting and intermittent colicky abdominal pain. X-rays reveal fluid levels and air in the biliary tree. What is the likely cause?

    (A) Abdominal adhesions
    (B) Gallstone ileus
    (C) Carcinoma of the right colon
    (D) Abdominal lymphosarcoma
    (E) Previous choledochoduodenostomy

Questions 79 and 80

A 40-year-old woman experiences flushing, diarrhea, and wheezing. On physical examination, she is found to have tricuspid valve insufficiency.

79. What is the most likely diagnosis?

    (A) Appendiceal carcinoid
    (B) Ileal carcinoid with liver metastasis
    (C) Gastric lymphoma
    (D) Small-bowel adenocarcinoma
    (E) Bronchial carcinoid

80. The most useful diagnostic finding is which of the following?

    (A) Elevated 5-hydroxyindoleacetic acid (5-HIAA) levels
    (B) Elevated blood sugar levels
    (C) Elevated serum gastrin levels
    (D) Elevated amylase levels
    (E) Elevated norepinephrine levels

81. A 56-year-old man has suffered from intermittent claudication for 5 years. He has recently developed cramping abdominal pain that is made worse by eating. He has a history of a 15-lb weight loss. What is the most likely diagnosis?

    (A) Chronic intestinal ischemia (intestinal angina)
    (B) Chronic cholecystitis
    (C) Esophageal diverticulum
    (D) Peptic ulcer
    (E) Abdominal aortic aneurysm

82. A 68-year-old male musician presents to the emergency department with a sudden onset of colicky abdominal pain and massive vomiting of 4-hour duration. Examination shows an elevated WBC of 13,200 with a HCT of 45%. Electrolytes and blood urea nitrogen (BUN) are normal. An erect film of the abdomen reveals dilatation of the stomach with distended loops of bowel. What is his clinical diagnosis?

    (A) Complete proximal intestinal obstruction
    (B) Incomplete proximal intestinal obstruction
    (C) Complete ileal obstruction
    (D) Incomplete ileal obstruction
    (E) Small-bowel perforation

83. What is true with reference to small-bowel physiology migrating motor complexes (MMC)?

    (A) They are increased after feeding.
    (B) They occur once every 10 minutes.
    (C) They continue throughout laparotomy.
    (D) They inhibit nutrient absorption.
    (E) They may explain diarrhea that occurs following vagotomy.

84. A 38-year-old man with a history of fever associated with abdominal pain of 3-week duration presents now with a sudden onset of abdominal pain and copious vomiting. Plain abdominal x-rays reveal air under a diaphragm. A CT scan shows mesenteric lymphadenopathy and splenomegaly is found. Laparotomy is performed and 3 feet of ileum resected. The luminal aspect of the resected bowel shows marked ulceration of Peyer's patches. What is the most likely diagnosis?

(A) Typhoid enteritis

(B) Tuberculosis enteritis

(C) Crohn's disease

(D) Primary peritonitis

(E) Ulcerative colitis

Questions 85 and 86

85. A 48-year-old man is admitted to hospital because of a 3-day history of mild abdominal pain, repeated vomiting, and marked abdominal distension. Immediately after the pain commenced, he had one small-bowel movement but no further passage of stool or flatus. An abdominal flat plate revealed marked distension of loops of bowel confined to the small bowel. A plain abdominal film shows loops of bowel that all extensively show valvulae conniventes. What is the most likely site of obstruction (Fig. 6–3)?

(A) High-small bowel

(B) Mid-small bowel

(C) Rectum

(D) Colon

(E) Duodenum

86. Following insertion of a nasogastric tube and appropriate rehydration and electrolyte correction, there is no change in clinical presentation. What should the next step involve?

(A) Barium reduction with controlled hydrostatic pressure

(B) Laparoscopy

(C) Colostomy

(D) Needle tap to deflate bowel

(E) Exploratory laparotomy

87. Following resection of the left colon, a 67-year-old obese woman develops left-sided leg edema due to deep-vein thrombosis. She is placed on anticoagulants, but after 2 weeks of warfarin (Coumadin), she develops a pulmonary embolus with slight hypoxemia. What should the next step in management involve?

(A) Increasing the dose of anticoagulants

(B) Discontinuing anticoagulants

(C) Use of an inferior vena cava (IVC) filter

(D) CT scan of the leg and abdomen

(E) Femoral vein ligation

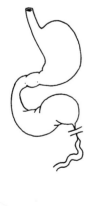 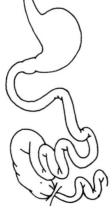 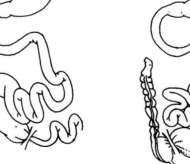 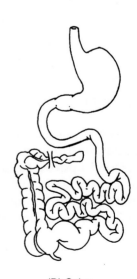

(A) High small bowel   (B) Mid-small bowel   (C) Distal small bowel   (D) Colon

Figure 6–3.
Intestinal obstruction. *(Reproduced, with permission, from Way LW: Current Surgical Diagnosis & Treatment, 10th ed. Appleton & Lange, 1994.)*

Questions 88 and 89

A 44-year-old female immigrant from India, and now resident in the US, has been treated for partial intestinal obstruction due to tuberculosis. There is no evidence of intestinal perforation.

88. What should the next step in treatment involve?

    (A) Laparoscopy
    (B) Laparotomy and bowel resection
    (C) A full course of antituberculous drugs
    (D) Steroids
    (E) Radiation therapy to the abdomen

89. What is the most likely outcome for the patient?

    (A) Full recovery
    (B) Rapid deterioration and possible death
    (C) Pneumonia
    (D) Empyema
    (E) Scrofula

90. A 64-year-old woman presents with a strangulated femoral hernia. At operation, what is the criterion used to determine the viability of a loop of bowel?

    (A) Increased peristalsis
    (B) Absent arterial pulsation
    (C) Venous engorgement
    (D) Intraoperative CT scan
    (E) Serum amylase

DIRECTIONS (Questions 91 through 98): Each set of matching questions in this section consists of a list of lettered options followed by several numbered items. For each numbered item, select the appropriate lettered option. Each lettered option may be selected once, more than once, or not at all.

Questions 91 and 92

    (A) Vitamin A
    (B) Vitamin C
    (C) Vitamin D
    (D) Vitamin E
    (E) Vitamin K

    (F) Vitamin B$_1$
    (G) Chyle
    (H) Sympathetic denervation
    (I) Failure of rectal muscles to contract
    (J) Gluten
    (K) Peptides
    (L) Bile salts
    (M) Meissner and Auerbach plexus deficiency
    (N) Vagus nerve excess
    (O) Inferior mesenteric ischemia

91. Steatorrhea and megaloblastic anemia, occurring in a patient after bowel resection, is caused by a failure to absorb what? SELECT ONE.

92. What does Hirschsprung's disease involve? SELECT ONE.

Questions 93

    (A) Spigelian hernia
    (B) Direct inguinal hernia
    (C) Femoral hernia
    (D) Richter's hernia
    (E) Appendix
    (F) Hydrocele
    (G) Sliding hernia
    (H) Bladder
    (I) Liver
    (J) Seminal vesicle
    (K) An adrenal metastasis
    (L) Ureter
    (M) Prostate
    (N) Pubic bone
    (O) Cowper's (bulbourethral) glands

93. An 84-year-old man has had a reducible hernia in the right groin for 17 years. One day before admission to the hospital, he complains of abdominal pain; because of the swelling, the hernia has become irreducible. At operation, part of the wall of the cecum is noted to form a portion of the hernia sac. What is the hernia?

Questions 94 through 95

    (A) Supralevator space
    (B) Perianal space

(C) Levator ani muscle

(D) Intermuscular space

(E) External sphincter

(F) Ischioanal space

(G) Submucous space above the levator ani muscle

(H) Marginal mucocutaneous space

94. A 25-year-old patient with a 2-cm painful abscess in perianal region for 1 day. The patient does not have fever or leukocytosis. Which space is this lesion in? SELECT ONE.

95. A 30-year-old patient presents with a 5-day history of pain to right buttock. A 7-cm firm area is noted on the right buttock. Patient also describes purulence from rectum and has a temprature 101°F. In which space is this lesion? SELECT ONE.

96. A 28-year-old woman recently treated as an out-patient for pelvic inflammatory disease presents with fever, leukocytosis, and deep rectal pain. In which space is this lesion? SELECT ONE.

Questions 97 and 98

(A) Pilonidal sinus

(B) Posterior perianal sinus

(C) Single anterior perianal sinus

(D) Multiple anterior perianal sinus

(E) Periurethral abscess

(F) Bartholin gland abscess

(G) Prostatic abscess

(H) Rectovaginal fistula

97. Which opens into the anal mucosa in the midline? SELECT ONE.

98. What has hair inside? SELECT ONE.

Answers and Explanations

1. **(C)** In uncomplicated appendicitis laparoscopic appendectomy can be performed with similar outcomes to an open technique. Studies reveal hospital stay and return to full feeding is similar. Wound complication and overall complication rates are the same. Procedure cost are higher owing to the use of additional equipment.

2. **(D)** Laparoscopic appendectomy does present the surgeon with several advantages. Although in hospital recovery is similar to the open technique, posthospital recovery can be shorter in uncomplicated appendicitis. In cases where the diagnosis of appendicitis is less certain the laparoscopic approach confers several advantages. In addition to accurately diagnosing appendicitis, the laparoscopic approach allows the surgeon the ability to inspect the entire abdominal cavity when a normal appendix is found. The laparoscopic approach can also be used to treat other intra-abdominal surgical pathologies and, therefore, reduces the need for extending or converting to a conventional laparotomy incision. Laparoscopic technique does result in a longer operative time for appendectomy with higher operative cost. Cosmesis is generally better with the laparoscopic technique owing to smaller wound size.

3. **(B)** The normal appendix should be removed to avoid future diagnostic confusion and appendicitis. The entire abdomen should be explored for other potential causes of the clinical presentation. If found, other pathologies, which are the cause of the presentation, may be treated surgically, either laparoscopically or open if indicated.

4. **(B)** Ulcerative colitis is a disease of unknown etiology, which involves the colon and rectum and spares the remainder of the GI tract. It's clinical course is variable with inflammatory changes and clinical symptoms ranging from mild to severe. The process is confined to the mucosa and the submucosa and does not extend through the full thickness of the bowel wall. Inflammatory changes are confluent with no skip areas. The risk of dysplasia and colorectal cancer is higher in ulcerative colitis than in the general population.

5. **(C)** Toxic megacolon is a fulminant exacerbation of ulcerative colitis, causing massive dilatation of the colon with perforation, fecal peritonitis, and death. Emergency total colectomy is indicated.

6. **(D)** Risk of dysplasia and colorectal cancer is higher in ulcerative colitis than in the general poulation. The severity, duration, and anatomic extent of the inflammation are risk factors for the development of dysplasia and cancer. These cancers do not seem to follow the adenoma carcinoma sequence and can arise in flat mucosa making them difficult to detect even with regular colonoscopies. After 8–10 years of colitis survellance colonoscopy should be performed with multiple random biopsies. The finding of dysplasia is an indiction for immediate total protocolectomy. Centers have reported up to 42% of colons removed for dysplasia also had colon cancer.

7. **(D)** The man likely has diverticulitis. The differential includes irritable bowel, appendicitis, inflammatory bowel disease, pyelonephritis,

ischemic colitis, and perforated carcinoma. Diverticulitis is an infectious complication of diverticulosis resulting from perforation of the colonic diverticulum. The resulting inflammation may be confined to the pericolonic tissue (incomplicated diverticulitis) or result in abscess, free perforation, fistulization, or obstruction (complicated diverticulitis). The clinical spectrum is correspondingly broad ranging from mild symptoms to peritonitis and sepsis. Patients with signs and symptoms of sepsis should be hospitalized and undergo diagnostic study. A CT scan is the best study to evaluate the extent of the inflammatory process as well as to exclude other pathology. Plain x-ray would not reveal specific pathology. Both barium enema and colonoscopy in the acute setting are risky and may cause free perforation and contamination of the peritoneal cavity there by converting a localized process to generalized peritonitis. Barium has the additional risk of a chemical peritonitis caused by the barium itself. Diagnostic laparoscopy is invasive and may risk spreading a localized process.

8. **(C)** Diverticulitis results from acute inflammation of a colonic diverticula. The process may extend into adjacent organs (e.g., the urinary bladder and a fistula between the colon and bladder colovesical fistula may ensue). This leads to passage of colonic gas and fecal material into the bladder and urine resulting in pneumaturitis and fecaluria. Sigmoid resection and repair of the bladder fistula is indicated.

9. **(A)** Uncomplicated diverticulitis is treated with broad spectrum antibiotics and bowel rest. Surgery is not indicated—either resection or diversion of the fecal stream by colotomy or ilestomy. Anti-inflamatory agents are not indicated in the therapy of diverticulitis. The risk of a second episode is less than 30%. After a second episode, the risk is greater than 50% and resection may be advised at this stage.

10. **(E)** This patient has sigmoid volvulus. Plain abdominal x-ray shows a massively distended loop in the right upper quadrant, because the sigmoid colon, as it progressively distends, as a result of the twist of its mesentery, has no space,

in the LLQ to occupy and flips over to the largest available area—namely the right upper quadrant. Given the clinical presentation and findings, the plain abdominal x-ray is diagnostic.

11. **(E)** Rigid sigmoidoscopy is effective in reduction and decompression of the volvulus, often resulting in a copious rush of gas and stool as decompression results. It also allows for evaluation of bowel viability. If the point of rotation is beyond the 25-cm rigid sigmoidoscopy, flexible endoscopy may be attempted by an experienced endoscopist using minimal inflation of air. A rectal tube should be placed to allow for bowel decompression. Laparotomy may occasionally be necessary in cases of perforation or compromised viability.

12. **(B)** Technetium sulfur colloid scans have the advantage of immediate availability but the patient must be bleeding when the isotope is injected as the isotope is quickly cleared by the reticuloendothelial system of the liver and spleen.

13. **(B)** Vasopressin can be selectively infused into a bleeding mesentric vessel. A bleeding rate of .5 per minute is necessary for a positive angiogram. Temporary success in stopping the bleeding will not obviate the need for surgery. The angiodysplasia of the colon is one of the most common causes of lower GI bleeding in elderly patients. With diverticular disease, 75% of the patients will have only a single episode of hemorrhage, whereas angiodysplasia patients are very likely to have recurrent episodes of variable severity.

14. **(C)** This patient has a T2Ni stage III colon cancer for colon cancer—staging is categorized by TNM system. Where, T is depth of penetration through bowel wall, N = nodal involvement, and M = metastatic disease.

T 1's	carcinoma in situ
T 1	invades submucosa
T 2	invades muscularis propria
T 3	through the muscularis propria
T 4	through visceral peritonuem
N 0	no lymph node involvement
N 1	1–3 positive nodes
N 2	4 or more pericolic nodes

N 3   any node along the main vascular
M 0   no metastasis
M1   distant metastasis

Staging is a follows:

T1 or T2 No Mo = stage I
T3 or T4 No Mo = stage II
Avg T N1 Mo = stage III
Avg T Avg N M1 = stage IV

15. **(D)** Patients with stage III colon cancer have 5-year survival ranging from 20% to 50%. Prognosis is largely related to lymph node involvement. Recurrence is usually in liver, peritoneal cavity, or lungs. Adjuvant chemotherapy with 5 FU based regimens have proven benefit in decreasing recurrence and improving survival. Capecitabine is an oral fluoropyrimidine, which is converted to 5 FU in tumor cells. It's role is still being defined in national clinical trials. Radiation therapy is not offered in stage III colon cancer as local failure is rare because adequate margins can be obtained.

16. **(A)** The small intestine arises from the midgut segment. The midgut segment extends between the ampulla of Vater and the distal transverse colon. It enters the physiological umbilical hernia at sixth week and returns to the peritoneal cavity by the tenth week. The vitellointestinal tract (site from which Meckel's diverticulum arises) is attached to the antimesenteric margin of the distal ileum. The urachus is attached to the bladder. The intestinal lymphatic drainage is directed to the preaortic glands.

17. **(D)** The small intestine commences to the *left* of the midline at Treitz's ligament and ends at the ileocecal junction. The mesenteric attachment is only 15 cm in length. It is supplied by the midgut vessel (superior mesenteric). The sympathetic and parasympathetic (vagus) nerves enter the mesentery to supply the vessels and gut wall.

18. **(C)** Crohn's disease differs from ulcerative colitis in that clinical improvement usually occurs when a diseased segment is excluded from the fecal stream. Crohn's disease involves the distal ileum in most patients, but almost any part of the alimentary tract could be affected. Steroids frequently result in improvement in patients with Crohn's disease and ulcerative colitis. In Crohn's disease, steroids are a double-edged sword, because they clearly allow initial improvement, but eventually their benefit is counteracted by adverse complications of steroids.

19. **(C)** The serosa appeared normal on inspection, but the colon mucosa was extensively involved. In ulcerative colitis, the distal rectum and colon are primarily involved in continuity to the proximal extent of the lesion. In Crohn's disease, a similar pattern may be found on rare occasions, but other features, such as small intestinal disease, transmural involvement, skip lesions, and fistula formation, favor Crohn's disease. The small bowel is not primarily involved in ulcerative colitis, but a "backwash" ileitis may be encountered.

20. **(D)** Gangrene of the bowel occurs before the ominous sign of intramural air can be detected. The stack-of-coins sign is seen in intestinal obstruction where the proximal small intestine folds are stacked to provide this characteristic feature on a plain x-ray of the abdomen.

21. **(C)** In a patient with small intestine infarction, the possibility of nonocclusive ischemic disease should be excluded by angiography. If there is no evidence of gangrene, then fluid resuscitation and intra-arterial superior mesenteric papaverine administration may be adequate, and surgical intervention may be avoided. Von Willebrand's disease is characterized by a mild to moderate fall in factor VIII levels (pseudohemophilia) but with a much milder bleeding tendency than in true hemophilia. It affects males and females equally.

22. **(C)** Most air that reaches the stomach and intestines comes from swallowed air. Air is nearly always seen in the small intestine on a plain film of the abdomen. Gas in the stomach is derived mainly from swallowed air, which has an oxygen content of 20% and nitrogen content of 80%. CO_2 is formed by organic fermentation and comprises 40% of the gases in the distal bowel. Nitrogen is absorbed so that it is reduced below

50% distally. Methane and hydrogen sulfide gases are added in the distal bowel.

23. **(D)** A plain film of the abdomen shows valvulae conniventes in jejunal (proximal) obstruction, a featureless bowel pattern in distal ileal obstruction, and haustra in colon obstruction.

24. **(A)** The initial management of intestinal obstruction is to correct fluid and electrolyte imbalance. Surgery is indicated if strangulation is anticipated or if the obstruction fails to respond to conservative management. Nasogastric suction is often effective in obstruction because of adhesions but is contraindicated when the obstruction is caused by a hernia and/or strangulation is suspected.

25. **(B)** In patients presenting with small-bowel obstruction, clinical examination can usually identify a groin swelling attributable to strangulated hernia. If external groin hernia is excluded, the presence of an abdominal scar would highly suggest that intestinal obstruction is caused by adhesions. Peritoneal metastasis and primary tumors, bands, Crohn's disease, and gallstone ileus must be excluded. The distention is mainly a result of swallowed air. If the obstruction is proximal, the onset is usually more severe and rapid.

26. **(D)** In a Richter hernia, only part of the circumference of the bowel wall has become trapped in the hernia sac, and normal bowel movements may still occur. In the presence of a reducible groin hernia, it is important on clinic examination to be certain that other pathologic conditions are not overlooked.

27. **(E)** Primary small-bowel volvulus is common in countries where the diet is high in bulk. Except for the neonatal variety (associated with malrotation), it is rare in the United States. Small-bowel volvulus secondary to adhesions is more common here. The ileum is more frequently involved than the jejunum. If a small-bowel resection is required, it is usually of a limited nature.

28. **(C)** The ileum is the exclusive site of bile salt absorption, and failure of its absorption contributes to the steatorrhea. Ileal resection, which

at times includes the ileocecal valve, is more commonly performed than is proximal resection. Over a longer period of time (2–3 years), megaloblastic anemia occurs.

29. **(A)** Transit time in the ileum is slower than that in the jejunum. Resection of equal lengths of intestine results in greater deterioration after ileal resection as the site of slower (and therefore more complete) absorption is removed. Jejunal resection is followed by hypertrophy of the residual villi in the ileum and functional compensation to a degree greater than in the jejunum after ileal resection.

30. **(B)** Massive resection occurs if more than 75–80% is resected (leaving less than 1 m of small bowel). The most common indications for major bowel resection are ischemia, Crohn's disease, volvulus, and trauma.

31. **(A)** In the blind loop syndrome, bacteria proliferate in an affected segment that fails to show appropriate peristaltic activity. It may be seen in surgery requiring jejunal or ileal bypass, small intestinal diverticular disease, scleroderma, diabetes mellitus, and intestinal carcinoma. Macrocytic anemia, caused by malabsorption of Vitamin B_{12} and folic acid, is a key diagnostic feature in its diagnosis.

32. **(C)** Intestinal obstruction due to a Meckel's diverticulum may result from a volvulus, band obstruction, or intussusception. Among children, bleeding and inflammation are seen more frequently. Meckel's diverticulum is a remnant of the vitellointestinal duct.

33. **(B)** Peutz–Jeghers syndrome is rare but should be considered if pigmented spots are found on the lips, mouth, or hands. Hamartomas are not neoplasms; the name is derived from the Greek *hamartos,* which refers to the misfiring of a javelin. The tissues appropriate to the site misfire and are arranged in an irregular order.

34. **(A)** Unfortunately, in most series, division of adhesions accounts for as much as 25% of postoperative intestinal fistulas. These cases usually involve sites that are not recognized at the time

of operation. The fistulas occurring after resection of the bowel in Crohn's disease are less likely to heal without surgical intervention. The small intestine is the most common site of intestinal fistula formation.

35. **(B)** Internal small-bowel fistulas are caused almost exclusively by small-bowel disease or surrounding visceral disease involving the small bowel. Crohn's disease is the most common cause of internal small-bowel fistulas, but neoplasia, lymphoma, and tuberculosis must be excluded. Internal fistula may be asymptomatic or cause serious malabsorption (proximal to distal fistulas) or infection (enterovesical fistulas).

36. **(C)** Both zinc and vitamin C (ascarbate) deficiency, impair wound healing. Vitamin A deficiency is also implicated in would healing and supplemental Vitamin A has been shown in experimental studies to prevent radiation included defects in wound healing. Incision through the same abdominal wall scar incision actually promotes wound healing, because the initial lag interval after creation of the wound is avoided (unless the whole scar of the incision is removed). Increase in local oxygen tension actually promotes wound healing.

37. **(A)** Doxorubicin cleaves diribonucleic acid (DNA) and has been shown to decrease wound healing. Treatment should be delayed at least 4 weeks. Wound healing will improve by reducing wound infection rates. This is the rational for the use of antibiotic prophylaxis. The use of mechanical cleansing alone will not reduce wound infection and may actually increase complications. Mechanical preparation with oral nonabsorbable antibiotics does reduce microbial flora and has been shown to reduce surgical infectious complications. Denervation of tissue surrounding the incision does not influence wound healing. Steroids delay the rate of wound healing and decrease protein synthesis.

38. **(D)** The omentum and peritoneal cavity seem to be less efficient in localizing the disease in these age groups. Appendicitis has a particularly high-complication rate in infants and the elderly. Delay in establishing the accurate diagnosis in these two age groups also contributes to a worse prognosis.

39. **(D)** In appendicitis, patients frequently note that the pain commences in the umbilical region and moves later to the right iliac fossa. Pain in the iliac fossa occurs when the overlying parietal peritoneum is involved. Patients with appendicitis typically indicate that they have anorexia. 70–80% of patients with appendicitis have vomiting.

40. **(C)** This is McBurney's point and often indicates the region where maximal tenderness can be elicited. In addition to tenderness, guarding and percussion tenderness should be sought to verify whether localized and/or general peritonitis exists.

41. **(B)** The mortality rate from appendicitis is 4/1,000,000 in the general population, which is a 20-fold decline from that reported 50 years ago. The mortality rate for ruptured appendicitis is 4–5% but increases to 9% in infants and 15% in patients above 65 years of age and those with serious underlying medical illness. The high rate of perforation is partly due to physician delay in establishing the diagnosis of acute appendicitis. The mortality rate of 0.1% in patients with nonruptured appendicitis highlights the fact that the condition remains a potentially lethal disease. The diagnosis of acute appendicitis is nearly always determined on clinical grounds without need to request a CT scan (Fig. 6–4).

42. **(C)** If the surgeon's records indicate that all operations on the appendix are abnormal, there is a real danger that a true appendicitis will be missed and that the criteria chosen are too rigid. On the other hand, if the rate of normal appendices removed is increased, the criteria selected for operation require further defining. Good clinical observation and appropriate laparoscopy in female patients will help achieve the goal of optimal incidence of accuracy with emergency appendectomy. After unwarranted appendectomy, complications include persistent pain from adhesions, inadvertent visceral trauma at operation, and small-bowel obstruction. In older patients in particular, the usual diverse complications of operations occur.

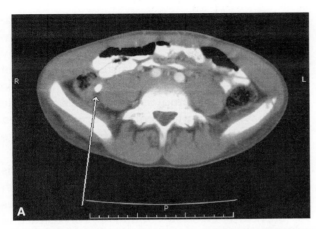

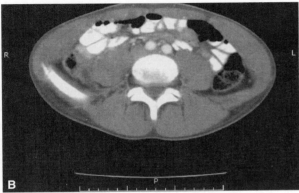

Figure 6–4.
A. CT scan shows a fecolith in the appendix. **B**. CT scan shows a dilated appendix with fluid.

43. **(A)** Rousing's sign is corroborative of acute appendicitis. The other signs are corroborative of appendicitis. Hyperesthesia is a useful sign provided that it is performed objectively. The area of hyperesthesia is a triangular area (base placed upward) in the right lower abdomen.

44. **(A)** The presence of a blind loop leads to malabsorption with steatorrhea, macrocytic anemia, and malabsorption. A blind loop is likely to occur if an antiperistaltic loop is created, and it is more than 3–6 inches in length. The antiperistaltic loop causes failure of adequate emptying of intestinal contents; this leads to stasis and overgrowth of bacteria.

45. **(C)** Irradiation of the abdominal cavity of more than 50 Gy is associated with a higher rate of complications. The incidence of symptomatic sigmoiditis may be as high as 75%, and histologically

abnormal rectal biopsy findings occur in 11% of patients undergoing treatment for pelvic malignancy. Previous surgery with possible adhesion formation increases the risk of irradiation damage.

46. **(E)** In most patients, ischemic colitis is a self-limiting illness that usually resolves within 7–10 days. Patients may manifest pyrexia and peritonitis, have persistent symptoms, and develop complications, such as stricture formation, perforation, and bleeding. Unlike small-bowel ischemia, the main vessels are characteristically patent.

47. **(A)** The mucosa is friable and bleeds readily. Ulcers vary in size and often tend to be transverse in position and surrounded by telangiectasis. They are often more prominent on the anterior wall around the anal verge. Rectal strictures usually are located about 8–12 cm above the anal verge. Rectovaginal fistula may develop in female patients. On barium enema, a narrow stricture is difficult to differentiate from a carcinoma.

48. **(D)** In 90% of cases with colonic ischemia, the patient is over 65 years of age. Precipitating causes, such as cardiac disease, are much less frequently encountered than in small-bowel ischemia. In 20% of patients, an underlying obstructive lesion of the colon is noted. Unlike small-bowel ischemia, the pain is often insidious in onset.

49. **(E)** The classic finding of thumbprinting may be missed if the barium enema study is deferred for more than 10 days after onset of symptoms. Unlike small-bowel ischemia, the main vessels are patent in most cases.

50. **(D)** After 10 years with ulcerative colitis, the chances of developing carcinoma increase fourfold. After 20 years, the cumulative risk is 12%, and at 25 years, it is 25%. Malignancy is often detected at a late stage and has a larger percentage of synchronous lesions as compared to that seen in patients with cancer who do not have ulcerative colitis. Patients with extensive disease and those in whom the disease occurs at an earlier age must undergo careful surveillance.

51. **(A)** Occurs more frequently than in the rest of the population. The cumulative risk of developing cancer in patients with extensive ulcerative colitis is greater than in those with more localized disease (42% at 25 years). Children are more likely to have extensive disease. Colon cancer occurs more frequently in the sigmoid and rectum in ulcerative colitis, but cancer is more likely to occur in patients who have universal disease. Synchronous carcinomas in patients without ulcerative colitis occur in 4%, compared to 25% in those with colitis. Lesions usually are flat, are frequently missed at examination, and have a worse prognosis than sporadic colon cancers found in normal risk patients. Adults developing cancer under the age of 45 have a poorer prognosis than those who develop it later.

52. **(C)** There has been an increase in incidence of colon cancer relative to that of the rectum in recent years. This observation may be related to the improved diagnostic techniques now available with colonoscopy. The higher mortality of some rectal cancer patients may be attributed to an incomplete resection of the tumor when it is close to the cut edge. Each year, 14,000 new cases are diagnosed and over 6000 deaths occur.

53. **(E)** Just under half of patients with local disease will also have associated metastatic disease. Patients with microscopic lymph node metastasis—adjacent as opposed to remote—and with one to three lymph nodes involved have a better prognosis than patients with more extensive disease.

54. **(B)** Synchronous malignant lesions (present in 4–5%) refer to those present at the time of surgery or found in investigations carried out within 6 months after operation. Metachronous lesions are those not detected during this period but subsequently identified. Metachronous carcinomas occur in about 5% of cases.

55. **(B)** Synchronous carcinoma and polyps, of all types, occur at sites in the colon not included in an anterior or sigmoid resection. Both synchronous carcinomas and benign polyps occur mainly at sites in the colon that would not be included in the definite resection for the primary carcinoma. Thus, it is important to try, whenever possible, to perform colonoscopy before colon resection to facilitate planning of the operation should a synchronous lesion be detected. If this study is omitted, it is advisable to have a complete colonoscopy performed within the first 2–3 months after resection.

56. **(C)** Dukes A lesions have an excellent prognosis of 90% 5-year survival compared to that with serosal extension (B2), particularly if lymph nodes are heavily involved. Around 70 % of obstructing lesions occur on the left side and 30% proximal to the hepatic flexure. The CEA level correlates with the extent of encirclement of the tumor, Dukes classification, and the likelihood of recurrence.

57. **(C)** The most common sites of obstruction are descending colon (21%), sigmoid (17%), and splenic flexure (15%). The percentages for cases with obstruction at a particular site are splenic flexure, 37%; sigmoid, 16%; and right colon, 14%.

58. **(A)** The ducts of the anal glands drain into the anus and are covered by the vertical columns of Morgagni. Infection of these glands may account for some cases of perianal abscess. The folds end distally at about the level of the dentate line. The lower third of the anus receives its nerve supply from the pudendal nerve (somatic). In order to minimize spread of infection, the local anesthetic should be confined to the skin immediately overlying the abscess. This should be performed in a hospital setting, in an operating room, with good lighting, in the lithotomy position, using a combination of IV sedation and local anesthesia. Protoscopy/sigmoidoscopy can be undertaken at he same time.

59. **(C)** CEA is useful in the follow-up care of patients with colon carcinoma after resection. The levels of this antigen usually come to normal after complete resection of the tumor. A subsequent elevation may suggest a recurrence of the tumor either at the resection margin or at distant sites. The sensitivity and specificity of CEA for diagnosis of colon carcinoma is poor. It has no implications for resectability of the lesion.

60. **(E)** Insidious development of a microcytic, hypochromic anemia is an important clue for the diagnosis of carcinoma of the right colon. Guaiac-positive stool with or without a palpable mass in the RLQ should raise the possibility. All the other possibilities listed may also cause lower GI bleeding but are characteristically associated with abdominal pain (peptic ulcer disease, Crohn's disease, ulcerative colitis). Bleeding in sigmoid diverticulosis usually is bright red and painless.

61. **(A)** Recurrent fistulas in ano are a feature of Crohn's colitis. The absence in the rectum eliminates the possibility of ulcerative colitis. Amebic colitis presents with recurrent episodes of diarrhea with bleeding. Ischemic colitis also presents with diarrhea.

62. **(D)** The picture described suggests large-bowel obstruction in a patient with a competent ileocecal valve. The most likely cause is an obstructing carcinoma. The site of obstruction is in the sigmoid colon above the level of sigmoidoscopy. Sigmoid volvulus, ischemic colitis, and diverticulitis will present some findings on sigmoidoscopy. Pseudo-obstruction of the colon will manifest as colonic distention down to the rectum (Fig. 6–5).

63. **(D)** Rectosigmoid injuries should promptly raise a high index of suspicion, warranting immediate sigmoidoscopy to confirm the diagnosis. Sigmoidoscopy, rigid or flexible, involves much manipulation and insufflation of air. This is hardly desirable or safe in the presence of a significant tear in the presence of a rectal foreign body, free air under the diaphragm, in a patient with an acute abdomen, is all that is necessary to warrant laparotomy. Following this, CT scan with gastrofin administered orally, will give the diagnosis. The best treatment is exteriorisation that is colostomy, at the perforated site. This will depend upon the location and extent of the perforation. If small and localized, colostomy at the site or proximally may be chosen. If the tear is massive, then resection with proximal colostomy and mucous fistula (Hartman) may be indicated.

64. **(C)** Volvulus of the sigmoid (secondary type) is common in elderly patients who are chronically

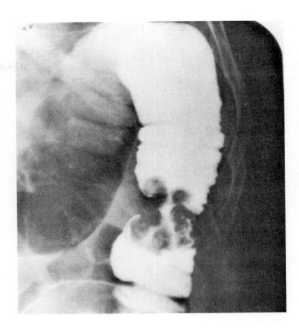

Figure 6–5.
Barium enema roentgenogram of an encircling carcinoma of the descending colon presenting an "apple core" appearance. Note the loss of mucosal pattern, the "hooks" at the margins of the lesion owing to undermining by the growth, the relatively short (6 cm) length of the lesion, and its abrupt ends. *(Reproduced, with permission, from Doherty GM: Current Surgical Diagnosis and Treatment, 12th ed. 721. McGraw-Hill, 2006.)*

constipated. Redundancy of the sigmoid and a narrow mesenteric attachment predispose for the twisting. In the large bowel, the sigmoid is the most common site. Abdominal distention and tenderness are the common presenting symptoms. Volvulus of the sigmoid colon can usually be detected on a supine and erect abdominal x-ray. Sigmoidoscopy and contrast barium studies may be helpful to differentiate carcinoma from volvulus (Fig. 6–6).

65. **(A)** The long history of bloody diarrhea should suggest a diagnosis of inflammatory bowel disease. The acute onset of abdominal pain together with the findings of an acute abdomen and systemic manifestations should raise the suspicion of a devastating complication. The picture is characteristic of acute toxic megacolon in ulcerative colitis. All the other possibilities listed may present with an acute abdomen, but the long history should point to ulcerative colitis.

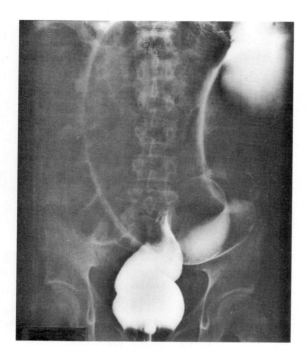

Figure 6–6.
Volvulus of the sigmoid colon. Barium enema taken with the patient in the supine position. Note the massively dilated sigmoid colon. The distinct vertical cease, which represents juxtaposition of adjacent walls of the dilated loop, points toward the site of torsion. The barium column resembles a "bird's beak" or "ace of spades" because of the way in which the lumen tapers toward the volvulus. *(Reproduced, with permission, from Doherty GM: Current Surgical Diagnosis and Treatment, 12th ed. 701. McGraw-Hill, 2006.)*

66. **(D)** In a patient with abdominal aortic aneurysm resection, the most worrisome complication is inadequate blood supply to the sigmoid colon through the marginal artery. Sigmoid ischemia should be ruled out by sigmoidoscopy. In the clinical picture described, sigmoidoscopy should be the most important test.

67. **(B)** The findings described on physical examination and CT scan are suggestive of acute diverticulitis of the sigmoid colon. The initial treatment of this condition is expectant with antibiotics with or without nasogastric drainage. An antibiotic with specificity against the *Bacteroides* species (third-generation cephalosporin, metronidazole, or clindamycin) should be part of the regimen. Steroids have no place in the treatment. Laparotomy is indicated only after failure of conservative treatment.

68. **(E)** The clinical picture of recurrent bright rectal bleeding that is not associated with abdominal pain is characteristic of diverticulosis of the colon. The bleeding in sigmoid carcinoma is often microscopic. Diverticulitis of the colon would present with associated pain. Adenomatous polyp may present with painless rectal bleeding, but the most common condition in this elderly age group is diverticulosis of the colon.

69. **(E)** Laparotomy and subtotal colectomy should be the preferred approach in a hypotensive patient. There is no time for trying to localize the site of bleeding by scans, mesenteric angiography, or colonoscopy. Although the common site of massive diverticular hemorrhage is the right colon, a blind right colon resection in an elderly woman with hypotension is fraught with the danger of recurrent bleeding from the left colon. The safest and most expeditious management is subtotal colectomy. The decision for anastomosis or proximal ileostomy will depend on the stability of the patient.

70. **(A)** A common cause of lower GI bleeding that is recurrent and painless is angiodysplasia of the colon. In the absence of diverticula or hemorrhoids, the suspicion is even higher for these lesions. Peptic ulcer and Meckel's diverticulum can cause predominantly lower GI bleeding. However, the bleeding is usually in the form of melena rather than bright red.

71. **(B)** Small-bowel turnover can be measured in rats by autoradiographic studies in which turnover of cells located in the crypts migrate along the villus toward the tip over a 2- to 3-day period. Intestinal villous mucosa undergoes hypertrophy and hyperplasia whenever an increased food load continuously enters the small intestine.

72. **(C)** All the choices listed except hyperplastic polyp are precancerous lesions. The carcinomas in ulcerative colitis and familial polyposis are multicentric. Large villous adenomas may have carcinomatous changes. Any patient with a colon carcinoma is predisposed to develop a metachronous lesion in the remaining colon,

hence the importance of regular follow-up examinations in these patients.

73. **(B)** All the clinical features mentioned and the strong family history should raise the possibility of familial polyposis. Although other possibilities listed may also cause rectal bleeding and abdominal pain, the strong familial history should give a clue to the diagnosis. The early onset of invasive carcinoma in these patients makes recognizing familial polyposis very important.

74. **(E)** Many patients who have metastasis to the liver or lung have resectable tumors. A reasonable disease-free interval has been reported after such resections, especially with carcinoma of the colon as the primary lesion.

75. **(A)** Cefizox is not effective against many strains of *Pseudomonas*. If the drug is used in

pseudomonas infection a higher dosage may be indicated, and the antibiotic should be changed if a quick response does not occur. Complications include cross reactions in patients who are allergic to penicillin. It does not seem to have nephrotoxic side effects.

76. **(A)** The presence of distended loops of bowel indicate bowel obstruction. The clinical features favor mechanical obstruction rather than paralytic ileus due to infection. Obstruction due to adhesions is more common than obstruction due to hernia.

77. **(A)** This is a relatively uncommon lesion. One sign that may be elicited with a mesenteric cyst is that the swelling moves freely in the direction between the left iliac fossa and the right hypochondria (i.e., perpendicular to the small-bowel mesentery axis) (Fig. 6–7).

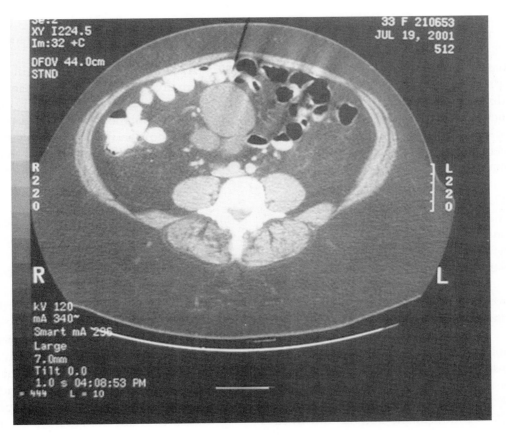

Figure 6–7.
CT scan a mesenteric unilocular appearance without associated solid component strongly suggest the diagnosis of benign cyst. *(Reproduced, with permission, from Brunicardi FC et al.: Schwartz's Principles of Surgery, 8th ed. 1325. McGraw-Hill, 2005.)*

78. **(B)** Gallstone ileus results in "tumbling" intestinal obstruction due to the intermittent nature of the condition. Previous choledochoduodenostomy could give air in the biliary tree but not obstruction.

79. **(B)** The carcinoid syndrome in patients with intestinal carcinoid tumors will occur only in the presence of hepatic metastasis. Approximately 40% of patients with hepatic metastasis from an ileal carcinoid will develop the syndrome.

80. **(A)** Patients with carcinoid tumor due to ovarian dermoid or pulmonary lesion may develop the syndrome with an elevated 5-HIAA, although hepatic metastasis are absent. The liver does not counteract the hormone in this instance, because the portal system is bypassed.

81. **(A)** Patients with underlying ischemic disease may develop acute intestinal infarction or intestinal angina, which is aggravated by eating.

82. **(A)** Mechanical obstruction implies a barrier that impedes progress of intestinal contents. Complete mid- or distal small-bowel obstruction presents with colicky abdominal pain, more marked abdominal distention but with vomiting that is less frequent and occurs at a later stage than that of proximal jejunal obstruction.

83. **(E)** MMC are isoperistaltic waves and occur approximately once every 90 minutes. Oral feeding inhibits the MMC for as much as 3–4 hours. The inhibition of the MMC in the stomach and intestine may account in part for nausea and vomiting occurring after surgery. The major force that drives chyme aborally is that of segmentation and not the MMC.

84. **(A)** Typhoid fever typically presents with initial symptoms. Small intestine complications are related to involvement of Peyer's patches of the small intestine, which result in bleeding and/or perforation in the second and third week after symptoms are noted.

85. **(B)** The absence of loops of colon makes a colonic site most unlikely as a cause of the current clinical presentation. Distention does not occur in high small-bowel obstruction.

86. **(E)** In view of the presence of bowel obstruction, surgery is indicated. In general, patients who have obstruction due to adhesions may undergo an initial short trial period of conservative management. Laparotomy is usually indicated in bowel obstruction due to other causes, where gangrene may be evident, and in all cases in which an initial period of conservative treatment fails.

87. **(C)** In general, failure (or inability) to continue anticoagulants is an indication to insert an IVC filter to minimize the possibility of serious and possibly fatal pulmonary embolus.

88. **(C)** Tuberculosis is the great mimicker of disease and, therefore, should always be considered in the differential diagnosis of different abdominal conditions. Surgical intervention will be required if the obstruction becomes complete.

89. **(A)** Although intestinal tuberculosis still remains relatively uncommon in the United States, it should be particularly excluded in the AIDS population. In these patients, the rarity of the condition may make its clinical detection particularly difficult. Always suspect tuberculosis in the differential diagnosis of fever without a clearly defined cause.

90. **(B)** The blood supply to a loop of ischemic bowel is determined by the presence or absence of arterial pulsation, peristalsis, and color of the bowel after resuscitation and relief of obstruction.

91. **(L)** The jejunum is the first part of the alimentary tract and, therefore, is the primary site of absorption of nearly all nutrients. It is unable to absorb vitamin B_{12} and bile salts, which are absorbed exclusively in the ileum. If the ileum is transposed between the duodenum and the jejunum, it undergoes compensatory hypertrophy and takes over the function of the jejunum and becomes the primary site of nutrient absorption.

92. **(M)** In Hirschsprung's disease, there is an absence of myenteric plexus in the upper anal

segment (i.e., the most distal portion of the cloaca). In 15%, the myenteric plexus involves only the upper anus; in 70%, the rectum is also involved; and in 15%, part of the colon is also involved. The abnormal segment is contracted; whereas, the dilated bowel is proximal to the diseased segment.

93. **(G)** In this variety, the hernia does not have a complete covering of peritoneum. It is called a sliding hernia. It is important that the surgeon does not attempt to remove peritoneum from the circumference bowel wall where it does not exist, because the bowel will become devascularized.

94. **(B)** Perianal abscess is most common type of anorectal abscess. It is superficial and lies in perianal space. Duration of symptoms is short and patient is unlikely to have fever or leukocytosis.

95. **(F)** Ischiorectal abscesses are often large, erythematous indurated, and tender. They are often associated with fistula.

96. **(F)** Supralovator abscesses are relatively rare. Most patients have a pelvic inflammatory condition such as salpingitis, diverticulitis or Crohn's, or have had recent pelvic surgery.

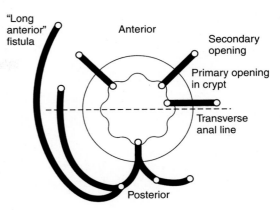

Figure 6–8.
Salmon–Goodsall rule. The usual relation of the primary and secondary openings of fistulas. When the external opening of a fistula is anteriorly situated, the internal opening is found internal to it in the same radial position; when the external opening of a fistula is posteriorly situated, the internal opening is found in the midline posteriorly. Note the exception to this rule of the far lateral (anterior) fistula. *(Reproduced, with permission, from Doherty GM: Current Surgical Diagnosis and Treatment, 12th ed. 754. McGraw-Hill, 2006.)*

97. **(B)** A single or multiple sinuses that has an external opening in the posterior half of the skin that surrounds the anus will have an internal opening in the midline on the distal anus if a fistula has formed (Fig. 6–8).

98. **(A)** The most common site for a pilonidal abscess to develop is in the midline posteriorly in the natal cleft posterior to the sacrum.

CHAPTER 7

Pancreas, Biliary Tract, Liver, and Spleen

Valerie L. Katz and Akella Chendrasekhar

Questions

DIRECTIONS (Questions 1 through 99): Each of the numbered items in this section are followed by five answers. Select the ONE lettered answer that is BEST in each case.

1. A 1-week-old infant is brought to the hospital because of vomiting. An upper gastrointestinal (GI) series reveals duodenal obstruction. On laparotomy, annular pancreas is found. Which of the following statements about annular pancreas is TRUE?

   (A) Resection is the treatment of choice.
   (B) It is associated with Down's syndrome.
   (C) Symptoms usually begin with back pain.
   (D) It is most likely due to abnormal rotation encircling the third part of the duodenum.
   (E) Symptoms begin in childhood.

2. A 60-year-old alcoholic is admitted to the hospital with a diagnosis of acute pancreatitis. Upon admission, his white blood cell (WBC) count is 21,000. His lipase is 500, blood glucose is 180 mg/dL, lactate dehydrogenase (LDH) is 400 IU/L, and aspartate aminotransferase (AST) is 240 IU/dL. Which of the following is TRUE?

   (A) This patient is expected to have a mortality rate of less than 5%.
   (B) The patient's lipase level is an important indication of prognosis.

   (C) This patient requires immediate surgery.
   (D) A venous blood gas would be helpful in assessing the severity of illness in this patient.
   (E) A serum calcium level of 6.5 mg/dL on the second hospital day is a bad prognostic sign.

3. A 19-year-old man is brought to the emergency department by emergency medical service (EMS) with a stab-wound to the right upper quadrant (RUQ) of the abdomen. A FAST scan shows free fluid, and the patient is taken to the operating room for an exploratory laparotomy. The findings are a nonbleeding laceration of the right lobe of the liver and a gallbladder laceration. Which of the following is TRUE?

   (A) The gallbladder injury can be treated with cholecystectomy.
   (B) Isolated gallbladder injuries are uncommon.
   (C) Bile is usually sterile.
   (D) The liver laceration does not require closed suction drainage.
   (E) A thorough exploration is not necessary if the bleeding is confined to the RUQ.

4. A 15-year-old female presents with RUQ abdominal pain. Workup reveals a choledochal cyst. Which of the following statements is TRUE?

   (A) Choledochal cysts are more common in men.
   (B) Laparoscopic cholecystectomy is the recommended treatment.
   (C) Patients with a choledochal cyst have an increased risk of cholangiocarcinoma.
   (D) All patients with a choledochal cyst have abdominal pain, a RUQ mass, and jaundice.
   (E) The etiology is infectious.

5. A 13-year-old female presenting with RUQ abdominal pain is suspected of having a chole-dochal cyst. Which of the following studies would be least helpful in confirming the diag-nosis in this case?

   (A) Computed tomography (CT) scan
   (B) Percutaneous transhepatic cholangiography
   (C) Endoscopic retrograde cholangiopancreatography
   (D) Magnetic resonance cholangiopancreatography (MRCP)
   (E) Upper GI series

6. An intraoperative cholangiogram is performed during an elective laparoscopic cholecystec-tomy on a 30-year-old woman. She has no pre-vious surgical history. There is a 0.8-cm filling defect in the distal common bile duct (CBD). The surgeon should:

   (A) Complete the laparoscopic cholecystectomy and check liver function tests (LFTs) postoperatively. If they are normal, no further treatment is needed.
   (B) Complete the laparoscopic cholecystectomy and repeat an ultrasound postoperatively. Observe the patient if no CBD stone is visualized.
   (C) Perform a CBD exploration either laparoscopically or open along with a cholecystectomy.

   (D) Complete the laparoscopic cholecystectomy, no further treatment is necessary.
   (E) Complete the laparoscopic cholecystectomy and plan for a postoperative hydroxy iminodiacetic acid (HIDA) scan.

7. An 85-year-old man is brought to the hospital with a 2-day history of nausea and vomiting. He has not passed gas or moved his bowels for the last 5 days. Abdominal films show dilated small bowel, no air in the rectum and air in the biliary tree. Which of the following statements is TRUE?

   (A) Air in the biliary tree associated with small-bowel obstruction suggests a diagnosis of gallstone ileus.
   (B) An enterotomy should be distal to the site of obstruction and the stone should be removed.
   (C) Gallstone ileus is more common in the young adults.
   (D) Cholecystectomy is contraindicated.
   (E) Small-bowel obstruction usually occurs in the distal jejunum.

8. A 45-year-old man with hepatitis C undergoes an uneventful percutaneous liver biopsy. About 6-weeks later, he complains of RUQ pain, is clin-ically jaundiced, with a hemoglobin of 9.2 mg/dL and is fecal occult blood positive. Which diagnosis best explains this patient's symptoms?

   (A) Hepatocellular carcinoma
   (B) Chronic hepatitis C
   (C) Colon carcinoma with liver metastasis
   (D) Hemobilia
   (E) Symptomatic cholelithiasis

9. A 40-year-old patient with a history of trauma to the RUQ presents with RUQ pain, clinical jaundice, and guaiac positive stools. Which one of the following studies would be most useful to confirm the patient's diagnosis?

   (A) Abdominal ultrasound
   (B) CT of the abdomen
   (C) Angiography

(D) HIDA scan

(E) Diagnostic laparoscopy

10. A 40-year-old female alcoholic is suspected of having a hepatic mass. Percutaneous ultrasound-guided liver biopsy is contraindicated in which of the following?

(A) Hepatocellular carcinoma

(B) Metastatic carcinoma

(B) Cirrhosis

(D) Hepatitis C

(E) Hepatic adenoma

11. A 20-year-old man is brought to the emergency department with a gunshot wound to the abdomen. His blood pressure is 70 systolic and his heart rate is 140 beats per minute (bpm). He is taken directly to the operating room for an exploratory laparotomy. A large, actively bleeding liver laceration is found. A pringle maneuver is performed as part of the procedure to control his bleeding. The pringle maneuver compresses which structures?

(A) Portal vein, hepatic vein, and hepatic artery

(B) Portal vein, hepatic artery, and cystic artery

(C) Portal vein and hepatic artery

(D) Portal vein, hepatic artery, and CBD

(E) Cystic artery, cystic duct, and CBD

12. A 22-year-old medical student is seen by the student health service prior to beginning school. Routine labs are drawn. The medical student immunized against hepatitis B in childhood will have which hepatitis profile?

(A) HbsAb+, HbsAg+, HbcAb+

(B) HbsAb+, HbsAg+, HbcAb–

(C) HbsAb–, HbsAg–, HbcAb–

(D) HbsAb+, HbsAg–, HbcAb–

(E) HbsAb–, HbsAg+, HcbAb–

13. A 36-year-old man presents to the emergency department after a motor vehicle crash. He is complaining of left-sided chest pain and abdominal pain. His blood pressure is 130/80 mm Hg. An electrocardiogram shows sinus rhythm with a heart rate of 95 bpm. A chest x-ray shows left 8, 9, and 10 rib fractures. An abdominal computed axial tomography (CAT) scan is obtained. It shows a 3-cm laceration in the upper pole of the spleen with a small amount of blood around the spleen. No other injury is identified. Which of the following statements is TRUE?

(A) This is a class I injury and it may be treated nonoperatively.

(B) This is a class II injury and it may be treated nonoperatively.

(C) This is a class II injury and it requires immediate laparotomy.

(D) The patient should be prophylactically transfused in anticipation of continued blood loss.

(E) Delayed splenic rupture is not possible with this injury.

14. A 38-year-old man undergoes excisional biopsy of a cervical lymph node. Pathology reveals Hodgkin's lymphoma. Which of the following statements about Hodgkin's disease is TRUE?

(A) Splenectomy is always required for accurate staging.

(B) Staging laparotomy involves liver biopsy, biopsy of the spleen, and periaortic lymph node dissection.

(C) Stage II disease involves disease on both sides of the diaphragm.

(D) If the spleen is involved, the patient has stage IV disease.

(E) Splenectomy is sometimes indicated for thrombocytopenia.

15. A 50-year-old woman complains of weakness, profuse watery diarrhea, and crampy abdominal pain. She reports a 10-lb weight loss. Her serum potassium is 2.8 mEq/L. Select the most likely diagnosis.

(A) Watery, diarrhea, hypokalemia, and achlorhydria (WDHA) syndrome

(B) Somatostatinoma

(C) Glucagonoma

(D) Insulinoma

(E) Multiple endocrine neoplasia type 1(MEN-1)

16. A 45-year-old man presents with an upper GI bleed. An upper endoscopy reveals multiple duodenal ulcers and an enlarged stomach. Select the most likely diagnosis.

   (A) WDHA syndrome
   (B) Glucagonoma
   (C) Zollinger-Ellison syndrome
   (D) Insulinoma
   (E) Somatostatinoma

17. A 35-year-old woman with epigastric pain, which did not improve on ranitidine, is found to have a nonhealing pyloric channel ulcer on upper endoscopy. Her serum calcium level is 12 mg/dL. Select the most likely diagnosis.

   (A) WDHA syndrome
   (B) MEN-1
   (C) MEN-2A
   (D) MEN-2B
   (E) Zollinger-Ellison syndrome

18. A 30-year-old man is noted to be anemic, with clinical jaundice and a palpable spleen on abdominal exam. Splenectomy is the only treatment for this patient's autosomal dominant disorder. Select the most likely diagnosis.

   (A) Thalassemia
   (B) Hereditary spherocytosis
   (C) Sickle cell disease
   (D) Idiopathic autoimmune hemolytic anemia
   (E) Thrombotic thrombocytopenic purpura (TPP)

19. The peripheral smear of a child with anemia shows hypochromic microcytic anemia with target cells. What is the child's diagnosis?

   (A) Thalassemia
   (B) Hereditary spherocytosis
   (C) Sickle cell disease
   (D) Idiopathic autoimmune hemolytic anemia
   (E) TTP

20. A woman with longstanding rheumatoid arthritis has neutropenia on routine labs and splenomegaly is noted on physical examination. Which is the most likely diagnosis?

   (A) Thalassemia
   (B) Hereditary spherocytosis
   (C) Sickle cell disease
   (D) Idiopathic autoimmune hemolytic anemia
   (E) Felty's syndrome

21. A 50-year-old woman underwent wide excision of a 2.5-cm infiltrating ductal carcinoma of the breast with axillary lymph node dissection followed by radiation and chemotherapy 2 years ago. The patient now complains of RUQ abdominal pain. A CAT scan reveals two masses in the right lobe of the liver. Select the most likely diagnosis.

   (A) Adenoma
   (B) Focal nodular hyperplasia
   (C) Hemangioma
   (D) Hepatocellular carcinoma
   (E) Metastatic carcinoma

22. A 35-year-old woman complains of RUQ pain after meals with nausea and vomiting. An ultrasound reveals cholelithiasis and an anechoic 3-cm mass on the inferior surface of the right lobe of the liver. Select the most likely diagnosis.

   (A) Nonparasitic cyst
   (B) Hydatid cyst
   (C) Hamartoma
   (D) Adenoma
   (E) Focal nodular hyperplasia

23. A 42-year-old man who consumed more than 3 bottles of vodka weekly over the past 20 years is admitted with upper abdominal pain radiating to the back, nausea, and vomiting. Serum amylase and lipase are elevated, and a diagnosis of pancreatitis is made. In determining his prognosis, which of the following factors would cause the greatest concern?

   (A) Hypercalcemia (Ca >12 mg/dL)
   (B) Age over 40 years
   (C) Hypoxemia

(D)   Hyperamylasemia (>600 U)

(E)   Elevated lipase

24.   A 24-year-old college student recovers from a bout of severe pancreatitis. He has mild epigastric discomfort, sensation of bloating, and loss of appetite. Examination reveals an epigastric fullness that on ultrasound is confirmed to be a pseudocyst. The swelling increases in size over a 3-week period of observation. What should be the next step in management?

(A)   Percutaneous drainage of the cyst

(B)   Laparotomy and internal drainage of the cyst

(C)   Excision of pseudocyst

(D)   Total pancreatectomy

(E)   Administration of pancreatic enzymes

25.   A 40-year-old alcoholic male is admitted with severe epigastric pain radiating to the back. Serum amylase level is reported as normal, but serum lipase is elevated. The serum is noted to be milky in appearance. A diagnosis of pancreatitis is made. The serum amylase is normal because

(A)   The patient has chronic renal failure.

(B)   The patient has hyperlipidemia.

(C)   The patient has alcoholic cirrhosis.

(D)   The patient has alcoholic hepatitis.

(E)   The diagnosis of pancreatitis is incorrect.

26.   A 52-year-old woman is admitted to the hospital with abdominal pain. She reports that she drinks alcohol only at social occasions. The amylase is elevated to 340 U. Which following x-ray finding would support a diagnosis of idiopathic pancreatitis?

(A)   Hepatic lesion on CT scan

(B)   Choledocholithiasis on ultrasound

(C)   Anterior displacement of the stomach on barium upper GI series

(D)   Large loop of colon in the RUQ

(E)   Irregular cutoff of the CBD on cholangiogram

27.   A 67-year-old woman is noted to have a gradual increase in the size of the abdomen. A CT scan reveals a large pancreatic mass. The lesion was excised; on pathology examination, it is shown to be a TRUE cyst. Which statement is correct regarding true cysts?

(A)   They are commonly seen in alcoholic pancreatitis.

(B)   They commonly occur after trauma.

(C)   They are frequently malignant.

(D)   They are associated commonly with choledochocele.

(E)   They have an epithelial lining.

28.   A 40-year-old man with a history of alcohol consumption of 25-year duration is admitted with a history of a 6-lb weight loss and upper abdominal pain of 3-weeks duration. Examination reveals fullness in the epigastrium. His temperature is 99°F, and his WBC count is 10,000. Which is the most likely diagnosis?

(A)   Pancreatic pseudocyst

(B)   Subhepatic abscess

(C)   Biliary pancreatitis

(D)   Cirrhosis

(E)   Splenic vein thrombosis

29.   A 58-year-old man with a 30-year history of alcoholism and pancreatitis is admitted to the hospital with an elevated bilirubin level of 5 mg/dL, acholic stools, and an amylase level of 600 U. Obstructive jaundice in chronic pancreatitis usually results from which of the following?

(A)   Sclerosing cholangitis

(B)   CBD compression caused by inflammation

(C)   Alcoholic hepatitis

(D)   Biliary dyskinesia

(E)   Splenic vein thrombosis

30. A 48-year-old woman is admitted with acute cholecystitis. The bilirubin level is elevated, as are the serum and urinary amylase levels. Which radiologic sign indicates biliary obstruction in pancreatitis?

    (A) Pancreatic intraductal calcification
    (B) Smooth narrowing of the distal CBD
    (C) Stomach displaced anteriorly
    (D) Calcified gallstone
    (E) Air in the biliary tree

31. A 62-year-old man is admitted with abdominal pain and weight loss of 5 lb over the past month. He has continued to consume large amounts of rum. Examination reveals icteric sclera. The indirect bilirubin level is 5.6 mg/dL with a total bilirubin of 6 mg/dL. An ultrasound shows a 4-cm pseudocyst. What is the most likely cause of jaundice in a patient with alcoholic pancreatitis?

    (A) Alcoholic hepatitis
    (B) Carcinoma of pancreas
    (C) Intrahepatic cyst
    (D) Pancreatic pseudocyst
    (E) Hemolytic anemia

32. A 42-year-old woman with a history of chronic alcoholism is admitted to the hospital because of acute pancreatitis. The bilirubin and amylase levels are in the normal range. An ultrasound reveals cholelithiasis. The symptoms abate on the fifth day after admission. What should she be advised?

    (A) To start on a low-fat diet.
    (B) To increase the fat content of her diet.
    (C) To undergo immediate cholecystectomy.
    (D) To undergo cholecystectomy during the same hospital stay as well as an assessment of her bile ducts.
    (E) That she will be discharged and now should undergo elective cholecystectomy after 3 months.

33. Following a motor vehicle accident a truck driver complains of severe abdominal pain. Serum amylase level is markedly increased to 800 U. Grey Turner's sign is seen in the flanks.

Pancreatic trauma is suspected. Which statement is true of pancreatic trauma?

    (A) It is mainly caused by blunt injuries.
    (B) It is usually an isolated single-organ injury.
    (C) It often requires a total pancreatectomy.
    (D) It may easily be overlooked at operation.
    (E) It is proved by the elevated amylase level.

34. A 40-year-old woman with severe chronic pancreatitis is scheduled to undergo an operation, because other forms of treatment have failed. The ultrasound shows no evidence of pseudocyst formation or cholelithiasis and endoscopic retrograde cholangiopancreatogram (ERCP) demonstrates dilated pancreatic ducts with multiple stricture formation. Which operation is suitable to treat this condition?

    (A) Pancreaticojejunostomy (Puestow procedure)
    (B) Gastrojejunostomy
    (C) Cholecystectomy
    (D) Splenectomy
    (E) Subtotal pancreatectomy

35. A 26-year-old woman with a known history of chronic alcoholism is admitted to the hospital with severe abdominal pain due to acute pancreatitis. The serum and urinary amylase levels are normal. On the day following admission to the hospital, there is no improvement, and she has a mild cough and and slight dyspnea. What is the most likely complication?

    (A) Pulmonary atelectasis
    (B) Bronchitis
    (C) Pulmonary embolus
    (D) Afferent loop syndrome
    (E) Pneumonia

36. A 30-year-old male is admitted with frequent episodes of hypoglycemia. Biochemical investigations confirmed an insulinoma. Localization studies were carried out. A CT scan and magnetic resonance imaging (MRI) of the abdomen failed to reveal a tumor in the pancreas. An endoscopic ultrasound, however, localized a 2-cm insulinoma in the tail of the pancreas. What should be the next step in the management of this patient?

(A) Somatostatin receptor scintigraphy (SRS) to confirm the insulinoma

(B) Exploratory laparotomy and total pancreatectomy

(C) Distal pancreatectomy

(D) Whipple pancreaticoduodenectomy

(E) Enucleation of the tumor

37. A 66-year-old man with obstructive jaundice is found on ERCP to have periampullary carcinoma. He is otherwise in excellent physical shape and there is no evidence of metastasis. What is the most appropriate treatment?

(A) Radical excision (Whipple procedure) where possible

(B) Local excision and radiotherapy

(C) External radiotherapy

(D) Internal radiation seeds via catheter

(E) Stent and chemotherapy

38. A 74-year-old man complains of epigastric discomfort. There is no jaundice evident, but an enlarged gallbladder is palpated. The bilirubin level is 13 mg/dL, the alkaline phosphatase level is 410 U, and the hematocrit is 35%. CT scan and MRI findings are shown in Fig. 7–1.

What is the most likely malignant tumor causing extrahepatic obstructive jaundice?

(A) Gallbladder

(B) Common hepatic duct

(C) Cystic duct

(D) Periampullary area

(E) Head of the pancreas

39. A 25-year-old female presents with episodes of bizarre behavior, memory lapse, and unconsciousness. She also demonstrated previously episodes of extreme hunger, sweating, and tachycardia. During one of these episodes, her blood sugar was tested and was found to be 40 mg/dL. Which of the following would most appropriately indicate a diagnosis of insulinoma?

(A) Demonstration of insulin antibodies in blood

(B) Abnormal glucagon level

(C) CT of the pancreas showing a mass

(D) Hypoglycemia during a symptomatic episode with relief of symptoms by intravenous glucose

(E) Decreased circulating C peptide in the blood

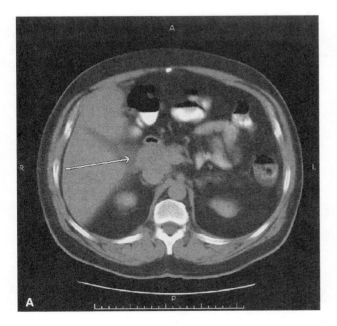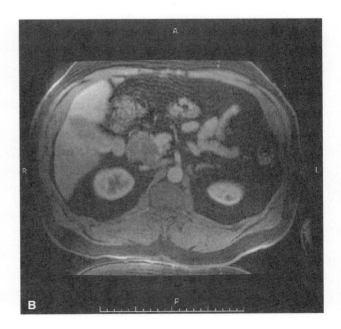

Figure 7–1.
A, CT scan shows dilated gallbladder, which in obstructive jaundice, suggests the presence of an underlying malignancy (Courvoisier's sign).
B, MRI at a lower level than **A** shows tumor (anterior and medial to that of the right kidney).

40. A 41-year-old woman is known to have multiple endocrine neoplasia syndrome. She has multiple family members who have had adenoma tumors removed from the parathyroid, pancreas, and/or pituitary glands. She has severe diarrhea associated with low gastric acid secretion and a normal gastrin level. Which of the following serum assays would be best to evaluate the possible cause of the diarrhea?

(A) Glucagon
(B) Vasoactive intestinal peptide (VIP)
(C) Cholecystokinin
(D) Serotonin
(E) Norepinephrine

41. A 45-year-old patient with chronic pancreatitis is suffering from malnutrition and weight loss secondary to inadequate pancreatic exocrine secretions. Which is TRUE regarding pancreatic secretions?

(A) Secretin releases fluid rich in enzymes.
(B) Secretin releases fluid rich mainly in electrolytes and bicarbonate.
(C) Cholecystokinin releases fluid, predominantly rich in electrolytes, and bicarbonate.
(D) All pancreatic enzymes are secreted in an inactive form.
(E) The pancreas produces proteolytic enzymes only.

42. A 48-year-old woman presents with severe recurrent peptic ulcer located in the proximal jejunum. Five years previously she underwent parathyroidectomy for hypercalcemia. Her brother was previously diagnosed as having Zollinger-Ellison syndrome. To confirm the diagnosis of Zollinger-Ellison syndrome, blood should be tested for levels of which of the following?

(A) Parathyroid hormone
(B) Histamine
(C) Pepsin
(D) Gastrin
(E) Secretin

43. A 50-year-old patient develops severe peptic ulcer disease that recurs despite gastric resection and vagotomy operations. She now presents with melena from a peptic ulcer located in the third part of the duodenum. To localize the gastrin-producing tumor, she should have which of the following?

(A) CT scan of the abdomen
(B) Ultrasound of the abdomen
(C) SRS
(D) MRI of the abdomen
(E) Barium meal and follow through

44. A 42-year-old accountant presents with recurrent RUQ pain of 3-year duration. He had undergone a laparoscopic cholecystectomy 2-years ago for presumed symptomatic cholelithiasis, but the pain persisted. An upper GI endoscopy is normal. A sonogram and CT scan of the abdomen are normal. An ERCP is performed, and the pressure in the CBD is 45-cm saline (normal bile duct pressure is 10–18-cm saline). What is the most likely diagnosis?

(A) Acalculous cholecystitis
(B) Emphysematous cholecystitis
(C) Biliary dyskinesia
(D) Cancer of the gallbladder
(E) Myasthenia gravis

45. In the emergency department, blood is taken from a 42-year-old man who presents with central abdominal pain of 12-hour duration. There is no history of alcohol abuse or gallstones. The serum is noted to be lactescent (milky appearance). To help elucidate the significance of the abdominal pain, which of the following tests should be requested?

(A) Amylase
(B) Hemoglobin electropheresis
(C) Creatinine kinase MB (CK-MB)
(D) Lipase
(E) Calcium

46. A 67-year-old woman is evaluated for obstructive jaundice. The cholangiographic findings indicate that she has a cancer of the lower end of the CBD. Clinical examination would most likely reveal which of the following?

(A) Enlarged gallbladder

(B) Shrunken gallbladder

(C) Enlarged pancreas

(D) Shrunken pancreas

(E) Palpable tumor

47. A 73-year-old woman is evaluated for obstructive jaundice after an injury to the CBD, 7 months previously at laparoscopic cholecystectomy. The alkaline phosphatase is elevated. In obstructive jaundice, which of the following statements is true regarding alkaline phosphatase?

(A) Its level increases before that of bilirubin.

(B) Its level is unlikely to be increased in pancreatic malignancy.

(C) Its elevation indicates bone metastasis.

(D) Its elevation excludes hepatic metastasis.

(E) Its level falls after that of the bilirubin, following surgical intervention.

48. A recently arrived emigrant from China develops jaundice, rigors, and high fever. Investigations revealed that he is suffering from oriental cholangiohepatitis. This condition is confirmed by detecting which of the following?

(A) Schistosomiasis (*Bilharzia*) parasite

(B) Ameba

(C) *Opisthorchis (Clonorchis) sinensis*

(D) Hydatid cyst (*Echinococcus*)

(E) Hookworm

49. A 48-year-old female travel agent presents with jaundice. Radiological findings confirm the presence of sclerosing cholangitis. She gives a long history of diarrhea for which she has received steroids on several occasions. She is likely to suffer from which of the following?

(A) Pernicious anemia

(B) Ulcerative colitis

(C) Celiac disease

(D) Liver cirrhosis

(E) Crohn's disease

50. A 40-year-old man underwent laparoscopic cholecystectomy 2 years earlier. He remains asymptomatic until 1 week before admission, when he complains of RUQ pain and jaundice. He develops a fever and has several rigor attacks on the day of admission. An ultrasound confirms the presence of gallstones in the distal CBD. The patient is given antibiotics. Which of the following should be undertaken as the next step in therapy?

(A) Should be discharged home under observation

(B) Should be observed in the hospital

(C) Undergo surgical exploration of the CBD

(D) ERCP with sphincterotomy and stone removal

(E) Anticoagulants

51. A 43-year-old woman undergoes open cholecystectomy. Intraoperative cholangiogram revealed multiple stones in the CBD. Exploration of the CBD was performed to extract gallstones. The CBD was drained with a #18 T-tube. After 10 days, a T-tube cholangiogram reveals a retained CBD stone. This should be treated by which of the following?

(A) Laparotomy and CBD exploration

(B) Subcutaneous heparinization

(C) Antibiotic therapy for 6 months and then reevaluation

(D) Extraction of the stone through the pathway created by the T-tube (after 6 weeks)

(E) Ultrasound crushing of the CBD stone

52. A 62-year-old woman who underwent chole-cystectomy and choledochoduodenostomy (CBD duodenal anastomosis) 5 years previously is admitted to the hospital with a 3-day history of upper abdominal pain, chills, fever, and dark urine. These symptoms are suggestive of ascending cholangitis. What is the laboratory finding that supports a diagnosis of ascending cholangitis?

    (A) Amylase elevation with normal findings on liver studies
    (B) Alkaline phosphatase elevation with normal or elevated normal bilirubin levels
    (C) Elevated serum glutamic oxaloacetic transaminase (SGOT) levels
    (D) Altered urea/creatinine ratio
    (E) Urobilin in urine

53. A 70-year-old male underwent a choledo-choduodenostomy for multiple common duct stones. The patient now presents with RUQ abdominal pain. What should be the initial test (least invasive with the best yield) to determine patency of the choledochoduodenostomy?

    (A) ERCP
    (B) Percutaneous transhepatic cholangiogram (PTC)
    (C) HIDA scan
    (D) CT scan of the abdomen
    (E) Ultrasound of the abdomen

54. An 70-year-old male presents with a clinical diagnosis of acute cholangitis. Which organism is most likely involved in the pathogenesis of ascending cholangitis?

    (A) *Clonorchis sinensis*
    (B) *Escherichia coli*
    (C) *Salmonella*
    (D) *Staphylococcus aureus*
    (E) *Clostridia*

55. Following admission to the hospital for intestinal obstruction, a 48-year-old woman states that she previously had undergone cholecystectomy and choledochoduodenostomy. The most likely indication for the performance of the choledochoduodenostomy was:

    (A) Hepatic metastasis were present.
    (B) Multiple stones were present in the gallbladder at the previous operation.
    (C) Multiple stones were present in the CBD at the previous operation.
    (D) The common hepatic duct had a stricture.
    (E) The small intestine was occluded.

56. In attempting to minimize complications during cholecystectomy, the surgeon defines the triangle of Calot during the operation. The boundaries of the triangle of Calot (modified) are the common hepatic duct medially, the cystic duct inferiorly, and the liver superiorly. Which structure courses through this triangle?

    (A) Left hepatic artery
    (B) Right renal vein
    (C) Right hepatic artery
    (D) Cystic artery
    (E) Superior mesenteric vein

57. A 64-year-old man complains of abdominal pain, pruritus, 4-lb weight loss, and anorexia. There are multiple scratch marks on the skin of the extremities and flank. The bilirubin is 1.0 mg/dL. To determine if the condition is due to cholestasis, blood should be tested for which of the following?

    (A) Direct and indirect bilirubin
    (B) Alkaline phosphatase
    (C) Serum glutamic-oxaloacetic transaminase (SGOT)
    (D) Serum glutamic-pyruvic transaminase (SGPT)
    (E) Bile pigments

58. A 49-year-old African American woman born in New York is admitted with RUQ pain, fever, and jaundice (Charcot's triad.) A diagnosis of ascending cholangitis is made. With regard to the etiology of ascending cholangitis, which of the following is TRUE?

(A) It usually occurs in the absence of jaundice.

(B) It usually occurs secondary to CBD stones.

(C) It occurs frequently after choledochoduodenostomy.

(D) It does not occur in patients with cholangiocarcinoma.

(E) It is mainly caused by the liver fluke.

59. A 43-year-old man is admitted with jaundice of 6-week duration. An ultrasound shows multiple small stones in the gallbladder and the presence of a CBD stone. A preoperative ERCP followed by a laparoscopic cholecystectomy is planned. The international normalization ratio (INR) is elevated to 3.1 What is the next step in management?

(A) Infusion of cryoprecipitate

(B) Oral vitamin K tablets to decrease prolonged INR

(C) Parenteral vitamin K to decrease prolonged INR

(D) Demonstration that urobilinogen is increased in the urine

(E) Demonstration that stercobilinogen is increased in the stool

60. A 65-year-old woman is admitted with RUQ pain radiating to the right shoulder, accompanied by nausea and vomiting. Examination reveals tenderness in the RUQ and a positive Murphy's sign. A diagnosis of acute cholecystitis is made. What is the most likely finding?

(A) Serum bilirubin levels may be elevated.

(B) Cholelithiasis is present in 40–60%.

(C) Bacteria are rarely found at operation.

(D) An elevated amylase level excludes this diagnosis.

(E) A contracted gallbladder is noted on ultrasound.

61. A surgeon is removing the gallbladder of a 35-year-old obese man. One week previously the patient had recovered from obstructive jaundice and at operation, numerous small stones are present in the gallbladder. In addition to cholecystectomy, the surgeon should also perform which of the following?

(A) Intraoperative cholangiogram

(B) Liver biopsy

(C) No further treatment

(D) Removal of the head of the pancreas

(E) CBD exploration

62. A 42-year-old man presents with recurrent RUQ pain for 2 years. A sonogram is negative for gallstones, and the CBD is normal. An upper GI endoscopy is also normal, and there is no peptic ulcer disease. Biliary dyskinesia is suspected, and the patient undergoes further evaluation. Which of the following will stimulate contraction of the gallbladder?

(A) Cholecystokinin

(B) Vagal section

(C) Secretin

(D) Epinephrine

(E) Gastrin

63. A 57-year-old previously healthy business executive presents with gradually increasing obstructive jaundice. An ultrasound of the liver shows dilated intrahepatic ducts, but the CBD is normal. An ERCP shows a filling defect at the level of the common hepatic duct. Endoscopic brush biopsies are taken, and histology confirms cholangiocarcinoma. In discussing these findings, the surgeon should inform the patient that

(A) This tumor affects men more commonly than women.

(B) The tumor is a result of gallstones.

(C) The tumor is best treated with a stent to relieve obstructive jaundice.

(D) Weight loss is common in this condition.

(E) The most common location of these tumors is at the ampulla of Vater.

64. A 38-year-old male lawyer develops abdominal pain after having a fatty meal. Examination reveals tenderness in the right hypochondrium and a positive Murphy's sign. Which test is most likely to reveal acute cholecystitis?

(A) HIDA scan
(B) Oral cholecystogram
(C) Intravenous cholangiogram
(D) CT scan of the abdomen
(E) ERCP

65. A 55-year-old white female undergoes a laparoscopic cholecystectomy for symptomatic cholelithiasis. The operation went well, and the patient was discharged home. One week later, she comes to your office for a routine postoperative follow-up. The final pathology report shows an incidental finding of a gallbladder carcinoma confined to the mucosa. In further advising the patient, you should inform her that

(A) She should undergo radiation therapy.
(B) She should undergo right hepatectomy to remove locally infiltrating disease.
(C) She should undergo regional lymphadenectomy.
(D) She requires systemic chemotherapy.
(E) She does not require any further therapy.

66. A 49-year-old man who recovered 7 years ago from acute viral hepatitis develops chronic active hepatitis and liver cirrhosis. He is seen in the office without any abdominal symptoms. An ultrasound reveals cholelithiasis and ascites. What treatment should be instituted?

(A) He should undergo percutaneous dissolution of stones.
(B) He should undergo cholecystectomy.
(C) He should undergo cholecystostomy.
(D) He should be placed on a diet that avoids fatty foods and discouraged from undergoing elective cholecystectomy.
(E) He should be treated with ursodeoxycholic acid.

67. A 48-year-old man is admitted to the hospital with severe abdominal pain, tenderness in the right hypochondrium, and a WBC count of 12,000. A HIDA scan fails to show the gallbladder after 4 hours. Acute cholecystitis is established. After diagnosis, cholecystectomy should be performed within which of the following?

(A) 3–60 minutes
(B) The first 2–3 days following hospital admission
(C) 8 days
(D) 3 weeks
(E) 3 months

68. A 60-year-old diabetic man is admitted to the hospital with a diagnosis of acute cholecystitis. The WBC count is 28,000, and a plain film of the abdomen and CT scan show evidence of intramural gas in the gallbladder. What is the most likely diagnosis?

(A) Emphysematous gallbladder
(B) Acalculous cholecystitis
(C) Cholangiohepatitis
(D) Sclerosing cholangitis
(E) Gallstone ileus

69. A 60-year-old woman is recovering from a major pelvic cancer operation and develops severe abdominal pain and sepsis. Following a positive HIDA scan, laparotomy is performed. The gallbladder is severely inflamed and removed. There is no evidence of gallbladder stones (acalculous cholecystitis). Cholecystectomy is performed. Which is true of acalculous cholecystitis?

(A) It is usually associated with stones in the CBD.
(B) It occurs in 10–20% of cases of cholecystitis.
(C) It has a more favorable prognosis than calculous cholecystitis.
(D) It is increased in frequency after trauma or operation.
(E) It is characterized on HIDA scan by filling of the gallbladder.

70. Following recovery in the hospital from a fracture of the femur, a 70-year-old nursing home female patient develops RUQ abdominal pain and fever. She has tenderness in the right subcostal region. There is evidence of progressive sepsis and hemodynamic instability. The WBC count is 24,000. A bedside sonogram confirms the presence of acalculous cholecystitis. What should treatment involve?

(A) Intravenous antibiotics alone
(B) ERCP
(C) Percutaneous drainage of the gallbladder
(D) Urgent cholecystectomy
(E) Elective cholecystectomy after 3 months

71. In designing a study related to gallbladder function, it should be noted that the healthy gallbladder mucosa selectively absorbs which of the following?

(A) Bile pigment
(B) Bile salts
(C) Cholesterol
(D) Sodium
(E) Free fatty acids

72. On a recent safari in Africa, a 39-year-old male engineer developed an acute diarrhea state requiring hospitalization and treatment with Flagyl. Six weeks after his return, he developed RUQ pain, fever and chills. A chest x-ray showed elevation of the right hemidiaphragm, and sonogram showed a large abscess in the right lobe of the liver.Which of the following statements is TRUE regarding this disease process?

(A) Satisfactory treatment is not readily available.
(B) Diagnosis is easily made by finding *Entamoeba histolytica* in stools in nearly all patients.
(C) Bloody diarrhea is always present.
(D) Anchovy-paste pus is usually present in the abscess cavity.
(E) Extensive surgical drainage is usually indicated.

73. A 45-year-old male is suspected of having an amebic abscess of the liver. Serum bilirubin is mildly elevated. The WBC is 11,000 but there is eosinophilia. The initial line of treatment involves which of the following?

(A) Cortisone
(B) Metronidazole (Flagyl)
(C) Surgical excision
(D) Sulfonamides and penicillin
(E) Colon resection

74. In performing hepatic resection, a knowledge of the different lobes and segments of the liver is mandatory. The right and left lobes of the liver are separated by an imaginary plane (Cantlie's line) that passes between the the inferior vena cava (IVC) and which of the following?

(A) Portal vein
(B) Falciform ligament
(C) Left margin of the quadrate lobe
(D) Gallbladder
(E) Left margin of the caudate lobe

75. A 32-year-old diabetic woman who has taken contraceptive pills for 12 years develops RUQ pain. CT scan of the abdomen reveals a 5-cm hypodense lesion in the right lobe of the liver consistent with a hepatic adenoma. What should the patient be advised to do?

(A) Undergo excision of the adenoma
(B) Stop oral contraceptives only
(C) Stop oral hypoglycemic medication
(D) Undergo right hepatectomy
(E) Have serial CT scans every 6 months

76. A 35-year-old woman is seen in the office with focal nodular hyperplasia. This condition is similar to hepatic adenoma, in that it does what?

(A) Frequently causes symptoms
(B) Tends to lead to liver rupture
(C) LFT and alpha fetoprotein (AFP) are normal
(D) Easily detected by CT scan of the liver
(E) Tends to undergo malignant changes

77. A 64-year-old man has mild upper abdominal pain. On contrast CT scan, a 5-cm lesion in the left lobe of the liver enhances and then decreases over a 10-minute period from without to within. The most likely lesion is which of the following?

    (A) Congenital cyst
    (B) Hemangioma
    (C) Fungal abscess
    (D) Focal nodular hyperplasia
    (E) Hepatic adenoma

78. A 16-year-old previously healthy male fell off his bicycle while riding back home from school. On examination there was mild tenderness in the RUQ. No other abnormality was detected. A sonogram showed a large solitary hypoechogenic cyst in the liver. The LFTs are normal, and there is no family history of cystic disease involving solid organs. What is the most likely cause?

    (A) Fungal abscess
    (B) Trauma
    (C) Developmental
    (D) Neoplastic
    (E) Pyogenic abscess

79. A healthy 64-year-old woman had a cancer of the left colon resected 4 years previously. During follow-up, an increased carcinoembryonic antigen (CEA) level lead to a CT scan of the abdomen, which revealed two discrete lesions in the left lateral lobe of the liver. Liver biopsy confirms that this is metastatic colon cancer. What is the most appropriate plan?

    (A) Inform the patient that there is no treatment, and that her expectation of life is limited.
    (B) Irradiation is recommended.
    (C) Local cauterization of the cancer is recommended.
    (D) Liver resection is recommended.
    (E) Chemotherapy is recommended.

80. A 42-year-old man undergoes a liver transplantation. There is rapid deterioration after the completion of the graft, and the patient dies within 12 hours. What is the most likely cause of death?

    (A) Massive pulmonary embolus
    (B) Graft rejection
    (C) Fat embolus
    (D) Massive hemorrhage
    (E) Subphrenic abscess

81. In discussing the treatment of a 42-year-old man with severe liver cirrhosis, the possibility of heterotopic transplantation is considered. Which statement about heterotopic liver transplantation is TRUE?

    (A) It implies removal of the recipient's liver.
    (B) It is preferable to orthotopic liver transplantation.
    (C) It should be done in the iliac vessels.
    (D) It is rarely associated with long-term survival.
    (E) Heterotopic auxiliary liver transplants require high-out flow pressures.

82. A 43-year-old man develops chronic hepatitis, which was attributed to a complication resulting from multiple blood transfusions for sickle cell anemia. He complains of chronic sweating, palpitation, and hunger attacks. What would be the most likely cause of these symptoms?

    (A) Hepatogenic hypoglycemia
    (B) Hemolytic anemia
    (C) Jaundice
    (D) Spontaneous hyperglycemia
    (E) Elevated bile salts in the blood

83. A 42-year-old man is admitted with bleeding from esophageal varices. Investigation reveals that he has an occlusion of the portal vein. There is no evidence of liver cirrhosis. Which test will most likely reveal an underlying predisposing factor for this condition?

    (A) Hepatitis screening
    (B) Isoamylase
    (C) Intravenous pyelogram to exclude hydronephrosis
    (D) Coagulation tests to include antithrombin III
    (E) CT of abdomen

84. A 9-year-old girl had multiple episodes of upper GI bleeding. Contrast enhanced CT scan showed multiple cavernous malformation surrounding the portal vein (Fig. 7–2). She is admitted with severe hematemesis and melena. At birth, she had developed an infection around the umbilicus. What is the most likely site of bleeding?

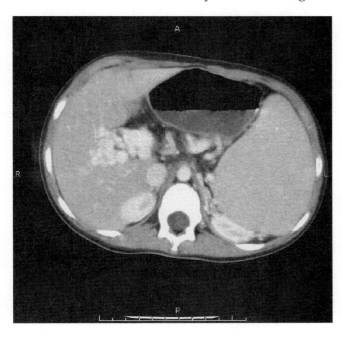

Figure 7–2.
Following portal vein thrombosis, massive cavernous malformations around the portal vein is demonstrated. Note large spleen.

(A) Meckel's diverticulum
(B) Esophageal varices
(C) Peptic ulcer
(D) Duodenal varices
(E) Mallory-Weiss tear of the lower end of the esophagus

85. A 49-year-old man with a history of cirrhosis is admitted with significant hematemesis. There is jaundice and clubbing of the fingers. His extremities are cold and clammy, and the systolic blood pressure drops to 84 mm Hg. The initial step in the management is to proceed with which of the following?

(A) Urgent endoscopy and sclerotherapy
(B) Sengstaken-Blakemore tube
(C) Infusion of intravenous crystalloids
(D) Intravenous pitressin
(E) Surgery to stop bleeding

86. A 42-year-old woman with a known history of esophageal varices secondary to hepatitis and cirrhosis is admitted with severe hematemesis from esophageal varices. Bleeding persists after pitressin therapy. What would the next step in management involve?

(A) Emergency portacaval shunt
(B) Emergency lienorenal shunt
(C) Insertion of Sengstaken-Blakemore tube
(D) Vagotomy
(E) Transjugular intrahepatic portasystemic shunt (TIPS)

87. A 12-year-old boy who underwent a previous splenectomy for thalassemia presents to the emergency room with fever, chills, and septic shock. The parents give a history of seemingly minor sore throat, which started only a few hours previously. The child is hypotensive and appears moribund. A diagnosis of overwhelming postsplenectomy infection (OPSI) is made. Which of the following statements about OPSI is TRUE?

(A) The condition is more common in children.
(B) The condition is more common after splenectomy for trauma.
(C) Prophylactic antibiotics have not been shown to improve outcome in children.
(D) Prophylactic vaccination against *Enterococcus* should be performed.
(E) The condition is very common after splenectomy.

88. A 43-year-old man with chronic hepatitis and liver cirrhosis is admitted with upper GI bleeding. He has marked ascites and shows multiple telangiectasias, liver palmar erythema, and clubbing. A diagnosis of bleeding esophageal varices secondary to portal hypertension is made. Portal pressure is considered elevated when it is above which of the following?

    (A) 0.15 mm Hg
    (B) 1.5 mm Hg
    (C) 12 mm Hg
    (D) 40 mm Hg
    (E) 105 mm Hg

89. A 23-year-old male college student has a history of liver cirrhosis due to Kimmelstiel-Wilson syndrome (abnormality in copper metabolism). He should be treated with which of the following?

    (A) Penicillamine as soon as the diagnosis is established
    (B) Penicillamine after variceal bleeding has occurred
    (C) A portocaval shunt
    (D) Sclerosis of the esophageal varices as a prophylactic measure
    (E) Splenorenal shunt

90. A 24-year-old woman presents with menorrhagia, an easy tendency toward bruising, and a history of prolonged bleeding after extraction of an impacted molar several years previously. A diagnosis of idiopathic thrombocytopenic purpura (ITP) is made after appropriate investigations. Her disease has failed to respond to steroid and immunoglobin therapy. She is scheduled to undergo splenectomy in 1 week, but her platelet count is 22,000. What should be the treatment of choice?

    (A) She should be given platelets daily and be scheduled for splenectomy when her platelet count is more than 75,000.
    (B) She should undergo bone marrow transplantation.
    (C) She should be treated with steroids only, and the operation should be canceled.

    (D) She should receive transfusion with 3 U of packed cells.
    (E) She should not be given platelets routinely before surgery.

91. Following a successful splenectomy, for thrombocytopenia, a 24-year-old patient notes that she was no longer prone to excessive bleeding. Her platelet count had become elevated. However, 2 years later, she developed further skin purpura, and her platelet count was reduced to 45,000. What should she undergo?

    (A) Radioactive technetium (^{99m}Tc) scan to see if a splenunculus is present
    (B) Radioactive (I^{135}) to see if a splenunculus is present
    (C) Exploratory laparotomy
    (D) Platelet transfusion
    (E) Red blood cell (RBC) fragility test

92. A 28-year-old woman is diagnosed with TTP. In addition to purpura and thrombocytopenia, studies will show which of the following?

    (A) Normal arterioles on biopsy of the spleen
    (B) Absence of infarction on biopsy of the spleen
    (C) Leukopenia
    (D) Elevated urea and creatinine levels
    (E) Suppression of reticulocytes

93. A 24-year-old African American man has sickle cell disease. He is admitted to the hospital because of a sickle cell crisis. His hemoglobin is 10 g/dL, and he complains of pain in the lower chest wall and legs. His further course of management should include which of the following?

    (A) Emergency splenectomy
    (B) Elective splenectomy
    (C) Admission to the hospital for hydration and given dehydromorphine as required
    (D) Administer steroids
    (E) Exchange transfusions to keep his hemoglobin at a normal level

94. A 24-year-old woman from the Caribbean is admitted to the hospital for severe lower chest and upper abdominal pain. Her hemoglobin is 9 g/dL. The findings on ultrasound of the abdomen and chest x-ray are normal. Her father has sickle cell disease. For her physician to establish the diagnosis of sickle cell trait or disease, she must undergo which procedure?

(A) A bone marrow study

(B) Injection of radioactive RBCs

(C) Red cell fragility studies

(D) Studies to determine her response to erythropoietin

(E) Blood smear and electrophoresis

95. Splenectomy is often indicated in the management of which of the following?

(A) Hereditary spherocytosis

(B) Hereditary neurofibromatosis

(C) Aplastic anemia

(D) Pheochromocytoma

(E) Hashimoto's disease

96. A 2-year-old African-American boy is diagnosed as having hereditary spherocytosis. His parents should be informed that this condition is which of the following?

(A) It is not associated with a marked increase in gallstones.

(B) It is transmitted as a recessive trait.

(C) It is diagnosed by showing RBCs undergo lysis at a higher osmotic pressure.

(D) It is characterized by a low reticulocyte count.

(E) It is infrequently treated by splenectomy.

97. A 67-year-old man is admitted to hospital with a diagnosis of polycythemia vera. He has considerable back pain and is diagnosed as having myeloid metaplasia. This condition is characterized by which of the following?

(A) Decrease of the connective tissue in the spleen

(B) Decrease in the blood elements of the spleen

(C) Aplastic anemia

(D) Deterioration after splenectomy

(E) A favorable response to alkylating agents

98. A 24-year-old woman with rheumatoid arthritis involving the sacroiliac joint and fingers is noted to have splenomegaly and neutropenia (Felty's syndrome). She is advised to have splenectomy, but she should be informed that

(A) Large-joint disease symptoms will lessen.

(B) Small-joint disease symptoms will lessen.

(C) Neutropenia responds to splenectomy.

(D) The joint symptoms will become worse.

(E) All symptoms will lessen.

99. A 10-year-old boy is hit by a truck while riding his bicycle home from school. A CT scan shows a tear of the spleen. His hematocrit is 32%, and he is in pain, although fully alert and oriented. His blood pressure is 110/60 mm Hg, and his heart rate is 104 bpm. The next step in management should be which of the following?

(A) Cross-match blood and transfuse appropriately

(B) Perform splenectomy as soon as possible

(C) Perform laparotomy, and suture the tear where possible

(D) Perform angiographic embolization of the spleen

(E) Avoid surgery, even if bleeding continues profusely after transfusion

Answers and Explanations

1. **(B)** Annular pancreas is a congenital anomaly; a band of pancreatic tissue encircles the second part of the duodenum. Annular pancreas is associated with Down syndrome as well as duodenal stenosis or atresia. Duodenojejunostomy and gastrojejunostomy are acceptable treatments. Resection is not an acceptable choice due to the high incidence of fistula In adults, annular pancreas usually presents with abdominal pain, nausea, and vomiting.

2. **(E)** The patient has three Ranson's criteria at the time of admission. The expected mortality rate is 15% with 3–4 Ranson's criteria. Amylase and lipase levels are not prognostic factors in acute pancreatitis. Calcium level <8 mg/dL within the first 48 hours is one of Ranson's criteria, as is arterial PO_2 <60 mm Hg.

3. **(B)** Most gallbladder injuries are associated with other injuries, most often to the liver, large intestine, and/or small intestine. Isolated gallbladder injuries are rare. A gallbladder injury can be treated with cholecystectomy or cholecystostomy. A nonbleeding liver laceration does not need further treatment. A careful search for injuries should be made during laparotomy.

4. **(C)** Choledochal cysts can involve the intrahepatic and/or extrahepatic biliary tree (see Fig. 7–3 for classification). Choledochal cysts present more commonly in infants and children, but may present in adults. They are more common in females. The classic triad of jaundice, RUQ mass and abdominal pain is found in less than a third of patients. There is an association between choledochal cysts and hepatobiliary cancers, most commonly cholangiocarcinoma. For most

types of choledochal cyst, excision of the cyst with a Roux-en-Y biliary enteric anastomosis is recommended. Laparoscopic cholecystectomy alone is not sufficient.

5. **(E)** An upper GI series would not visualize the cyst. Ultrasound may diagnose a choledochal cyst, showing size and location, but is not always diagnostic. CAT scan and MRCP can show size, location, and extent of disease. ERCP visualizes the distal duct anatomy well, while PTC is better at visualizing the proximal ductal anatomy.

6. **(C)** The intraoperative cholangiogram is suggestive of a CBD stone. Normal LFTs do not rule out choledocholithiasis. Patients with choledocholithiasis often have dilatation of the CBD on ultrasound; the stones may be visualized, but a normal ultrasound does not rule out CBD stones. A HIDA scan is unlikely to be helpful. An exploration of the CBD is indicated (either laparoscopically or open) along with a cholecystectomy.

7. **(A)** Gallstone ileus usually results from formation of a cholecystoenteric fistula and is seen more often in elderly patients. Obstruction occurs most often at the terminal ileum. Treatment is laparotomy and removal of the stone through an enterotomy proximal to the obstruction; cholecystectomy should be done if the patient can tolerate the additional surgery.

8. **(D)** Hemobilia should be suspected in a patient with a history of liver trauma who later develops GI bleeding and abdominal pain. Hemobilia usually appears weeks after the injury; pain is often intermittent and melena or hematemesis may occur. In this case, the injury is the result of

Type I   Type II   Type III

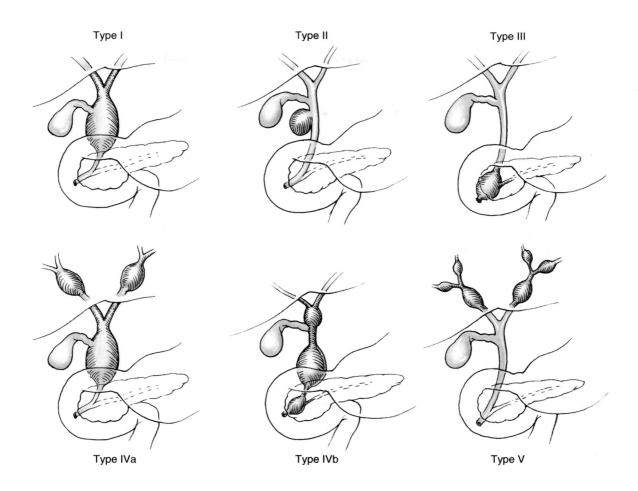

Type IVa   Type IVb   Type V

Figure 7–3.
Classification of choledochal cysts. Type I, fusiform or cystic dilations of the extrahepatic biliary tree, are the most common type, making up over 50% of all choledochal cysts. Type II, saccular diverticulum of an extrahepatic bile duct, is rare, comprising <5% of choledochal cysts. Type III, bile duct dilations within the duodenal wall (choledochoceles), make up about 5% of choledochal cysts. Types IVa and IVb, multiple cysts, make up 5–10% of choledochal cysts. Type IVa affects both extrahepatic and intrahepatic bile ducts, while type IVb cysts affect the extrahepatic bile ducts only. Type V, intrahepatic biliary cysts, are very rare and make up only about 1% of choledochal cysts. *(Reproduced, with permission, from Brunicardi FC et al.: Schwartz's Principles of Surgery, 8th ed. 1210. McGraw-Hill, 2005.)*

the melena and hematemesis may occur. In this case, the injury is the result of the biopsy. The other diseases listed are less likely to explain all of the findings listed.

9. **(C)** Once again hemobilia should be suspected, with the history of trauma to the liver and guaiac positive stools and RUQ abdominal pain. Angiography can be diagnostic as well as therapeutic. The source of bleeding can be identified and embolized. Ultrasound is unlikely to identify the bleeding source; it would identify cholelithiasis or a liver tumor. A CAT scan likewise would identify a tumor. A HIDA scan documents patency of the cystic duct and would not be useful in this case. Laparoscopy would be unlikely to identify the communication between a hepatic vessel and the biliary tree.

10. **(E)** Tru-cut needle liver biopsy allows pathologic diagnosis of liver lesions. Needle biopsy is contraindicated if hemangioma is suspected and in adenomas, because of the risk of bleeding. Other potential complications of percutaneous needle biopsy are pain, pneumothorax, and bile peritonitis. Needle biopsy can diagnose posthepatic and postnecrotic cirrhosis, malignant tumors, and hepatitis, and can determine the need for treatment in hepatitis C.

11. **(D)** Pringle's maneuver is occlusion of the porta hepatis. The portal vein, hepatic artery, and the CBD are the structures of the porta hepatis.

12. **(D)** Hepatitis B vaccine is made from genetically engineered hepatitis B surface antigen particles. Vaccination produces hepatitis B surface antibodies but not hepatitis B core antibodies. Hepatitis B surface antigen will not be present.

13. **(B)** A laceration to the parenchyma of the spleen 1–3 cm deep is a class II injury. A class I injury is a nonexpanding subcapsular hematoma involving less than 10% of the surface area of the spleen. Nonoperative management may be attempted for both of these injuries. This patient is hemodynamically stable and does not require emergency laparotomy. A class III injury is a major parenchymal injury. Prophylactic transfusion is not indicated. Delayed splenic rupture may occur within 2 weeks or more of a blunt splenic injury in 10–15% of patients.

14. **(E)** Staging of Hodgkin's disease is often done nonoperatively. Staging laparotomy consists of wedge biopsy of the liver, splenectomy, examination and biopsy of peraortic lymph nodes, as well as biopsy of mesenteric and hepatoduodenal nodes. Stage I Hodgkin's lymphoma is limited to one anatomic area, while Stage II involves 2 or more areas of the same side of the diaphram. Stage III disease involves both sides of the diaphram limited to lymph nodes, Waldyer's ring or the spleen. Stage IV disease involves organs other than lymph nodes, Waldyer's ring, or the spleen. Splenectomy may improve thrombocytopenia and allow chemotherapy to be administered.

15. **(A)** WDHA or vasoactive intestinal polypeptide (VIPoma) is characterized by voluminous diarrhea, 5 L or more daily, rich in potassium, which looks like watery tea. The diarrhea is secretory and if refractory to antidiarrheal agents. Patients are weak, with metabolic acidosis and hypokalemia. Octreotide decreases diarrhea volume. The pancreatic tumor should be excised. Secretory diarrhea also occurs in some patients with Zolliger-Ellison syndrome (ZES), and is the only complaint in less than 10% of ZES patients.

More than 90% of ZES patients have peptic ulcer disease. Unlike the diarrhea associated with ZES, the diarrhea of WHDA continues with fasting and continuous nasogastric tub suctioning. 15% of patients with glucagonoma have diarrhea; glucagonoma is associated with migratory necrotizing dermatitis.

16. **(C)** Gastrinoma, or Zollinger-Ellison syndrome, should be suspected in patients with peptic ulcer disease refractory to medical treatment, or in patients with multiple ulcers or ulcers in uncommon locations. Gastrin secretion by the tumor, most commonly found in the pancreas, results in hypersecretion of gastric acid. Common patient complaints are epigastric pain, melena, hematemesis, diarrhea, and weight loss. ZES may occur as part of the MEN-1 syndrome; this patient presents with only atypical peptic ulcer disease. The treatment of choice involves the identification and resection of the gastrinoma. Preoperative treatment may include treatment of the ulcers with omeprazole.

17. **(B)** Multiple endocrine neoplasia syndrome type 1 (MEN-1, or Werner's syndrome), and autosomal dominant disorder, involves tumors or hyperplasia of two or more glands, most commonly parathyroid, pancreas, and pituitary glands. Hyperparathyroidism is most common, followed by various pancreatic isle cell tumors and pituitary adenomas. MEN-2A (Sipple's syndrome) consists of pheochromocytoma, medullary carcinoma of the thyroid, and often hyperparathyroidism. MEN-2B is characterized by medullary carcinoma of the thyroid, pheochromocytoma, neuromas, and marfinoid body habitus. MEN 2-A and 2-B are also autosomal dominant.

18. **(B)** Hereditary spherocytosis is the most common symptomatic familial hemolytic anemia, and is transmitted as an autosomal dominant trait. A defect in the red cell membrane causes increased trapping in the spleen and hemolysis. Anemia, jaundice, and splenomegaly are clinical findings. Splenectomy is the only treatment. Thalassemia is transmitted as a dominant trait; anemia is the result of a defect in hemoglobin synthesis. Thalassemia major, or

homozygous thalassemia, is associated with anemia, icterus, splenomegaly, and early death. Transfusions are usually required. Splenectomy may reduce hemoloysis and transfusion requirements. Sickle cell anemia is hereditary hemolytic anemia. Serum bilirubin may be mildly elevated. Splenomegaly often precedes autoinfraction. Splenectomy may be indicated for chronic hypersplenism or acute splenic sequestration.

19. **(A)** In thalassemia, intracellular hemoglobin precipitates, or Heinz bodies, damage red cells and contribute to early destruction. Cells are small, thin, misshapen, and resistant to osmotic lysis. Diagnosis is made by peripheral smear. Nucleated red cells, or target cells, are present. Distorted red cells, or target cells, are present. Distorted red cells of different shapes and sizes are found. In sickle cell disease, characteristic sickle cells are seen on peripheral smear. In hereditary spherocytosis, the peripheral smear shows small, thick, nearly spherical red cells. Cells have increased osmotic fragility.

20. **(E)** The triad of rheumatoid arthritis, splenomegaly, and neutropenia is known as Felty's syndrome. Gastic achlorhydria is common. Thrombocytopenia and mild anemia are sometimes seen. Splenectomy is sometimes used to treat the neutopenia in patients with serious infections, anemia requiring transfusions, or severe thrombocytopenia.

21. **(E)** Breast cancer commonly metastasizes to bone, lung, soft tissues, liver, and brain. The patient should be worked up for local recurrence as well as other distant metastasis. The presence of masses in the liver should lead to the diagnosis of metastatic cancer.

22. **(A)** Benign liver cysts can be single or multiple. Solitary nonparasitic cysts usually contain clear, watery fluid. These cysts are more common in the right lobe. They are most likely congenital and most are asymptomatic; many are found incidentally. An anechoic area on ultrasound is suggestive. Hydatid cysts, caused by *Echinococcus*, are also more common in the right lobe. The colorless fluid in the cyst is under high pressure, unlike parasitic cysts. Ultrasound will show internal echoes. Hemangiomas can have a variable echogenic pattern on ultrasound; focal nodular hyperplasia is often hypodense. Hepatocellular carcinoma and metastasis have a characteristic sonographic appearance different from benign nonparasitic cysts.

23. **(C)** Ranson's criteria allow for early identification of patients who have severe pancreatitis. Mortality increases with increasing number of Ranson's criteria score. The five criteria of poor prognosis at the time of admission are age >55, WBC >16,000, blood glucose >200 mg/dL, AST >250, LDH >350. During the following 48 hours, six additional criteria may develop. These include hypoxemia with arterial PO_2 <60 mm on room air, base deficit >4, fluid requirement >6 L, hematocrit fall >10%, blood urea nitrogen (BUN) increase >8 mg/dL, and serum Ca <8 mg/dL. Amylase and lipase elevation may focus attention on the appropriate diagnosis, but amylase levels fail to correlate with prognosis

24. **(A)** Pseudocysts frequently are encountered on ultrasound examination early after an acute attack of pancreatitis. In most cases, the pseudocyst resolves, but if it enlarges, it may compress the stomach anteriorly. An enlarging pseudocyst is an indication to attempt percutaneous drainage. If percutaneous drainage is unsuccessful, internal drainage into the stomach should be performed at an appropriate interval to allow the pseudocyst wall to mature (Fig. 7–4).

25. **(B)** In pancreatitis, the serum amylase level may be normal. The causes include: (a) hyperlipidemia, which interferes with chemical determination of amylase; (b) increased urinary excretion of amylase; and (c) near complete destruction of pancreatic parenchyma as a result of chronic pancreatitis. On the other hand, the serum amylase level may be elevated in the absence of pancreatitis (for example, perforated peptic ulcer, gangrenous cholecystitis, small-bowel strangulation or chronic renal failure.)

26. **(C)** If a large pseudocyst is present, it may cause displacement of the transverse colon, duodenum, or stomach (anteriorly). Other radiologic signs in pancreatitis include pseudocyst on

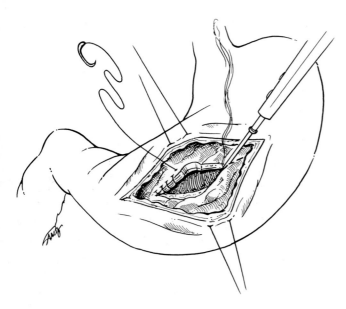

Figure 7–4.
After cyst evacuation, the opening is enlarged to 3- to 4-cm diameter. Adherent posterior gastric and anterior cyst wall is sewn with nonabsorbable suture. *(Reproduced with permission, from Maingot's Abdominal Operations, 10th ed. 2023. Appleton & Lange, 1996.)*

ultrasound or CT scan, downward displacement of transverse colon, dilated pancreatic duct on pancreatogram, and smooth tapering of the CBD on cholangiogram (if the head of the pancreas is diseased). The irregular tapering of the common duct is suggestive of neoplasm. The looping of the colon in the RUQ is seen with sigmoid volvulus.

27. **(E)** True epithelial-lined cysts in the pancreas are extremely rare. They should not be confused with the more common pseudocyst (no epithelial lining), benign cystadenoma, or malignant cystadenoma of the pancreas. Pseudocysts are more common in men, but cystadenocarcinoma occurs more frequently in women.

28. **(A)** The presence of an epigastric mass 2–3 weeks after the onset of acute pancreatitis strongly favors a pancreatic pseudocyst. The history of alcoholism points to pancreatitis as a possible etiologic factor in the differential diagnosis. Pseudocysts develop in 10% of patients following acute pancreatitis. Most of these, however, resolve spontaneously. They may also develop in patients with chronic pancreatitis or after pancreatic trauma.

29. **(B)** Fibrosis in the head of the pancreas as a result of chronic inflammation may lead to compression of the CBD. In pancreatitis, the narrowing of the CBD is smooth on x-ray studies. There is no association with pancreatitis and sclerosing cholangitis. Alcoholic hepatitis is the most common cause of jaundice, but it most frequently is not of an obstructive nature. Pseudocysts and carcinoma of the head of the pancreas are other recognized causes of obstructive jaundice in patients with chronic pancreatitis.

30. **(B)** The passage of small stones through Vater's ampulla often results in pancreatitis. It is important to perform cholecystectomy after pancreatitis has subsided but during the same hospital stay in patients with documented gallstone pancreatitis (to avoid recurrence of symptoms). Smooth tapering of the common duct is usually seen with stones obstructing the common duct. Pancreatic intraductal calcification is consistent with chronic pancreatitis, and air in the biliary tree is consistent with gallstone ileus.

31. **(A)** A recent increase in alcohol consumption explains the jaundice secondary to alcoholic hepatitis in the majority of such patients. Carcinoma of the pancreas is relatively rare but often causes difficulty in the differentiation from pancreatitis. A pseudocyst measuring 4 cm is not likely to be associated with nonobstructive jaundice in this patient.

32. **(D)** Patients who develop acute pancreatitis as a result of cholelithiasis should have gallbladder surgery performed during the same hospital stay to avoid recurrence. An assessment of the bile ducts should be performed either preoperatively or intraoperatively after the resolution of the pancreatitis. Elective cholecystectomy should be avoided during the actual phase of pancreatitis.

33. **(D)** Because of its protected retroperitoneal location, pancreatic injury occurs with deep penetrating wounds or with significant blunt trauma to upper abdomen. Blunt trauma accounts for less than 20–30% of all pancreatic injuries. The most common site of injury is at the neck of the pancreas where the pancreatic tissue is compressed against the spine.

Associated visceral and vascular injuries occur commonly and together with the delay in diagnosis account for the high morbidity and mortality. Fistulae, pseudocyst, infection, and secondary (delayed) hemorrhage are common complications. Pancreatic injuries frequently are overlooked initially, and their detection requires a high index of suspicion. Elevation of amylase after trauma is nonspecific.

34. **(A)** If the pancreatic duct is dilated and symptoms persist, a longitudinal pancreaticojejunostomy (Puestow) is performed (Fig. 7–5). In this operation, the pancreatic duct is slit open and anastomosed side-to-side to the cut end of the divided jejunum with a Roux-en-Y anastomosis. Resection of the pancreas is reserved for patients without a dilated duct (<6 mm). In these cases, a distal pancreatectomy is performed when the disease primarily involves the body and tail of the pancreas; whereas, a

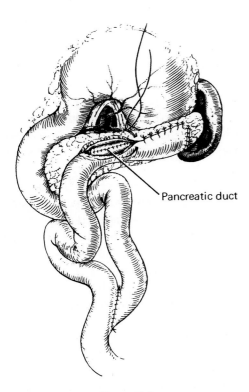

Figure 7–5.
Lateral pancreaticojejunostomy (Puestow) for chronic pancreatitus. (*Reproduced, with permission, from Doherty GM: Current Surgical Diagnosis and Treatment, 12th ed. 618. McGraw-Hill, 2006.*)

Whipple operation is performed when the disease is confined to the head.

35. **(A)** Atelectasis is partly due to a factor released from the pancreas that alters pulmonary surfactant. The other conditions listed are not specifically related to pancreatitis.

36. **(E)** Most insulinomas are small (<2 cm), solitary, and benign. Therefore, simple enucleation is adequate. Less than 10% of cases are malignant and require resection in the form of either pancreaticoduodenectomy or distal pancreatectomy (depending upon the location of the tumor). Ten percent of insulinomas are associated with MEN I syndrome, and in these cases, the tumors are multiple. Partial pancreatic resection may be required for these patients. Total pancreatectomy is almost never required for the removal of insulinomas. Somatostatin receptors are not always present on insulinoma cells, and, therefore, SRS is less useful for localization of this tumor.

37. **(A)** Carcinoma of the head of the pancreas is treated with radical excision of the head of the pancreas along with the duodenum. Continuity of the biliary and GI tract is established by performing hepaticojejunostomy, pancreaticojejunostomy, and gastrojejunostomy (Fig. 7–6). The 5-year survival rate is higher for periampullary carcinoma (30%) than that for pancreatic head lesions (10%). Most centers do not give irradiation routinely before or after surgery, because pancreatic cancers do not respond well to radiotherapy. Endoscopically placed stents alone are used only in palliative circumstances in patients with limited life expectancy.

38. **(E)** Cancer of the head of the pancreas is the most common cause of obstructive jaundice. In cholangiocarcinoma of the common hepatic duct, the gallbladder will be empty and not distended. Anemia may occur as a result of bleeding into the duodenum in periampullary cancer, but this is relatively rare. Carcinoma of the gallbladder results in jaundice only after the tumor invades the adjacent biliary tree.

39. **(D)** The characteristic features of insulinomas include: (a) hypoglycemic symptoms; (b)

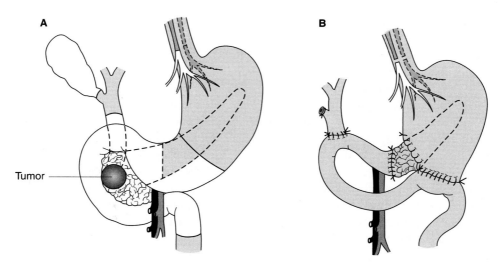

Figure 7–6.
Pancreaticoduodenectomy (Whipple procedure). **A:** Preoperative anatomic relationships showing a tumor in the head of the pancreas. **B:** Postoperative reconstruction showing pancreatic, biliary, and gastric anastomoses. A cholecystectomy and bilateral truncal vagotomy are also part of the procedure. In many cases, the distal stomach and pylorus can be preserved, and vagotomy is then unnecessary. *(Reproduced, with permission, from Doherty GM: Current Surgical Diagnosis and Treatment, 12th ed. 623. McGraw-Hill, 2006.)*

blood glucose <50 mg/dL during the symptomatic episodes; and (c) relief of symptoms by intravenous injection of glucose (Whipple's triad). Diagnosis is confirmed by demonstration of fasting hypoglycemia in the presence of inappropriately elevated levels of insulin in the blood. A ratio of plasma insulin/glucose >0.3 is diagnostic. Circulating levels of C-peptide are usually elevated in patients with insulinoma but not in patients with such other causes of hypoglycemia as tumors of mesenchymal origin and liver tumors. Patients who surreptitiously administer insulin develop insulin antibodies.

40. (B) VIP producing tumors (VIPomas) are usually malignant, although benign tumors and hyperplasia may also occur. Increase of VIP results in the WDHA syndrome. Diarrhea is severe and results in fluid and electrolyte disturbances. Treatment is directed to removal of the pancreatic tumor. Gastrinoma is more common but is associated with increased gastrin level in the blood.

41. (B) Secretin releases fluid rich mainly in electrolytes and bicarbonate. Both cholecystokinin and vagal stimulation result in fluid with a high content of enzymes. Among the pancreatic enzymes, amylase and lipase are released in their active forms; whereas, the proteolytic enzymes (trypsinogen, chymotrypsinogen) are secreted as inactive zymogens. Their activation occurs in the duodenum, where the zymogens are exposed to enterokinase.

42. (D) Zollinger-Ellison syndrome is caused by secretion of excessive amounts of gastrin by islet cells of the pancreas (gastrinoma). It should always be thought of in patients with peptic ulcer disease, whose ulcers are severe, refractory to management, recurrent or located distally, beyond the first part of the duodenum. Gastrin levels in the blood are increased markedly and can be raised further by secretin injection (paradoxical response). The source of gastrin level in the blood may arise from hyperplasia, adenoma, or most commonly carcinoma of the islets. Most gastrinomas are sporadic, but 25% of patients have a family history of multiple endocrine neoplasia.

43. (C) Because most gastrinomas are small, preoperative localization of the tumor may be difficult. A nuclear scan may be performed using radiolabeled somatostatin (octreotide) analogue. This binds with the somatostatin receptors present on the gastrin-producing cells which identifies the tumor. Endoscopic (not transcutaneous) ultrasound is also useful in localizing these lesions in the pancreas and in the duodenum. The combined accuracy of SRS and endoscopic ultrasound in preoperative localization of gastrinomas is 93%.

44. **(C)** Patients with biliary dyskinesia present with typical symptoms of gallstone disease, but investigations fail to reveal cholelithiasis or choledocholithiasis. Ironically, many patients will have undergone cholecystectomy for incidentally found gallstones but without relief of pain. ERCP with measurement of sphincter pressure will reveal basal sphincter pressure above 40 cm of water. Calcium channel blockers may be tried initially to relieve the spasm of the sphincter of Oddi, but many patients will require an endoscopic sphincterotomy.

45. **(D)** Lactescent serum is sometimes seen soon after an acute attack of pancreatitis. Lipase level should be elevated to show pancreatitis as the cause of the abdominal pain. Hypertriglyceridemia artificially lowers serum amylase levels. If the blood specimen appears milky, the serum should be diluted; after dilution, serum amylase levels may become elevated. Other uncommon causes of pancreatitis include steroids, thiazide diuretics, lasix, sulfonamides, protein deficiency, hypercalcemia, familial, traumatic, idiopathic, and anatomic anomalies such as stricture, or pancreas divisum of the pancreatic duct.

46. **(A)** The gallbladder is enlarged (Courvoisier's sign) in most cases of obstructive jaundice attributable to malignancy. In obstructive jaundice attributable to gallstones, the gallbladder is usually shrunken, owing to the previous inflammatory condition affecting the gallbladder.

47. **(A)** Alkaline phosphatase level usually is more sensitive than the bilirubin level for indicating cholestatic jaundice. It also is more likely to fall before the bilirubin level when the obstruction has been relieved. If an unexplained alkaline phosphatase elevation exists (even in the presence of a normal bilirubin), biliary pathology must be excluded. Elevation of the alkaline phosphatase from a possible source in bone disease can be excluded by measuring isoenzymes.

48. **(C)** Oriental cholangiohepatitis is thought to be caused by the Chinese liver fluke (*C. sinensis*). It is encountered mainly in China (Canton) and Hong Kong, and among Chinese who have emigrated elsewhere. There are multiple strictures in the biliary tree, and the intrahepatic ducts are dilated. Secondary infection supervenes. Schistosomiasis causes liver fibrosis, ameba causes liver abscess. *Echinococcus*, causes hydatid liver cysts, and hookworm causes anemia.

49. **(B)** Sclerosing cholangitis is rare and occurs mainly in the third and fourth decades of life. Unlike most autoimmune disorders, it affects men more commonly. It may occur without any other abnormal pathology or may be associated with ulcerative colitis or retroperitoneal fibrosis. The CBD is converted to a thickened cord whose lumen is almost completely obliterated. The prognosis is guarded, and the mean survival is only 5–6 years.

50. **(D)** The patient described has the features of Charcot's triad-jaundice, abdominal pain, and rigors, which indicates the presence of ascending cholangitis in a patient with obstructive jaundice. The patient should be treated with broad spectrum IV antibiotics and undergo ERCP, sphincterotomy, and stone extraction. If this fails, surgical exploration of the CBD will be required.

51. **(D)** If a stone is detected, the T tube should be left in place for 6 weeks to allow the tract to mature. At this time, the T tube can be removed, and the stone can be extracted by using a Dormia basket under fluoroscopy. This approach is indicated only when a T-tube larger than 16 has been inserted. If this approach is not feasible, the stone can be extracted by retrograde endoscopic techniques or CBD exploration.

52. **(B)** In the presence of previous gallbladder surgery, the possibility of cholestatic jaundice must be excluded. Elevation of alkaline phosphatase (with normal or elevated bilirubin level) strongly supports this diagnosis. The dark urine

results from increase in conjugated bilirubin (regurgitated jaundice). Urobilin is excreted in the urine in hepatocellular jaundice but is absent in the urine in obstructive jaundice, because this pigment forms only if bile reaches the small intestine.

53. **(C)** A HIDA scan will show excretion of the radiolabeled isotope into the biliary tree, but there will be no flow into the duodenum, indicating that the biliary-enteric anastomosis is occluded. If an upper GI study with barium is performed, visualization of the common bile duct would indicate patency of the choledocho-duodenal anastomosis.

54. **(B)** Gram-negative bacilli including *E. coli*, *Klebsiella*, and *Proteus* are the organisms most commonly involved in ascending cholangitis. Anaerobic bacteroids should also be excluded, especially in elderly patients. Intravenous hydration and early institution of appropriate antibiotics is indicated. The antibiotics selected should be effective against the isolated organisms. Combined therapy with an aminoglycoside, penicillin, and an antibiotic targeted specifically against anaerobic organisms should be administered initially until blood culture results are available.

55. **(C)** Multiple stones were present in the CBD at the previous operation. During exploration of the CBD, most stones can be removed by using Desjardin's forceps or under direct vision using a choledochoscope and Dormia basket. However, if there are multiple stones impacted in the lower part of the CBD, a drainage procedure may be indicated. The CBD must be dilated before considering performing a choledochoduodenostomy at the time of gallbladder surgery (Fig. 7–7). If a stone is present in a dilated CBD after previous cholecystectomy, a choledochoduodenostomy is performed, because the rate of recurrent jaundice is high (>20%). Alternatively ERCP and sphincterotomy could be considered.

56. **(D)** The cystic artery courses through the triangle of Calot. The identification of the triangle is therefore important in the performance of a cholecystectomy.

57. **(B)** Pruritus occurs frequently in untreated obstructive jaundice. Bile salt elevation is a possible cause of pruritus. Patients with generalized pruritus should have alkaline phosphatase levels determined; if levels are elevated, the possibility of cholestatic jaundice should be considered. Bilirubin is not always elevated in obstructive jaundice.

58. **(B)** Any obstruction to the biliary tree (stones and benign, malignant, or anastomotic strictures) can lead to infection and cholangitis. It may also occur after trauma to the biliary tree. In ascending cholangitis, there is fever, jaundice, and rigors (Charcot's triad). Suppurative cholangitis is suspected when additional signs of deterioration in mental status and hypotension are present in addition (Reynold's pentad). This entity requires immediate biliary decompression either endoscopically or surgically. *C. sinensis*, the liver fluke, causes suppurative cholangitis in the Far East.

59. **(C)** Vitamin K requires bile salts for efficient absorption from the gut, as do the other fat-soluble vitamins—A, D, and E. Therefore, the oral route is not suitable to administer patients with obstructive jaundice. If intramuscular vitamin K is given, correction will occur if there has been no hepatocellular damage. When emergency surgery is required in this circumstance, the coagulation defect due to hepatic disease may be corrected with fresh-frozen plasma (FFP). Urobilinogen usually is absent in the urine in obstructive jaundice, because its presence depends on a patent biliary–enteric circulation. Stercobilinogen will be absent in fecal examination.

60. **(A)** Stones are found in the gallbladder in over 90% of patients with cholecystitis. Bacteria are cultured in bile in about half the patients undergoing surgery; however, many patients have previously received antibiotics. The gallbladder is usually distended in patients with acute cholecystitis but contracted in chronic cholecystitis.

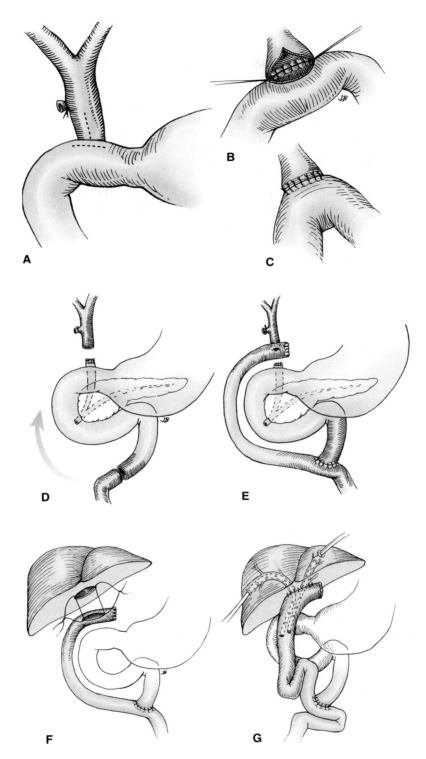

Figure 7–7.
Treatment for invasive gallbladder cancer is cholecystectomy and a wedge resection of the liver along with a regional lymphadenectomy. The wedge resection of the liver is illustrated. Segments 4 and 5 together with the lymph node regions should be removed. *(Reproduced, with permission, from Greenfield: Surgery: Scientific Principles & Practice, 2nd ed. 957. Lippincott, 1996.)*

61. **(A)** If there is a recent history of jaundice, although the CBD is not dilated, intraoperative cholangiography must be performed to exclude CBD stones. Other indications for intraoperative cholangiogram include a recent history of ascending cholangitis, dilated CBD on preoperative sonogram, or suspicion of a "missing" stone in the gallbladder (i.e., as detected by ultrasound or other observations). Elevated bilirubin and alkaline phosphatase are other indications that a CBD stone may be present.

62. **(A)** A cholecystokinin stimulated HIDA scan should be performed. Failure of the gallbladder to contract after stimulation by cholecystokinin may suggest dyskinesia. This is an indication for cholecystectomy, even though stones are not demonstrated. Secretin is the duodenal hormone that stimulates exocrine pancreatic secretion. Gastrin, released mainly from the antrum, increases gastric acid secretion that is high in bicarbonate and electrolytes.

63. **(A)** Unlike most biliary disease conditions, cholangiocarcinoma condition affects men more commonly than women. Primary sclerosing cholangitis, *C. sinensis,* and choledochal cysts may play an etiological role in some cases, but gallstones are not involved in the pathogenesis of this tumor. Patients present with obstructive jaundice; pain, and weight loss are less common. Proximal tumors (Klatskin) are most common, and they require excision of hepatic duct bifurcation and reconstruction with a Roux-en-Y limb of jejunum. Tumors of the distal duct can be resected by performing a Whipple pancreatoduodenectomy. Patients who are not operative candidates (those with advanced disease or those who cannot withstand a major operation) should undergo palliative endoscopic stent placement to relieve the obstruction.

64. **(A)** The HIDA scan is most accurate in establishing a diagnosis of acute cholecystitis. After injection, the technetium-labeled imminodiacetic acid radioisotopes are taken up by the liver and excreted into the biliary tree. If the cystic duct is obstructed (as in patients with acute cholecystitis) the gallbladder will not be visualized. Ultrasound may show ductal dilation, the presence of wall thickening (<3 mm), or pericholecystic fluid, which is highly suggestive of acute cholecystitis.

65. **(E)** She does not require any further therapy. In instances where gallbladder carcinoma is discovered incidentally during cholecystectomy and is shown to have only invaded the mucosa and submucosa it is classified as stage I. The 5-year survival for these patients is 100% and no further treatment is required as for more advanced lesions, that is, those penetrating the muscular layer or with lymph node involvement (stages II & III). Here there is a higher incidence of local and regional spread to the liver and porta hepatis lymph nodes, respectively. For these patients an en bloc resection of segments 4 and 5 of the liver is performed along with dissection of celiac axis and porta hepatis lymph nodes. For more advanced lesions (stage IV), the prognosis is very poor, and further resection is not indicated. Gallbladder carcinoma responds poorly to radiotherapy or chemotherapy.

66. **(D)** The morbidity and mortality of cholecystectomy is markedly increased in the presence of cirrhosis. The prognosis is particularly grave in patients with decompensated liver disease. Most gallstones in patients with cirrhosis are pigment stones, and hence dissolution with ursodeoxycholic acid is not an acceptable option of treatment.

67. **(B)** Early after the onset of acute cholecystitis, the plane of dissection may be facilitated because of early inflammatory response. Between the seventh and fourteenth day after admission, surgery may be extremely difficult because of resolving infection and adhesions. Where possible surgery should be avoided during this period.

68. **(A)** Emphysematous cholecystitis is caused by gas-forming organisms. On a plain x-ray of the abdomen, gas may be seen within the wall of the gallbladder. Clinically, the patient has rapidly progressive sepsis, RUQ pain, fever, and hemodynamic instability. The disease primarily affects diabetic men. Treatment with laparotomy and

cholecystectomy is urgent to avoid complications. Air within the biliary tree (not gallbladder wall) may be seen in gallstone ileus, after biliary-enteric anastomosis or after sphincterotomy.

69. **(D)** Acute acalculous cholecystitis is most commonly encountered in critically ill patients after trauma, other unrelated surgical operations, burns, sepsis, and multiorgan failure. The HIDA scan fails to visualize the gallbladder, and a sonogram may show a distended gallbladder with wall thickening and pericholecystic fluid. Acalculous cholecystitis carries a mortality rate of 10–30%. Delay in diagnosis and hence treatment is accompanied by severe complications, such as gangrene and perforation of the gallbladder in a patient who usually has other debilitating illnesses.

70. **(C)** Obstruction of the cystic duct may be caused by factors other than stones. Acalculous cholecystitis carries a high mortality, because it occurs in patients who are already critically ill. Furthermore, the establishment of the diagnosis is often delayed. Urgent cholecystostomy should be performed. In recent years, percutaneous cholecystostomy under CT or ultrasonography (US) guidance is performed more commonly than surgical cholecystectomy, because it carries a lower operative mortality rate. In a stable patient, cholecystectomy may be considered.

71. **(D)** Sodium chloride and water are selectively absorbed by the gallbladder mucosa. Bile salts and pigments are concentrated in the bile. Mucus also is secreted into the bile to function in a protective capacity. The presence of cholesterol crystals in biliary drainage material warrants further investigation, although the biliary system is normal.

72. **(D)** This patient has an amebic liver abscess. In most patients, the antecedent intestinal phase has subsided by the time patient presents with fever, chills, and a painful, tender enlarged liver. Amoebae are found in examination of fresh stools in 15% of cases, but the indirect hemagglutination test is almost always positive. Amebic abscess responds rapidly to treatment with metronidazole (Flagyl). Surgery should be avoided when possible and is indicated only when medical treatment has failed or complications, such as perforation, have occurred.

73. **(B)** Amebic liver abscess almost always responds to treatment with metronidazole (Flagyl). Occasionally, percutaneous aspiration is required when there is no response to Flagyl or if the abscess is secondarily infected. Amebic lever abscess affects mainly middle-aged men. Complications of amebic liver abscess include secondary infection in 20% and rupture into pleural, peritoneal, or pericardial cavity in 10% of cases.

74. **(D)** The hepatic artery, portal vein, and hepatic bile duct are distributed equally between both lobes of the liver divided by Cantlie's line. This line passes between the inferior vena cava posteriorly and the gallbladder fossa anteroinferiorly. The falciform ligament does not divide the liver into a right and left lobe; it divides the true left lobe into medial and lateral segments. The caudate and quadrate lobes are part of the left lobe, and, thus, Cantlie's line passes along their right (and not left) margins.

75. **(A)** Hepatic adenomas are associated with an increased incidence in patients receiving oral contraceptives, diabetes, and pregnancy. Most patients are symptomatic with pain and bleeding. Because of the real risk of intraperitoneal or intratumoral bleeding as well as malignant transformation, excision of the adenoma is recommended. Tumors are removed by enucleation or with a narrow rim of normal parenchyma, and major liver resection is not required.

76. **(C)** Unlike hepatic adenomas, these lesions do not usually cause symptoms. Unlike hepatic adenomas, focal nodular hyperplasia does not tend to cause intramural bleeding with rupture into the peritoneal cavity. CT or US scan may frequently miss the lesion, because it is so dense. There is no definite relationship with oral contraceptives. Focal nodular hyperplasia lesions are not well encapsulated and have a central stellate scar. Malignant changes have not been reported. LFT and AFP are normal in both conditions.

77. **(B)** Hemangioma is the commonest nodule in the liver. On intravenous contrast CT or MRI, a liver hemangioma shows initial centripetal enhancement followed by decrease in dye over 10 minutes from without to within. Hemangiomas occur more frequently in women. Most lesions are asymptomatic, discovered incidentally, and require no treatment. Larger hemangiomas may cause pain because of stretching of liver capsule or thrombocytopenia due to platelet trapping. These tumors may occasionally require resection.

78. **(C)** Congenital cysts are more frequently encountered than those that are acquired, which are caused by trauma, inflammation, or parasitic disease. Most congenital cysts tend to be asymptomatic and require no treatment. Larger cysts may cause pain and occasionally require radiologically guided percutaneous drainage or operative unroofing to prevent recurrence. Fungal abscesses, encountered mainly in immunosupressed patients, tend to be multiple. Pyogenic abscesses tend to be symptomatic with fever and pain, whereas, tumors are generally not hypoechoic.

79. **(D)** Before performing the left hepatic lobectomy, any extrahepatic metastasis should be ruled out. If lung, bone, adrenal, or skin metastasis were present, then subjecting the patient to a major operation would not be warranted in most cases. Moreover, before proceeding with surgery, it must be ascertained that control of the primary tumor has been achieved and that the patient's physical condition will allow such a major operation. Surgical excision of hepatic metastasis results in 25%, 5-year survival. Patients not treated by hepatic resection do not usually survive into the first year after clinical detection. Chemotherapy would be offered if resection were not indicated.

80. **(D)** Massive hemorrhage. Hemorrhage is a major cause of death after liver transplantation. Subphrenic infection and other intra-abdominal and intrahepatic infections may occur later in the postoperative period. Graft rejection is mainly a problem at a later period.

81. **(D)** Is rarely associated with long-term survival. Heterotopic (to a remote position) auxiliary transplantation is only occasionally indicated where orthotopic transplantation cannot be carried out. Long-term survival with this procedure is limited (2 of 69 cases). Hetrotopic auxiliary liver transplants require low outflow pressure and are, therefore, most likely to succeed if placed proximally as close to the heart as possible. One advantage of this procedure is that the procedure is technically easier, because the patient's liver is not disturbed.

82. **(A)** The liver plays a role in glucose formation from various glucogenic amino acids and other substances. Hepatic disease removes this source of glucose supply. In insulin hypoglycemia, there is enhanced rapid uptake of glucose by fat tissue and muscle.

83. **(D)** Antithrombin III counteracts excess of thrombin formation. The excess of thrombin facilitates conversion of fibrinogen to fibrin. Portal vein thrombosis will lead to portal hypertension but not hepatic congestion, as seen in Budd-Chiari syndrome. Portal vein thrombosis may occur in cirrhosis, trauma, in patients on contraceptive tablets, and in those who have an increased propensity for thrombus formation. It is also a direct complication of periumbilical infection in the neonate.

84. **(B)** Umbilical infection at birth is associated with ascending infection along the remnant of the left umbilical vein in the round ligament. This vein communicates with the left portal vein. Portal hypertension occurs because of portal vein thrombosis. In general, LFTs are normal, because the site of portal obstruction is outside the liver. Other causes of portal vein thrombosis include chronic pancreatitis, carcinoma of the pancreas, surgical intervention in this region, and diseases associated with an increased tendency toward clot formation. (See Answer 65.)

85. **(C)** As in any patient with upper GI bleeding, the initial intervention following clinical evaluation requires appropriate resuscitation. Blood transfusion may be required. Liver functions must be assessed, and coagulopathy

should be corrected with FFP or vitamin K injection. After resuscitation is completed, every attempt should be made to perform an upper GI endoscopy as soon as possible. These patients may be bleeding from varices, portal hypertensive gastropathy, peptic ulcer, or Mallory-Weiss tear, and early endoscopy will provide a higher diagnostic yield as to which lesion is actually bleeding.

86. **(E)** TIPS refers to an implantable, expandable metal stent placed radiologically through the hepatic parenchyma to establish a tract between the hepatic and portal vein. A portal systemic shunt is, therefore, created, and the varices are decompressed. Because of the high incidence of complications (esophageal perforation, aspiration, airway obstruction) associated with the Sengstaken-Blakemore tube, it is only used as a last ditch attempt to control exsanguination. In >50% of cases, bleeding recurs after the tube is deflated.

87. **(A)** The condition is more common in children. Splenectomy predisposes the patient to OPSI characterized by fulminant bacteremia, meningitis, or pneumonia. The mortality of this condition is high. The risk is greatest in children under 4 and for those undergoing splenectomy for thalassemia or lymphoma. The risk is lower in adults and those undergoing splenectomy for trauma than for ITP. All patients undergoing elective splenectomy should receive vaccination against pneumococcus and *H. Influenzae* about 2 weeks before surgery. Vaccination should be repeated every 5 years. In addition, children should be given penicillin prophylactically until they are 18 years of age. Postsplenectomy patients should seek medical attention at the first sign of even seemingly mild upper respiratory tract infection and should be advised to wear a Medic Alert tag indicating their asplenic state.

88. **(C)** Portal hypertension is suspected clinically if esophageal varices are detected, hypersplenism occurs, or ascites develop. Normal portal venous pressure is 5–10 mm Hg. Pressure may be measured indirectly by using hepatic venous wedge pressure (occlusive hepatic wedge pressure). About two-thirds of patients with portal hypertension will develop varices of which one-third will bleed.

89. **(A)** Penicillamine counteracts the adverse effects of copper on the liver in patients with Kimmelstiel-Wilson syndrome. This has been demonstrated in both humans and animals afflicted with this disease. Portocaval shunt and esophageal varices are not indicated prophylactically.

90. **(E)** Platelets should not be given before splenectomy, but arrangements should be made to have them available immediately before the operation. They should be used only if bleeding occurs and after the spleen has been removed. ITP is a hemorrhagic disorder characterized by a low platelet count with bone marrow findings that show normal or increased megakaryocytes. The female/male ratio is 3:1. This diagnosis implies that no other systemic disease or past history of drug intake could account for these changes. Some cases may be caused by an autoimmune response.

91. **(A)** Radioactive technetium (^{99m}Tc) scan to see if a retained accessory spleen (splenunculus) is present, which may account for postoperative thrombocytopenia. Radioactive technetium (not I^{135}) is used to localize splenic tissue. Patients with ITP have petechiae, ecchymosis, and/or bleeding. Splenectomy performed initially for ITP is likely to be successful in 80% of patients, but is less effective in older patients.

92. **(D)** Features of TTP include fever, thrombocytopenic purpura, hemolytic anemia, neurological manifestations, and renal disease. The exact cause of TTP has not been determined. Histologically, there is diffuse hyalinization of arterioles and capillaries, with occlusion and infarction. The disease may follow a rapid and fulminant course, with death occurring secondary to cerebral hemorrhage or renal failure. Treatment includes steroids, plasmapheresis, and splenectomy. Approximately, 1/20 cases occur in pregnancy, but unlike ITP, TTP is not improved by termination of pregnancy.

93. **(C)** Sickle cell disease is relatively common in African-Americans and certain ethnic communities in the United States. Most patients with sickle cell disease respond favorably to rehydration and analgesia for each attack. The patient must avoid unnecessary exposure to infections, hypoxemia, and dehydration. In most patients with sickle cell disease, there is autoinfarction of the spleen. Splenectomy is rarely indicated, except for patients with sickle cell disease with a massively enlarge spleen, where trapping of RBCs is demonstrated.

94. **(E)** Sickle cell disease is diagnosed by peripheral smear showing sickle-shaped red cells and HbS on electrophoresis. The pathogenesis of the disease is characterized by microinfarction in different parts of the body. This can lead to serious (and in some instances fatal) outcome.

95. **(A)** In hereditary spherocytosis, the abnormally shaped erythrocytes fail to pass through the splenic pulp and are more prone to earlier destruction. In hereditary elliptocytosis, the erythrocyte membrane also is abnormal. Children with spherocytosis should undergo splenectomy around their fourth birthday. Other less common hematological indications for splenectomy are thalassemia, sickle cell anemia, autoimmune anemia, and an enlarged spleen that becomes a major site of red cell sequestration.

96. **(C)** Characterized by RBCs that undergo lysis at a higher osmotic pressure. Gallstones are frequently encountered as a result of increased production of bilirubin. Hereditary spherocytosis

is transmitted as an autosomal-dominant trait. Because of a fault in the RBC membrane, the cells are smaller and round and undergo lysis in a minor vessel, which results in a relative obstruction to flow.

97. **(E)** Alkalating agents must be given cautiously, because patients with myeloid metaplasia are sensitive to these agents. The connective and hemopoietic tissues in the spleen and liver are increased. Polycythemia vera, myelogenous leukemia, and idiopathic thrombocytosis must be excluded. Splenectomy is often of value.

98. **(C)** Felty's syndrome is characterized by splenomegaly, neutropenia, and rheumatoid arthritis. Steroids are used initially, but their effect usually is transient. Splenectomy favorably alters the leukocyte count; it does not alter the clinical course of rheumatoid arthritis. As with all patients undergoing elective splenectomy, this patient must be given pneumovax, as well as haemophilus and meningiococcal vaccines before surgery.

99. **(A)** The risk of infection after removal of the spleen as well as the good results of conservative treatment should encourage a nonoperative approach in children. In adults, surgery is usually recommended, but when possible, the spleen should be repaired and not removed. If the spleen is to be removed on an elective basis, pneumovax and prophylactic vaccine against *H. influenza* are given about 2 weeks before surgery. (See Answer 69.)

CHAPTER 8

Hernia

Max Goldberg and Nanakram Agarwal

Questions

DIRECTIONS (Questions 1 through 21): Each of the numbered items in this section is followed by five answers. Select the ONE lettered answer that is BEST in each case.

1. A 6-month-old boy presents with an inguinal hernia, first noticed 2 weeks after birth. What is the best treatment choice?

   (A) Observation
   (B) Laparotomy
   (C) Surgical repair when the child is fully grown
   (D) Surgical repair of the affected side
   (E) Surgical repair of the affected side and exploration of the nonaffected side to search for and repair a sac that was not previously detected by clinical means

2. A 60-year-old male presents with an inguinal hernia of recent onset. Which of the following statements are TRUE?

   (A) The hernia is more likely to be direct than indirect.
   (B) Presents through the posterior wall of the inguinal canal, lateral to the deep inguinal ring.
   (C) Is covered anteriorly by the transversalis fascia.
   (D) Is more likely than a femoral hernia to strangulate.
   (E) The sac is congenital.

3. A 70-year-old cigarette smoker presents with a right inguinal mass that has enlarged and has caused discomfort in recent months. He complains of recent difficulty with micturition and nocturia. The swelling, which does not extend to the scrotum, reduces when resting. What is the likely diagnosis?

   (A) Direct inguinal hernia
   (B) Strangulated indirect inguinal hernia
   (C) Hydrocele
   (D) Aneurysm of the femoral artery
   (E) Cyst of the cord

4. A 65-year-old female requires emergency surgery for a strangulated inguinal hernia. Which of the following is correct?

   (A) The sac is formed by an unobliterated processus vaginalis.
   (B) The hernia is direct rather than indirect.
   (C) Such herniae never contain small intestine.
   (D) Strangulation never results in bowel ischemia and gangrene requiring resection.
   (E) Indirect inguinal herniae are never found in female patients.

5. An otherwise healthy, 60-year-old male has been advised to undergo surgical treatment for a left inguinal hernia. Which of the following are acceptable standards of surgical treatment?

(A) Traditional surgical repair under general or local anesthesia

(B) Repair of the hernia and ipsilateral orchiectomy, in order to better assure closure of the inguinal canal and reduce the possibility of recurrence

(C) Laparotomy to perform a retroperitoneal repair

(D) Surgical exploration of the contralateral groin to search for an occult hernia sac and to remove it before a hernai develops

(E) The patient should be advised to wear a truss postoperatively, in order to reduce the incidence of recurrence

6. A 62-year-old male presents with an irreducible swelling and severe pain in the left groin. He had a known reducible hernia for 15 years prior to this. He had a bowel movement while in the emergency room. At surgery, a Richter's hernia was found. Which of the following statements is TRUE?

(A) It presents lateral to the rectus sheath.

(B) It presents through the lumbar triangle.

(C) It presents through the obturator foramen.

(D) It contains a Meckel's diverticulum.

(E) It may allow normal passage of stool.

7. At surgery for a right inguinal hernia, a 72-year-old man is found to have a hernia sac that is not independent of the bowel wall. The cecum forms part of the wall of the sac (Fig. 8–1). Such a hernia is properly referred to as which of the following?

(A) Incarcerated

(B) Irreducible

(C) Sliding

(D) Richter's

(E) Interstitial

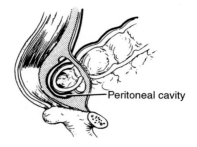

Figure 8–1.
Hernia has entered internal inguinal ring. Note that one-fourth of the hernia is not related to the peritoneal sac. *(Reproduced, with permission, from Way LW: Current Surgical Diagnosis & Treatment, 10th ed. 176. Appleton & Lange, 1994.)*

8. The following structures may be injured during surgery to repair an inguinal hernia:

(A) The ilioinguinal, genitofemoral, iliohypogastric, and lateral femoral cutaneous nerves

(B) The femoral nerve

(C) The popliteal nerve

(D) The nerve to the psoas major muscle

(E) The pudendal nerve

9. Which of the following structures would be encountered during repair of an inguinal hernia in a male?

(A) Spermatic cord, cremaster muscle, transversalis fascia, deep epigastric vessels, conjoined tendon

(B) Round ligament

(C) Obturator nerve

(D) Symphysis pubis

(E) Nerve to the adductor muscles of the thigh

10. In repair of a femoral hernia, the structure most vulnerable to major injury lies:

(A) Medially

(B) Laterally

(C) Anteriorly

(D) Posteriorly

(E) Superficially

11. A 28-year-old professional football player has sudden pain and swelling in the right groin when attempting to intercept a pass. He is admitted to the local emergency department. On examination, there is a tender swelling in the right groin. The scrotum and penis show no abnormality. What is the next step in management?

  (A) Needle aspiration to exclude hematoma
  (B) Forceful manual reduction
  (C) Laparotomy within 20 minutes
  (D) Preoperative preparation and exploration of the groin with hernia repair
  (E) Morphine and reevaluation within 12 hours

Questions 12 and 13

A 70-year-old woman presents with a tender irreducible mass immediately below and lateral to the pubic tubercle. Plain abdominal x-ray shows intestinal obstruction.

12. What is the likeliest diagnosis?

  (A) Small-bowel carcinoma
  (B) Large-bowel carcinoma
  (C) Adhesions
  (D) Strangulated inguinal hernia
  (E) Strangulated femoral hernia

13. Treatment with a nasogastric tube and intravenous fluids is initiated. What is the next step in treatment?

  (A) Sedation to relax the patient and allow spontaneous reduction of the mass
  (B) Sedation and surgery scheduled for the next elective surgical appointment
  (C) Sedation and manual taxis (reduction)
  (D) Emergency surgery on the left groin
  (E) Emergency laparotomy for intestinal obstruction and hernia repair from the peritoneal cavity

14. A 2-year-old African American boy presents with a reducible umbilical hernia, under 2-cm diameter. This is best managed by:

  (A) Immediate surgery and repair with mesh
  (B) Immediate surgery repair without mesh
  (C) Laparoscopic repair with mesh
  (D) Laparoscopic repair without mesh
  (E) Periodic observation and evaluation

15. A 55-year-old woman, who recently had been dieting with a weight loss of 20 lb, presents with a small-bowel obstruction and pain, which radiates down the inside of her thigh to the knee. She has no past history of abdominal surgery. Which of the following is the likely diagnosis?

  (A) Strangulated obturator hernia
  (B) Obstructing neoplasm of the ileum
  (C) Gallstone ileus
  (D) Strangulated femoral hernia
  (E) Fracture of the pubic bone

16. A 50-year-old man presents with a complaint of a 1-cm moderately painful, tender mass situated one-third of the way between the xiphisternum and the umbilicus (Fig. 8–2). What is the most likely diagnosis?

  (A) Fibrosarcoma of the abdominal wall
  (B) Omphalocele
  (C) Spigelian hernia
  (D) Fat necrosis
  (E) Epigastric hernia

17. A 70-year-old, moderately obese, male presents with a large, midline incisional hernia. One year previously, he underwent a colon resection for adenocarcinoma. Colonoscopy, metastasis workup and carcinoembryonic antigen (CEA) are normal. Which of the following statement is TRUE?

  (A) Repair with mesh can be performed laparoscopically.
  (B) Strangulation is uncommon because the neck is narrow.
  (C) Recurrence is common, even with the use of mesh of improved quality.
  (D) Surgical repair is simple to perform under local anesthesia.
  (E) Patients remain very uncomfortable, even with an adequate repair.

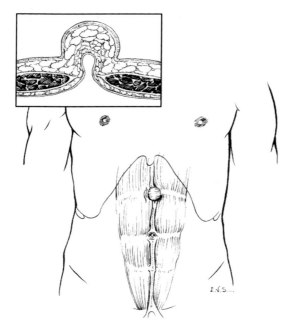

Figure 8–2.
Epigastric lesion. *(Reproduced, with permission, from Doherty GM: Current Surgical Diagnosis and Treatment, 12th ed. 774. McGraw-Hill, 2006.)*

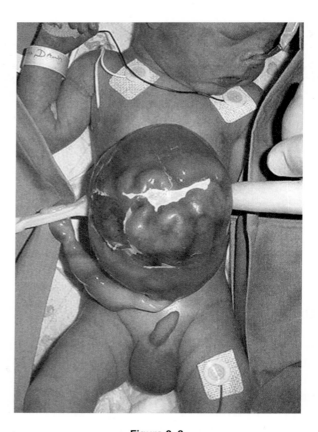

Figure 8–3.
Giant omphalocele in a newborn male. *(Reproduced, with permission, from Brunicardi FC et al.: Schwartz's Principles of Surgery, 8th ed. 1503. McGraw-Hill, 2005.)*

18. Following laparoscopic preperitoneal repair of an inguinal hernia, a 50-year-old male complains of severe burning pain, which radiates down the lateral side of the ipsilateral thigh. The most likely cause is injury to which of the following:

    (A) Ilioinguinal nerve
    (B) Iliohypogastric nerve
    (C) Genitofemoral nerve
    (D) Femoral nerve
    (E) Lateral femoral cutaneous nerve

19. A male neonate is born with an omphalocele (shown in Fig. 8–3). This entity can be distinguished from gastroschisis, because in an omphalocele, the protrusion is:

    (A) Not covered by a sac
    (B) A defect in the abdominal musculature
    (C) Associated with an umbilicus attached to the abdominal wall musculature
    (D) Associated with partial or complete malrotation of the bowel
    (E) Really contains abdominal viscera

20. What is true of Spigelian hernia?

    (A) It occurs exclusively in males.
    (B) It involves part of the circumference of the bowel wall.
    (C) It is best repaired by the classical Bassini technique of inguinal ligament repair.
    (D) It occurs at the lateral edge of the linea semilunaris.
    (E) It always contains the vermiform appendix.

21. A 56-year-old man is scheduled to have a left indirect hernia repaired. He is asymptomatic. Before surgical treatment, he should have which of the following?

    (A) Rectal examination alone
    (B) Rectal examination and sigmoidoscopy
    (C) Barium enema
    (D) Colonoscopy
    (E) Intravenous pyelogram

Answers and Explanations

1. **(E)** Inguinal hernias in infancy are almost always congenital and indirect and are often bilateral. Bilateral exploration is recommended, except when the surgery is performed for incarceration.

2. **(A)** Hernias, which present in adult life are most often direct and aquired, rather than indirect. They protrude through the transversalis fascia, which forms the medial half of the posterior wall of the inguinal canal and is located medial to the deep inguinal ring and deep epigastric vessels. Strangulation of direct inguinal herniae is uncommon, probably because the neck of the sac tends to be wide, rather than narrow and constricting

3. **(A)** Direct hernias are more common in older patients. There is an increased incidence in patients with a chronic cough and prostatic obstruction. They are rarely encountered in children and women. This type of hernia does not extend to the scrotum and rarely undergoes strangulation.

4. **(A)** Indirect inguinal hernia sacs are found less commonly in female patients. They are formed by the unobliterated processus vaginalis of the peritoneum and allow for the entry of intraperitoneal viscera, such as loops of small intestine, omentum, and the likes. Compromise of blood supply by constriction leads to strangulation.

5. **(A)** Traditional hernia repair is performed under local or general anesthesia. Laparoscopic repair, in general, is performed under general anesthesia. Combinations of local anesthesia and intravenous sedation are in routine use. Orchiectomy, though occasionally used in special circumstances, is by no means a routine part of hernia repair. Exploration of the opposite groin, though recommended in infants, does not apply to adults.

6. **(E)** In Richter's hernia, part of the bowel wall is entrapped in the hernia sac. This results in a partial occlusion of the lumen and bowel movement remains possible, despite strangulation and gangrene of the entrapped portion. Evaluation at surgery, of the viability of the full-bowel wall must always be carried out before returning the entrapped segment to the peritoneal cavity.

7. **(C)** The term *sliding* refers to the peritoneum that slides along with the hernia in its passage along the cord (Fig. 8–4). The viscus forms part of the wall of the sac. The peritoneum should not be removed from the bowel wall, because devascularization may occur.

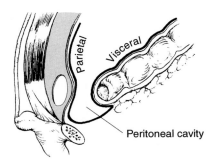

Figure 8–4.
Note cecum and ascending colon sliding on fascia of posterior abdominal wall. *(Reproduced, with permission, from Doherty GM: Current Surgical Diagnosis and Treatment, 12th ed. 771. McGraw-Hill, 2006.)*

8. **(A)** Any of these nerves may be devided, crushed, or entrapped by suture or mesh during repair of a groin hernia. The lateral femoral cutaneous nerve is vulnerable especially during laparoscopic hernia repair.

9. **(A)** All are normal and constant anatomic structures of the inguinal canal.

10. **(B)** The femoral vein lies immediately lateral to the femoral canal. Careful attention to this structure is essential in repair of femoral herniae.

11. **(D)** Unexplained recent onset of swelling in the groin, that is not reducible, should be considered to be a strangulated inguinal or femoral hernia until proved otherwise. Needle aspiration may cause fecal perforation and forceful manual reduction may result in the return of gangrenous bowel to the peritoneal cavity.

12. **(E)** Strangulated femoral hernia is located below and lateral to the pubic tubercle and is more common in females. Inguinal hernias occur in similar frequency in females, but compared to femoral hernias, they are less likely to undergo strangulation.

13. **(D)** This patient has a strangulated femoral hernia. Emergency surgery after appropriate resuscitation is the correct treatment. Gangrene of strangulated bowel may be present. No attempt at manual reduction should be made, because gangrenous bowel may be returned to the peritoneal cavity.

14. **(E)** As many as 90% of umbilical herniae up to 1.5 cm in diameter will not be clinically evident by the age of 5 years.

15. **(A)** Strangulation of a bowel loop may occur at the obturator fossa, classically following weight loss, which results in loss of the fat pad that covers the area, superiorly, where the obturator membrane is deficient. This allows entry and strangulation of a bowel loop. Compression of the obturator nerve causes the pain down the medial side of the thigh. CT scan with contrast may show the level of obstruction.

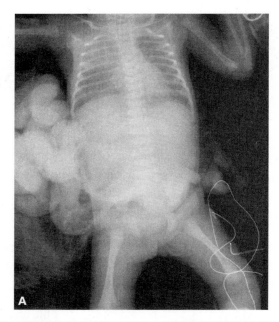

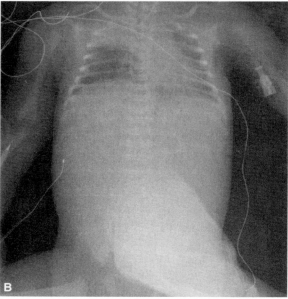

Figure 8–5.
Radiograph shows large swelling due to gastroschisis. (**A:** Multiple loops of bowel lying on the right side and outside of the abdomen. **B:** Bowel loops wrapped in synthetic bag to reduce bowel sequentially.)

16. **(E)** Epigastric hernia is a defect in the linea alba between the umbilicus and the xiphisternum. It usually contains preperitoneal fat rather than omentum or bowel. It may cause pain and is commonly encountered in older patients. Sometimes it is located on either side of the midline. Spigelian hernia occurs lateral to the linea semilunaris.

17. **(A)** Repair can be performed laparoscopically, under general anesthesia, following adequate preoperative medical preparation. Patients are more comfortable following adequate repair. Modern mesh is of much improved quality and recurrence has become much less common.

18. **(E)** The lateral femoral cutaneous nerve is visible in the laparoscopic approach to hernia repair. This nerve can be injured in placement of the mesh used for repair, especially if staples are used. Great care must be taken to avoid this injury, which causes severe burning pain and paresthesia of the thigh and is very disabling. Injury is not likely if staples are not inserted lateral to the deep inguinal ring.

19. **(D)** In omphalocele (see Fig. 8–5), the swelling is covered by a membrane formed by the peritoneum, Wharton's jelly, and amnion. The membrane is transparent, and underlying intestine can be seen. The other features listed are characteristic of gastroschisis. In gastroschisis, the protrusion is not covered by a membrane and the other features listed apply.

20. **(D)** Spigelian hernia occurs at the semilunar line, which extends along the lateral border of each rectus abdominis muscle. The posterior rectus sheath is deficient at the level of the arcuate line (semicircular line) about one-third of the distance between the umbilicus and the pubic symphysis; this is the most common site for Spigelian hernia to occur through the linea semilunaris. It occurs in both sexes. The Bassini technique refers to inguinal hernias only. A hernia that involves part of the bowel wall is known as a Richter's hernia. The appendix may or may not form part of the contents of the sac.

21. **(B)** Patients who have symptoms suggestive of change in bowel habits will require a barium enema or colonoscopy. It is important not to overlook an underlying carcinoma, which could cause the patient to strain and induce a hernia. Carcinoma and/or polyps may be overlooked if this approach is ignored.

CHAPTER 9

Male and Female Genitourinary Systems

Sean Fullerton and Albert Samadi

Questions

DIRECTIONS (Questions 1 through 59): Each of the numbered items in this section is followed by five answers. Select the ONE lettered answer that is BEST in each case.

Questions 1 and 2

1. A 62-year-old African American male attorney presents to a prostate-screening clinic during National Awareness Week. On careful questioning, he has noted slight urgency, frequency nocturia, and a decrease in the force of micturition. He is referred to have blood tests to include which of the following?

   (A) Carcinoembryonic antigen (CEA)
   (B) Prostatic acid phosphatase
   (C) Alkaline phosphatase
   (D) Prostate-specific antigen (PSA)
   (E) Lactic dehydrogenase (LDH)

2. General examination from his urologist is noncontributory. A rectal examination reveals hemorrhoids and a left-sided irregular mass in the prostate. Following normal blood tests, he should have which of the following?

   (A) Computed tomography (CT) scan of the pelvis
   (B) Magnetic resonance image (MRI) of the prostate
   (C) Colonoscopy and biopsy of the prostate under general anesthetic
   (D) Biopsy of the nodule
   (E) Bone scan

3. A 62-year-old postal officer develops minimal urinary symptoms. His PSA level is elevated and continues to increase during a 6-month period of observation. The next step in evaluation, if transrectal ultrasound (TRUS) prostate biopsy (Fig. 9–1) were positive for adenocarcinoma of prostate, would be:

   (A) Refer to oncologist for chemotherapy
   (B) Metastatic evaluation including CT and bone scans
   (C) Repeat PSA and biospy
   (D) Evaluation by radiation oncologist
   (E) Start hormonal ablation treatment

4. Because of positive biopsy findings and negative workup, he undergoes a radical prostatectomy. The pathology report reveals Gleason score 9/10 and involvement of several pelvic lymph nodes. Which is the most likely site for prostatic cancer metastasis?

   (A) Liver
   (B) Kidney
   (C) Lung
   (D) Bone
   (E) Brain

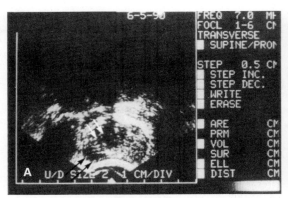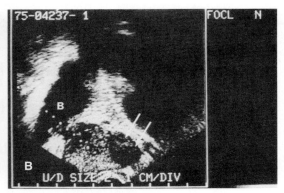

(Reproduced, with permission, from Doherty GM: *Current Surgical Diagnosis & Treatment*, 12th ed. 1047. McGraw-Hill, 2006.)

Figure 9–1.
Transrectal ultrasound of the prostate. Sagittal plane showing large hypoechoic prostate cancer at arrows. *(Reproduced, with permission, from Way LW: Current Surgical Diagnosis & Treatment, 10th ed. Appleton & Lange, 1994.)*

5. A 79-year-old man is examined for severe pain in the iliac crest. Metastatic disease from prostatic cancer is confirmed. What is the treatment offered initially to most patients with metastatic prostatic cancer?

(A) Cortisone and pituitary ablation

(B) Radical prostatectomy

(C) Luteinizing releasing hormone (LRH) agonist (Leuprolide)

(D) Local irradiation and testosterone

(E) Hyperthermia

6. During her eighth month of pregnancy, a 29-year-old woman is noted to have polyhydramnios. Further testing shows anencephalus. Polyhydramnios in this patient is caused by which of the following?

(A) Impairment of the fetus's swallowing mechanism

(B) Tumor of the fetus's brain

(C) A secretory peptide from the placenta

(D) Excess antidiuretic hormone (ADH) from the fetus

(E) Renal agenesis

7. Several weeks after lifting a heavy object, a previously healthy 34-year-old man continues to complain of heaviness in his left groin. Which of the following statements is true of testicular cancer?

(A) It is the most common solid tumor in men over 50 years of age.

(B) It is not associated with a higher incidence of infertility.

(C) It presents as a painless mass in the scrotum in more than 70% of patients.

(D) It accounts for 10% of malignant tumors in men.

(E) It rarely metastasizes.

8. During a workup for infertility, a 34-year-old man is noted to have a solid tumor in the anterior aspect of his right testis. What is the most likely diagnosis?

(A) Torsion of the testis

(B) Cyst of the epididymis

(C) Lipoma of the cord

(D) Cancer of the testis

(E) Epididymo-orchitis

9. Improved survival after lymphadenectomy for testicular tumors occurs after which of the following?

(A) Seminoma

(B) Embryonal cell carcinoma

(C) Leydig cell tumor

(D) Sertoli cell tumor

(E) Lymphoma

10. A 38-year-old woman presents with shortness of breath and abdominal distention. Workup reveals presence of ascites and hydrothorax. What is the name of this condition?

(A) Brenner tumor
(B) Dysgerminoma
(C) Wolffian duct remnant
(D) Krukenberg's tumor
(E) Meigs's syndrome

11. A 41-year-old man requests information concerning vasectomy for sterilization. In this prcedure, which of the following statements is true?

(A) The incidence of sexual dysfunction is not influenced in those with dependent personalities.
(B) The success rate in reestablishing continuity of the vas deferens is greater than 80% at 10 years.
(C) The failure rate occurs in 1/400 patients.
(D) Recanalization of the vas deferens does not occur.
(E) The procedure is difficult and requires laparotomy.

12. A 6-month-old boy was born with hypospadias. This condition is due to failure in the development of which of the following?

(A) Urogenital fold
(B) Müllerian system
(C) Genital tubercle
(D) Urachus
(E) Vitelline duct

13. A 64-year-old woman notes an ulcer on her left labia majora. Biospy reveals squamous cell carcinoma. What is the treatment?

(A) Wide local excision
(B) Radiotherapy
(C) Preoperative radiotherapy followed by wide local excision

(D) Wide excision and unilateral groin dissection
(E) Radical vulvectomy and bilateral groin dissection

14. A 6-year-old healthy appearing girl is brought for evaluation of bloody vaginal discharge. The most likely diagnosis is:

(A) Squamous cell carcinoma
(B) Sarcoma botryoides
(C) Carcinosarcoma
(D) Clear cell adenocarcinoma
(E) Lymphoma

15. A healthy appearing, 8-year-old boy is evaluated for an abdominal mass, felt by his mother during a bath. What is the most likely diagnosis?

(A) Lymphoma
(B) Rhabdomyoscarcoma
(C) Wilms' tumor
(D) Neuroblastoma
(E) Renal cell carcinoma

16. In repair of a third-degree perineal laceration, which structure shown in Fig. 9–2 is least likely to be divided?

(A) Bulbocavernosus muscle
(B) Vaginal mucosa
(C) Superficial transverse perineal lmuscle
(D) External anal sphincter
(E) Ischiocavernosus muscle

17. A 24-year-old man had been treated for gonorrhea 2 months previously. He developed an ulcerative lesion in the glands of the penis that is noted to be condylomata lata. The etiology of condylomata lata is which of the following?

(A) Mixture of organisms
(B) *Haemophilus ducreyi*
(C) *Herpesvirus hominis*, type II
(D) *Treponema pallidum*
(E) *Neisseria gonorrhoeae*

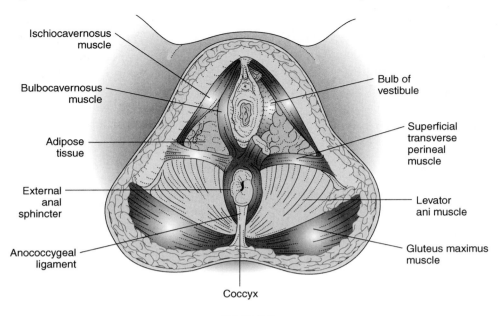

Ischiocavernosus muscle

Bulbocavernosus muscle

Adipose tissue

External anal sphincter

Anococcygeal ligament

Bulb of vestibule

Superficial transverse perineal muscle

Levator ani muscle

Gluteus maximus muscle

Coccyx

Figure 9–2.
Skin and subcutaneous tissues removed to reveal structures in perineum. *(Reproduced, with permission, from DeCherney AH et al.: Current Diagnosis & Treatment Obstetrics & Gynecologic, 10th ed. McGraw-Hill, 2007.)*

18. A 23-year-old woman has a cesarean section in which a Pfannenstiel incision (Fig. 9–3) is used. In the Pfannenstiel incision, which of the following is TRUE?

   (A) The recti and fascia are separated transversely.
   (B) The recti and fascia are separated vertically.
   (C) Fascia lata graft is used.

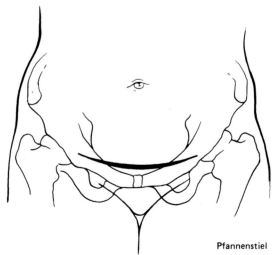

Pfannenstiel

Figure 9–3.
Pfannenstiel incision.

   (D) A prosthetic graft is used.
   (E) The upper abdomen can readily be explored.

19. What is the most common cause of failure of radiotherapy for stage II cervical carcinoma?

   (A) Liver metastasis
   (B) Bone metastasis
   (C) Para-aortic node metastasis
   (D) Resistance of the central tumor
   (E) Undifferentiated tumor histology

20. Twelve years after menopause, a 60-year-old woman undergoes laparotomy for an ovarian carcinoma. The ovarian tumor that is most likely to respond to radiotherapy is which of the following?

   (A) Dysgerminoma
   (B) Krukenberg's tumor
   (C) Arrhenoblastoma
   (D) Granulosa cell tumor
   (E) Brenner tumor

21. A 24-year-old woman has been unsuccessful becoming pregnant. She is admitted with abdominal pain; her blood pressure is 90/60 mm Hg,

her pulse rate is 102 beats per minute (bpm), and her hematocrit (HCT) is 28%. Features of ectopic pregnancy include which of the following?

(A) Elevated blood pressure on assuming an erect position
(B) Pulsus paradoxus
(C) Tenderness below the right subcostal margin (Murphy's sign)
(D) Pain referred to the supraclavicular region
(E) Ecchymosis around the umbilicus

22. After undergoing a partial cystectomy for carcinoma of the rectum, a 76-year-old woman develops a vesicovaginal fistula. The repair will have a higher chance of success if which of the following occurs?

(A) Scare tissue is not excised
(B) The bladder wall is closed under tension
(C) Repair is performed more than 6 months after the causative operation
(D) Repair is performed within 7–14 days of the onset of symptoms
(E) Urethral catheters removed within 7 days

23. After being treated for ovarian carcinoma, a 65-year-old woman develops complications attributed to cisplatin (*cis*-diamminedichloro-platinum). What is a common side effect of cisplatin?

(A) Multiple lipoma
(B) Ankylosing spondylitis
(C) Megaloblastic anemia
(D) Pulmonary fibrosis
(E) Peripheral neuropathy

24. A 33-year-old woman is seen for evaluation of infertility. She complains of dyspareunia. On vaginal examination, tender nodularity along the uterosacral ligaments is noted. What is the diagnosis?

(A) Adenomyosis
(B) Diethylstilbestrol (DES)-related disease
(C) Subserosal fibroids

(D) Endometriosis
(E) Adrenogenital syndrome

25. Following a radical nephrectomy, a 60-year-old, diabetic male develops necrotizing fasciitis. After treating the infection, the plastic surgeon places an omental graft, which is based on blood supply from which of the following?

(A) Omental branch of the abdominal aorta
(B) Middle colic artery
(C) Gastroepiploic artery
(D) Middle sacral artery
(E) Epigastric artery

26. An otherwise healthy, 30-year-old man is brought to the emergency department after being thrown off the back of a motorcycle. During the assessment, blood is noted at the urethral meatus. Which of the following statement is TRUE?

(A) A foley catheter should be inserted immediately.
(B) Dislocation of the sacroiliac joint is usually associated with a fracture of the pubic ramus or separation of the symphysis.
(C) Open lavage is a useful indication for the need to perform laparotomy.
(D) Fracture of the coccyx requires surgical excision in most patients.
(E) Pain is relieved on walking.

27. A 62-year-old woman with cardiac disease undergoes a pudendal nerve block to remove a tumor from the vulva. Fibers forming the pudendal nerve originate from which of the following?

(A) L2–L4
(B) L3–L5
(C) L4, L5, S1
(D) S1–S3
(E) S2–S4

28. A 42-year-old man has recurrent cystitis. Cystoscopic examination and biopsy confirm the presence of locally muscle invasive (T2) carcinoma of the bladder (Fig. 9–4)?

    (A) Repeat cystoscopic resection
    (B) Cystoscopic fulguration
    (C) Partial cystectomy
    (D) Radical cystoprostatectomy
    (E) Radiotherapy

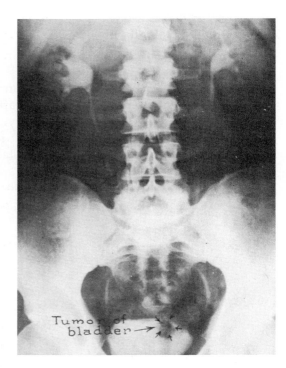

Figure 9–4.
Excretory urogram showing space-occupying lesion (transitional cell carcinoma) on the left side of the bladder. The upper tracts are normal. *(Reproduced, with permission, from Doherty GM: Current Surgical Diagnosis and Treatment, 12th ed. 1043. McGraw-Hill, 2006.)*

29. A healthy, 45-year-old woman undergoing abdominal hysterectomy and salpingo-oophrectomy for benign disease. The right ureter is accidentally cut. To minimize injury to the ureter, the surgeon should recognize what about this structure?

    (A) It enters the pelvis at the level of the aortic bifurcation.
    (B) It passes posterior to the iliac vessels.
    (C) It passes above the uterine artery.

    (D) It enters the pelvis 4-cm medial to the bifurcation of the common iliac artery.
    (E) It enters the pelvis immediately distal to the common itiac artery bifurcation.

30. A 56-year-old woman is admitted to the emergency department complaining of upper abdominal pain. An ultrasound of the abdomen reveals a thin-walled gallbladder filled with fluid and a solid, left renal mass. What should be the next test ordered?

    (A) Hydroxy iminodiacetic acid (HIDA) scan
    (B) Intravenous pyelogram (IVP)
    (C) CT scan of the abdomen and pelvis
    (D) Oral cholecystogram
    (E) Upper gastrointestinal (GI) series

31. A kidney graft between identical twins is likely to survive for which period of time?

    (A) 1–6 weeks
    (B) 7–52 weeks
    (C) 1–10 years
    (D) 11–25 years
    (E) more than 25 years

32. A 32-year-old woman with chronic renal failure undergoes successful renal transplantation. Tests carried out after the operation indicates the presence of cytomegalovirus (CMV). What is TRUE of this condition?

    (A) It cannot be measured by immunofluorescent assay.
    (B) It is detected in most patients after surgery.
    (C) It should not cause additional problems with regard to tissue rejection.
    (D) It results in infection that usually is fatal.
    (E) CMV infection occurs only in CMV positive donor.

33. A 4-year-old girl has a yellow, blood-tinged, foul-smelling, vaginal discharge. On examination, the external genitalia are red, and a malodorous, blood-tinged discharge is noted. The most likely cause of these findings are:

(A) Chlamydia trachomatis

(B) Gonorrhea

(C) Treponema

(D) Foreign body

(E) Vaginal cancer

34. A 46-year-old man is on a waiting list to secure a renal transplant. The genetic locus of transplant antigens in humans is known as which?

(A) Rhesus (Rh)

(B) Ig (Immunoglobulin) A and IgM

(C) Human leukocyte antigen (HLA)

(D) ABO

(E) Hepatitis B surface antigen (HBsAg)

35. A 64-year-old man underwent transplantation, which was complicated by graft-versus-host reaction. He had undergone a transplantation of which of the following?

(A) Kidney

(B) Skin

(C) Bone marrow

(D) Cornea

(E) Liver

36. In evaluating the role of the autonomic nervous system related to urinary incontinence that developed in a 67-year-old man after prostatectomy, it is determined that the sympathetic nerves are injured. What is the natural hormone in the catecholamine pathway?

(A) Norepinephrine

(B) Dopamine

(C) Vasoactive intestinal peptide (VIP)

(D) Isoproterenol

(E) Acetylcholine

37. During evaluation of the cause of varicocele in a 36-year-old man, attention is directed to the method of drainage of the left testicular vein, which usually enters which of the following?

(A) Left adrenal vein

(B) Left renal vein

(C) Left inferior mesenteric vein

(D) Inferior vena cava (IVC)

(E) Left inferior epigastric vein

38. A 42-year-old man presents with cancer of the left testis. To exclude lymphatic metastasis, which is the site that should be initially examined?

(A) Vertical chain of inguinal glands

(B) Horizontal chain of inguinal glands

(C) Retrorectal glands

(D) Para-aortic glands

(E) Obturator nodes

39. As a result of a motor vehicle crash, a 42-year-old female has a pelvic fracture, confirmed on x-ray of the pelvis. What does she require?

(A) Surgical repair under local anesthesia

(B) Open lavage and, if positive, immediate laparotomy

(C) Immobilization of the pelvis in a plaster cast

(D) Analgesics and observation

(E) Skeletal traction

40. A 42-year-old woman involved in a traffic accident presents to the emergency room complaining of flank pain and gross hematuria, she is hemodynamically stable. The next step in management is:

(A) Exploratory laparotomy

(B) Open lavage and, if positive, immediate laparotomy

(C) Immobilization of the pelvis

(D) Computed axial tomography (CAT) scan with the use of intravenous contrast

(E) Skeletal traction

41. A 62-year-old woman with metastatic cancer had mild chronic renal disease. Renal excretion of antineoplastic drugs is least likely to be affected by which of the following?

    (A) Nonsteroidal anti-inflammatory drugs (NSAIDs)
    (B) Probenecid
    (C) Aspirin
    (D) Alkalinizing urine
    (E) Aminoglycosides

42. A 62-year-old farmer had received chemotherapy for cancer of the head and neck. He has developed classical multidrug resistance (MDR) to which of the following?

    (A) Alkylating agents
    (B) Antimetabolites
    (C) Bleomycin
    (D) Vinca alkaloid
    (E) Cyclosporine

Questions 43 and 44

A 32-year-old female has chronic pyelonephritis with chronic renal failure. She is scheduled to have a renal transplantation. The donor kidney will be obtained from her brother-in-law, and left laparoscopic nephrectomy is planned. The donor kidney operation will be performed in a separate operating room under general anesthesia.

43. Where will the donor kidney be placed?

    (A) In the groin
    (B) Right iliac fossa
    (C) At site of bifurcation of aorta
    (D) Into the portal system
    (E) Inferior vena cava

44. With reference to the donor kidney, which of the following statement is TRUE?

    (A) The left side is preferred, because the left renal artery is larger than that on the right.
    (B) The left renal vein passes posterior to the aorta.

    (C) Renal arteries are end arteries.
    (D) Anomalous arteries are a contraindication for elective use in transplantation.
    (E) Renal fascia separates segments of kidney.

45. A 64-year-old male is admitted to the emergency department following a car accident. His pulse is 94 bpm, blood pressure 95/60 mm Hg, and HCT 30%. Severe hematuria is evident. Following resuscitation, his blood pressure is elevated to 120/80 mm Hg. A CT scan reveals extensive contusion confined to the left kidney and perirenal fat. His blood pressure declines to 80/40 mm Hg, and urgent laparotomy is performed via?

    (A) Through a left flank incision
    (B) Through a midline abdominal incision
    (C) Through an Gibson incision
    (D) Through a thoracoabdominal incision
    (E) Through an inguinal incision

46. A 42-year-old male presents with a solid swelling in the left testis of 2-month duration. Biopsy reveals this to be a Leydig cell tumor. The function of the Leydig cell is to produce what?

    (A) Follicle-stimulating hormone (FSH)
    (B) Inhibin
    (C) Testosterone
    (D) Luteinizing hormone (LH)
    (E) Progesterone

47. A 63-year-old male has had declining ability to achieve an erection over the past 18 months. He received a prescription of sildenafil (Viagra), which works via which route?

    (A) It prevents the breakdown of cyclic guanosine monophosphate (cGMP).
    (B) It is a nonspecific inhibitor of phosphodiesterase.
    (C) It stimulates the production of nitric oxide, a gaseous neurotransmitter.
    (D) It enhances proerectile signaling in the brain.
    (E) It inhibit phosodiesterase (PDE)-2.

48. A 65-year-old male patient complains of loss of libido and is found to have a low free and total testosterone level. Treatment is commenced with testosterone supplemental therapy. What is the next step in management after testosterone administration?

    (A) Check PSA levels
    (B) Testosterone levels are decreased
    (C) Decrease in size of benign prostatic tissue lesions occurs
    (D) Decrease in size of prostatic cancer occurs
    (E) Anemia occurs

49. A 45-year-old male CIA employee presents with a 3-week history of a tumor in the scrotum. The patient has a known history of diabetes controlled by diet. There is minimal discomfort. On examination, the lesion is located posteriorly and does not transilluminate to light. Both testes are clinically normal. What is the most likely diagnosis?

    (A) Spermatocele
    (B) Teratoma
    (C) Adenomatoid lesion of the epididymis
    (D) Varicocele
    (E) Torsion of a testicular appendiceal cyst

50. A 63-year-old man undergoes a peripheral vascular procedure under general anesthesia. A decrease in urine formation and excretion are noted. Decreased urine flow under general anesthesia occurs because of which of the following?

    (A) Vasopressin
    (B) Aldosterone suppression
    (C) Depression of glucocorticoid
    (D) Depression of thyroid function
    (E) Specific effect of anesthesia on renal tubules

51. A 32-year-old athletic long distance runner complains of severe pain in the left flank. There is no radiation of the pain to the groin. Examination reveals mild tenderness in the left flank. Investigations confirm the presence of renal calculi. The stone is most likely which of the following?

    (A) Cystine
    (B) Ammonium magnesium phosphate (struvite)
    (C) Calcium oxalate
    (D) Uric acid
    (E) Calcium phosphate

52. What characteristic of struvite (ammonium magnesium phosphate) stones makes antibiotics ineffective when treatment is being performed?

    (A) Resistant bacteria
    (B) Poor excretion of antibiotics
    (C) Ineffective antibiotics
    (D) Bacteria inaccessible to antibiotics
    (E) Antibiotics inactivated by the stone

53. Following nonsurgical management of the stone, the patient is readmitted with severe colicky pain radiating to the left groin. There is minimal tenderness in the left abdomen. An x-ray shows a stone in the ureter at the level of the L-5 vertebra. Surgical intervention should be considered for which reason?

    (A) For all ureteric stones
    (B) If analgesics are required
    (C) If urinary tract infection is present
    (D) For uric acid stones
    (E) If impaired renal function occurs

Questions 54 and 55

A 42-year-old female seeks advice concerning dyspareunia, dysuria, and urinary incontinence. Symptoms were mild for the past 3 years but have become more troublesome in the past 6 months. She has had five full-term deliveries. Symptoms are worse with coughing and sneezing. Pelvic exam reveals a suburethral mass, which is confirmed on transvaginal sonogram.

54. Which of the following statements is true concerning this condition?

    (A) It occurs in 5% of woman over the age of 50.
    (B) It is most likely due to interstitial cystitis.
    (C) It causes urgency incontinence if due to a urinary fistula.
    (D) It is suggestive of a urethral diverticulum if a suburethral mass is present.
    (E) Kegel pelvic muscle exercises would aggravate this condition.

55. Treatment for urinary incontinence for this 41-year-old involves which of the following?

    (A) Should exclude Kegel pelvic muscle exercises
    (B) Kegel pelvic muscle exercises, involving exclusively the thigh and abdominal wall muscles
    (C) Is by routine hysterectomy
    (D) Includes cholinergic drugs
    (E) Is by transabdominal or transvaginal surgical repair

56. A 32-year-old female had been unable to become pregnant for 6 years. Three weeks previously, she missed her period. She was admitted to hospital with left-side lower abdominal pain and nausea. Her B subunit human chorionic gonadotropin (HCG) and pelvic ultrasound confirms an ectopic pregnancy. Treatment includes which of the following?

    (A) Immediate laparotomy and salpingectomy
    (B) If unruptured, the fallopian tube should be spared

    (C) Avoid incidental appendectomy
    (D) If stable, avoid surgery
    (E) Transfer embryo to uterus

57. A 34-year-old woman who is G4P2 complains of abdominal pain, nausea, and vomiting. During her first trimester of pregnancy, laboratory findings reveal elevated levels of Bata HCG (>100,000 mIU/dL) and pelvic ultrasound shows a "snowstorm" appearance. Which of the following statements is TRUE about gestational trophoblastic disease?

    (A) It always leads to malignancy.
    (B) It is more common in multiple pregnancy.
    (C) Gestational trophoblastic disease has complete moles that are diploid and have a 20% risk of malignancy.
    (D) Gestational trophoblastic disease has partial moles that are triploid and always undergo neoplasia.
    (E) Gestational trophoblastic disease with hydatiform mole is then treated by hysterectomy.

58. Which of the following changes would be most consistent with the diagnosis of choriocarcinoma?

    (A) Increased B-HCG
    (B) Increased alpha-fetoprotein (AFP)
    (C) Increased thyroid-stimulating hormone (TSH)
    (D) Decreased AFP
    (E) Decreased thyroxine (T4)

59. In evaluating the menstrual cycle, which is TRUE?

    (A) Estrogen secretion predominates during week prior to menstruation.
    (B) Ovulation follows a surge in LH.
    (C) Progesterone predominates the first week after menstruation.
    (D) FSH is released at midcycle.
    (E) Basal body temperature raises during mild follicular phase.

DIRECTIONS (Questions 60 through 70): Each set of matching questions in this section consists of a list of lettered options followed by several numbered items. For each numbered item, select the appropriate lettered option. Each lettered option may be selected once.

Questions 60 through 63

(A) Ulcerative colitis
(B) Rheumatoid arthritis
(C) Hemolytic anemia
(D) Cancer of the thyroid
(E) Crohn's disease
(F) Behçet's syndrome
(G) Glomus tumor
(H) Renal agenesis
(I) Granuloma inguinale
(J) Schistosomiasis (Bilharzia)

60. A 44-year-old woman complains of pain in the perineum. On vaginal examination, she is noted to have a 2-cm ulcer on the posterior wall of the vagina. The most likely cause of vulvar ulcer with associated perineal fistula and/or a weeping pustular lesion is? SELECT ONE.

61. A 45-year-old man presents with two painless beefy red ulcers in the inguinal region, a biopsy and Giemsa stain reveal Donovan bodies, these findings are most consistent with? SELECT ONE.

62. A 35-year-old male presents with painful oral ulcers, photophobia and hazy vision along with ulcers of the penis and scrotum, he has been treated with topical corticosteroids which provide temporary symptomatic relief, his symptoms are most consistent with? SELECT ONE.

63. A 65-year-old man from Egypt presenting with gross hematuria is diagnosed with squamous cell carcinoma of the bladder. The most likely cause is? SELECT ONE.

64. A 46-year-old man has a swelling in the scrotum. It shows clear transillumination anterior to the testis when a light is applied to the scrotum in a dark room. This physical exam is most consistent with?

(A) Cyst of the epididymis
(B) Torsion of testis
(C) Hydrocele
(D) Direct inguinal hernia
(E) Hematocele

65. A 25-year-old male diagnosed with testicular cancer undergoes radical orchiectomy followed by retroperitoneal lymphadenectomy complains of azoospermia, his symptoms ae most likely secondary to?

(A) Impotence
(B) Failure of ejaculation
(C) Loss of sensation in the scrotum
(D) Absent bulbocavernous reflex
(E) Splanchnic nerve denervation

66. A 20-year-old female complains of vaginal bleeding. Diagnostic workup reveals clear cell adenocarcinoma of the vagina. A maternal history should be obtained for use of?

(A) Thalidomide
(B) Oral DES
(C) Loss of sevsation in the scrotum
(D) absent bulbocavernous refl
(F) Richter's hernia
(G) torsion of testis
(H) Fournier's gangrene of the scrotum

67. A 42-year-old premenopausal woman noted to have a questionable pelvic mass on examination. Ultrasound revealed a small left ovarian cyst. Plan x-rays show no evidence of calcification. The most likely cause is?

(A) Hydatid cyst
(B) Psuedocyst
(C) Corpus luteum
(D) Dermoid cyst
(E) Granulosa-theca cell tumors

68. A 55-year-old man with history of alcohol abuse recently started on oral medication for benign prostatic hyperplasia, after several weeks of use he complains of decrease in his semen volume. Which of the following medications is responsible for ejaculatory dysfunction?

(A) Doxazosin
(B) Finasteride
(C) Tamsulosin
(D) Dutasteride
(E) Alfuzosin

69. A 65-year-old man with history of hypertension (blood pressure-130/90 mm Hg) is recently diagnosed with benign prostatis hyperplasia. Which of the following α-blockers does not lower blood pressure in men and uncontrolled hypertensison

(A) Terazosin
(B) Doxazosin
(C) Tamsulosin
(D) Prazosin
(E) Phenoxybenzamine

70. A 75-year-old man with history of benign prostatic hyperplasia, hypertension, and diabetes, on finasteride (proscar) for 2 years with a PSA level of 4 ng/mL would most likely, if he were not taking finasteride, have a PSA value of:

(A) 2 ng/mL
(B) 6 ng/mL
(C) 8 ng/mL
(D) 12 ng/mL
(E) 4 ng/mL

Answers and Explanations

1. **(D)** According to American Cancer Society, all men over the age of 50 years should undergo annual PSA measurement and digital rectal examination (DRE). This recommendtion is further supplemented by the guidelines from American Urological Association to start screening 10 years earlier in high-risk individuals (caucasians with family history of prostate cancer and African Americans).

2. **(D)** At any time during prostate cancer screening, if either the PSA or the DRE is abnormal, recommendation is referral to a urologist to perform TRUS guided biopsy of prostate.

3. **(B)** Typical workup after a positive TRUS biopsy would be evaluating the common metastatic sites (pelvic lymph nodes and bone). CT scan of abdomen and pelvis with and without contrast is performed to also rule out other GU abnormalities (i.e., renal mass, renal stone, and so forth) in addition to pelvic lymphadenopathy. Bone scan, however, is typically not indicated for PSA <20 mg/mL.

4. **(D)** Bone metastasis is a characteristic feature of prostatic cancer. The lesions are typically osteoblastic on x-ray, and the serum acid phosphatase level becomes elevated.

5. **(C)** Previously, androgen ablation was achieved by bilateral orchiectomy. However, total androgen ablation is accomplished by oral administration of antiandrogens for 2 weeks followed by injection of LRH angonist.

6. **(A)** Anencephalus is due to failure of the cephalic part of the neural tube to close off. This condition happens in 1/1000 pregnancies, is four times more common in whites than blacks, and is four times more common in females than males.

7. **(C)** Testicular cancer accounts for 1–2% of all malignant tumors in men. There are two categories of testicular tumors—lymphomas (which occur in individuals <10 or >50 years of age) and nonhematogenous tumors, that is germ cell and nongerm cell tumors (which occur in 15–35 year old individuals). Typically, the patient presents few weeks or months after a vague recollection of heavy activity or local trauma.

8. **(D)** Nonhematogenous testicular tumors are divided into two categories—germ cell tumors (seminoma, nonseminoma, i.e., embryonal, choriocarcinoma, teratoma, teratocarcinoma, yolk sac tumors) and nongerm cell tumors (Leydig cell or Sertoli cell). There is no mass within the testis with torsion. Epididymitis presents within painful tender testis.

9. **(B)** Embryonal cell carcinoma should be treated by retroperitoneal lymph node dissection (RPLND), if tumor is not spread beyond peritoneal cavity. About 30% of patients will have lymph node metastasis at the time of diagnosis. Seminoma and embryonal cell carcinomas account for about 70% of all testicular tumors.

10. **(E)** This patient is suffering from Meigs's syndrome. Treatment would be removal of a benign ovarian fibroma. Brener tumor is a fibroepithelial tumor of the ovary with low-malignant potential. Dysgerminomas contain germ cells and infiltration with lymphocytes. Krukenberg's tumor is

metastasis of a primary alimentary tract adeno-carcinoma to the ovary.

11. **(C)** The failure rate of 1/400 patient has been reported. Since there is no alteration in the level of testosterone production, there is no reported sexual dysfuntion attributed to vasectomy. The success rate for reversal of vasectomy greatly depends on the time since the vasectomy was performed. Failure rates for vasovasostomy has been reported to be >80% after 10 years.

12. **(A)** Embryologically, the genital tubercule develops into the penis. The edge of the cloacal membrane forms the urogenital fold and by the process of invagination forms the urethral groove and finally the penile urethera. The severity of hypospadias depends on the location of the anomalous opening onto the penile urethra. The mildest degree is where the opening is on the glans and the most severe form at the peno-scrotal junction.

13. **(E)** Similar to penile cancer, radical vulvectomy and bilateral groin dissection have improved survival in patients with carcinoma of the vulva. The deep and superficial nodes are removed. If the lymph nodes are not involved, the cure rate exceeds 70%. The overall survival is approximately 50%. Radiotherapy has not offered additional benefit pregnancy.

14. **(B)** Sarcoma botryoides usually occurs as a grape-like polypoid mass in the vagina of young girls. Clear-cell adenocarcinoma occurs at an older age, in the second decade of life. It is associated with the administration of DES to patient's mother's during pregnancy. Squamous carcinoma is the most common tumor of the vagina in postmenopausal patients. However, malignant tumors of the vagina are rare in children.

15. **(C)** Typically Wilms' tumor is noted in well appearing children in the second half of their first decade of life. These masses are usually felt or visually noted by parents during routine daily activities. Children with neuroblastoma are usually younger and appear quite sick. Although unlikely, renal cell carcinoma has been reported in children and diagnosis is only

based on final pathology results. Lymphoma should be ruled out based on CT scan findings and subsequent needle-guided biopsy, since treatment is usually nonsurgical.

16. **(E)** Ischiocavernous muscle is not involved in third degree perineal lacerations. This muscle originates at the ischial tuberosity and inserts at the base of the clitoris.

17. **(D)** Condylomata lata are a manifestation of secondary syphilis. The treatment is intramuscular injection of penicillin. They are distinguished from condylomata acuminata; in that the latter are velvety and filiform in appearance and are result of infection with human papilloma virus (HPV).

18. **(B)** In the Pfannenstiel incision, the rectus muscles and the peritoneum are separated in a vertical fashion after the skin is incised transversely.

19. **(C)** In stage II cervical cancer, the incidence of nodal involvement is 25%–40%. Most tumors are not radioresistant, and distant metastasis (i..e., a more advanced stage) are a late complication of more advanced stages of the disease.

20. **(A)** Dysgerminoma (like seminoma in men) is very radiosensitive. The Krukenberg's tumor is a metastatic tumor to the ovary and is not treated by radiation. The other tumors are best treated by surgery. The Brenner tumor is most often a benign tumor. Arrhenoblastomas and granuloso cell tumors are hormone-producing tumors.

21. **(D)** Free bleeding in the peritoneal cavity results in pain referred to the right supraclavicular region due to diaphragmatic irritation. Patients who present with abdominal pain and (usually) a history of missed menstruation should undergo a pregnancy test after hospital admission.

22. **(C)** Repair of vesicovaginal fistula is recommended after enough time has passed, to allow a reduction in the inflammatory reaction and even spontaneous closure to occur. To promote spontaneous closure, a Foley catheter is inserted

for bladder drainage. It is advised to perform meticulous repair, excision of previous fistulous tract, and tension-free anastomosis. Frequently an omental interposition helps to separate overlapping suture lines.

23. **(E)** Peripheral neuropathy, ototoxicity, and nephrotoxicity may be encountered following cisplatinum treatment. Nephrotoxicity can be minimized by hydrating the patient well prior and during the treatment.

24. **(D)** Tender uterosacral ligament usually are a sign of endometriosis. Although the other conditions listed may be associated with some form of pelvic pain, they do not produce tender uterosacral ligaments.

25. **(C)** The greater omentum is supplied by the right and left gastroepiploic arteries. There is no omental branch from the aorta. The middle sacral artery is a pelvic artery that does not supply the omentum, and the epigastric arteries supply the anterior abdominal wall.

26. **(B)** Initially, advanced trauma life support (ATLS) protocol requires that airway, breathing, and circulation (ABC) to be maintained. Blood at the urethral meatus is an indication of lower urinary tract (bladder, urethra, penis) injury. Foley catheter should not be inserted until the integrity of urethra is assessed (usually by performing a retrograde urethrogram). Trauma x-ray panel includes a pelvic study to evaluate the extent of injury to to pelvic brim and pubic symphysis. Fracture of the pubic rami or diastasis of pubic symphysis are commonly associated with dislocation of the sacroiliac joint as well as direct or indirect injury to the bladder and bulbous urethra.

27. **(E)** The pudendal nerve is formed from the fibers of S2–S4. In males, this nerve supplies the scrotum and penis. In females, the clitoris, distal vigina, and more than 80% (posterior part) of the vulva are innervated by the pudendal nerve. Pudendal nerve block with local anesthetic infiltration may be offered to patients during vaginal delivery and/or repair of episiotomy.

28. **(D)** The main type of bladder cancer in this country is trasitional cell carcinoma (TCC). Persistent irritative voiding symptoms in men and women, as well as microscopic hematuria, should prompt the physician to refer the patient for more detailed workup including cystoscopic evaluation. Any bladder lesion must be appropriately biopsied and removed (usually by either cold-cup biopsy and transurethral resection of bladder tumor [TURBT]). Muscle invasive bladder cancer is usually treated with radical cystoprostatectomy (in men) or anterior exenteration (in women). Extensive pelvic lymph node dissection should be performed at the time of surgery for appropriate staging purposes.

29. **(E)** It is very important to be familiar with the ureter's course in the pelvis, in order to be able to minimize injury to this structure during pelvic and colon operations. The ureter enters the pelvis immediately distal to the bifurcation of the common iliac artery. It then passes (posterior to the ovary) towards the bladder, where it travels *inferior to* the uterine artery (water under the bridge)—about 12 mm lateral to the cervix and upper vagina.

30. **(C)** The ultrasound findings of the gallbladder are normal. However, the renal mass requires further imaging. Pre- and postcontrast CT scan of abdomen and pelvis will indicate if the tumor enhances and is thus more likely to be malignant. Hilar lymphadenopathy and possibility of metastatic disease can also be assessed.

31. **(E)** Immunosuppression will not be required after grafting between identical twins (isograft). These grafts have survived the longest. Although with current immunosuppressive agents the survival of renal allografts have improved, cadaveric grafts still have the highest rejection rate followed by living unrelated, living related (parents and children), and siblings.

32. **(C)** CMV infection may cause serious disease in immunosuppressed patients. In general, the CMV titer is elevated before transplantation in the recipient and only occasionally is attribued to transmission from the donor kidney. Although over one-half of patients with kidney allografts

have a positive CMV titer, only a small fraction develops serious disease.

33. **(D)** The possibility of sexual assault must always be considered in the differential diagnosis of a child presenting with an unexplained vaginal discharge.

34. **(C)** HLA was one of the first studied antigens. The transplant antigen is located on the surface. The strongest transplant antigen is known as the major histocampatibility complex (MHC) and is found in humans on chronomosome 6. The higher the number of MHC matches, the better chance of survival for the allograft. However, zero MHC-matched grafts have been placed due to overwhelming demands. On the other hand, mismatch in ABO and Rh group results in hyperacute rejection are elevated.

35. **(C)** Normal bone marrow cells are destroyed readily by drugs and ionizing irradiation; the red blood cell (RBC) stem cell in particular is sensitive to damage. The marrow is not destroyed by the host if transplanted into an immunosuppressed host. The transplanted bone marrow develops mature stem cells, which have immunologic competence that now reject those of the host (graft-versus-host reaction). Diarrhea, dermatitis, weight loss, and infection occur.

36. **(A)** The metabolic pathway of catecholamines is initiated by conversion of tyrosine to dopa, which in turn, forms dopamine. Dopamine forms norepinephrine, which is the precursor of epinephrine. Epinephrine is the main amine secreted during life and is concerned with the "fight or flight" reaction.

37. **(B)** The left testicular vein empties into the left renal vein, and the right testicular vein empties into the IVC. Partial occlusion of the right renal vein is an uncommon cause of varicocele and may signify an associated retroperitoneal malignancy.

38. **(D)** The right testis lymphatic drainage is to paracaval, interaortocaval, and para-aortic nodes. Lymphatic drainage is crucial to the understanding of metastatic spread of testicular cancer. The left testis drains mainly to the para-aortic and interaortic lymph nodes. However, crossover drainage from right to left is more common and, therefore, the right testis drains to paracaval, interaortocaval, preaortic, and para-aortic lymph nodes. The right testicular vein drains directly into the vena cava and the left vein into the left renal vein. Both testicular arteries arise from the aortia between the renal and mesenteric arteries.

39. **(B)** The patient that has a hemoperitoneum following a pelvic fracture need to be explored immediately. Surgical repair under local anesthesia is not feasible nor is immobilization and a plaster cast. Anelgesics and observation might be possble if the patient were a child and a CAT scan revealed a clinical and a liver injury. Local traction would not be effective in stopping the bleeding.

40. **(D)** In all patients in automobile accidents, the pelvis should be examined for local tenderness, and appropriate x-rays should be ordered when a fracture is suspected. Open lavage in fracture of the pelvis does not differentiate between a simple pelvic fracture and one associated with visceral injury. CAT scan with the use of intravenous contrast material is the preferred imaging study for renal trauma. In all patients in automobile accidents, the pelvis should be examined for local tenderness, and appropriate x-rays should be ordered when a fracture of the pelvis does not differentiate between a simple pelvic fracture and one associated with visceral injury.

41. **(A)** NSAIDs may decrease renal blood flow. Probenecid and aspirin inhibit excretion of methotrexate.

42. **(D)** The hallmark of classic MDR is the development of cross-resistance to several drugs after exposure to a single drug such as dactinomycin, anthracycline, vinca alkaloid, or doxorubicin; the mechanism is a glycoprotein transmitter (Pgp) that is a result of the MDR-1 gene. Cyclosporine and verapamil block the effect of Pgp.

43. **(B)** In general, the left external iliac vessels of the recipient are chosen for anastomosis of the renal artery and renal vein of the recipient. The ureter of the donor kidney is anastomosed directly to the bladder.

44. **(C)** In general, there are five segmental arteries supplying each kidney. Segmental arteries are end arteries and, therefore, occlusion of a segmental will lead to infarction of the affected segment. The segmental arteries arise from the main renal artery. In about 70% of normal kidneys, there is a single renal artery arising from the aorta to supply each kidney. In 30%, multiple arteries arise from the aorta. In 10% of cases, there are at least two veins draining into the IVC on the right side. Duplication of venous drainage on the left side occurs much less frequently. The left renal vein passes anterior to the aorta and is of longer length, which offers advantage for the selection of the left kidney as a donor organ. If a kidney is in an abnormal location, vascular anomalies are encountered more frequently.

45. **(B)** After entering the abdominal cavity the inferior mesenteric vein is isolated to the left of the fourth part of the duodenum and Treitz's suspensary ligament. An incision is made between the fourth part of the duodenum and the inferior mesenteric vein lateral to the aorta. This approach exposes the left renal hilum and allows early and accurate exposure and control of the left renal hilum. The approach allows exposure of the left kidney and enables the surgeon to determine if a renal repair or nephrectomy is needed. It also allows exposure to the opposite kidney.

46. **(C)** LH released from the anterior pituitary acts on Leydig cells to synthesize testosterone. Testosterone is a paracrine mediator and with FSH acts on the Sertoli cells to promote spermatogenesis. Testosterone inhibits release of Gn RH from the hypothalamus. It also has a direct effect in preventing release of LH from the anterior pituitary. The Sertoli cells releases inhibin, which inhibits FSH secretion from the anterior pituitary.

47. **(A)** Sildenafil citrate (viagra) is a selective inhibitor of PDE-5, the enzyme that breaks down cGMP. Sildenafil enhances the effect of nitric oxide on corporeal arterial and sinusoidal smooth muscle by inhibiting catabolism of cGMP by PDE-5. When nitric oxide enters a vascular smooth muscle cell it stimulates the enzyme guanylate cyclase to convert cGTP to cGMP.

48. **(A)** PSA levels can increase because both benign and malignant prostatic tissue are sensitive to testosterone (hormonal) therapy. There is increased prostatic growth with elevation of PSA and possible polycythemia.

49. **(C)** Adenomatoid is the most common tumor of the epididymis. The epididymis is posterior, and a cyst of the epididymis transilluminates to light. A hydrocele also transilluminates, but it is anterior to the testis. A cyst of the testis is a remnant of the proximal part of the paramesonephros (Müller's) duct. In the presence of a normal FSH, testicular biopsy would most likely confirm normal sperm formation.

50. **(A)** The ADH vasopressin (released from the posterior pituitary) is secreted to a large extent when a patient is under anesthesia. Thus, urine formation is suppressed. The metabolic response to anesthesia and surgery tends to be retention of fluids; therefore, one must be careful to avoid administering large amounts of fluid to patients with early or overt heart failure during this period.

51. **(C)** More than 70% of renal calculi are calcium oxalate stones. Nearly half of calcium oxalate stones contain phosphate in addition to oxalate. Calcium containing stones are radiopaque and can be visualized on plain x-rays. Struvite (ammonium magnesium phosphate) and cystine stones may also be radiopaque.

52. **(D)** Bacteria inaccessible to antibiotics. Stuvite calculi harbor infective bacteria within their interstices. Effective therapy must be directed to eradicate associated infection. Struvite stones are the second most common type of renal calculi after calcium oxalate stone.

53. **(E)** Surgical intervention by endoscopic percutaneous or open surgical procedure is indicated for stones more than 5 mm in diameter that cause persistent obstruction, intractable pain, impaired renal function, or persistent urinary tract infection. In over 90% of cases, a ureteric stone <4 mm will pass naturally.

54. **(D)** Patients with urethral diverticulum show a triad of dysuria, dyspareunia, and dribbling of urine The commonest form of urinary incontinence, called stress incontinence, is due to multifactorial causes, and frequently there is an anatomic defect of the bladder neck. Urge incontinence is attributed to detrusor bladder instability and may be associated with neurological causes such as Parkinson's disease. The urethral syndrome and intestitial cystitis are sensory bladder disorders usually occurring in younger patients who do not have urinary infection.

55. **(E)** Initial treatment for urinary incontinence revolves around well-planned Kegel pelvic floor muscles and sympathomimetic drugs (to increase urethral pressure). Surgery includes the Marshall Marchetti retropubic urethropexy. Transvaginal correction is equally effective.

56. **(B)** If unruptured the fallopian tube should be spared; laparoscopic surgery is indicated, on the side of the ectopic pregnancy. An incision is made into superior (antimesenteric) border of the fallopian tube and the products of conception removed by gentle traction. Preserving the fallopian tube may improve the chances of future conception. The appendix should be removed to avoid possible confusion of the diagnosis at a subsequent date.

57. **(C)** Complete moles are diploid and have a 20% risk of malignancy. Partial moles are triploid and do not as a rule undergo malignant change. Gestational trophoblastic disease is divided in (a) hydatiform mole (partial or complete); and (b) gestational trophoblastic neoplasia. Hydatiform moles are from paternal and maternal origin. Hydatiform moles are treated by suction curettage through the cervix.

58. **(A)** Gestational trophoblastic disease may involve hydatidiform mole, choricarcinoma, or placental trophoblastic tumor. Trophoblastic tissue produces B-HCG and thus B-HCG is elevated in all these conditions. AFP is increased in neural tube defect setting when screening at 15–18 weeks gestation. AFP may be decreased in Down syndrome.

59. **(B)** The proliferative (follicular) phase (estrogen) is between the first days of menstrual bleeding to ovulation. If fertilization does not take place, progesterone release results in the endometrial proliferative phase. FSH stimulates the cycle of follicular proliferation.

60. **(E)** Crohn's disease usually causes perineal fistulas, and suppurative hidradenitis can cause weeping pustular lesions. Carcinoma, syphilis, Crohn's disease, hidradenitis, granuloma inguinale, and Behçet's syndrome are some of the more common causes of ulcerative lesions of the vulva.

61. **(I)** Granuloma inguinale is a lesion related to a contagious, sexually transmitted disease. Identification of Donovan bodies in tissue prepared with Giemsa stain establishes the diagnosis. Treatment is with tetracycline.

62. **(E)** Behçet's syndrome is characterized by oral and genital ulcers, ocular inflammation, disorders of the skin resembling erythema nodosum or multiforme, and disturbances of the central nervous system (CNS). Arthritis and thrombophlebitis are not commonly associated with this condition. The etiology is not well understood, and it may be an autoimmune disease. Cortisone has been used as treatment with variable results.

63. **(J)** In Egypt, the majority of these tumors are associated with schistosoniasis infection. Squamous cell Ca, usually presents as a higher clinical stage lesion and prognosis is generally poorer than transitional cell Ca.

64. **(C)** In adults, this is diagnostic, but in children, transillumination is also seen in an indirect

inguinal hernai. As epididymal cyst may transilluminate but is posterior to the the testis.

65. **(B)** Infertility and failure of ejaculation occur because of sympathetic denervation. Infertility is found in many patients with testis cancer. In retroperitoneal dissection (and any surgery in the region of the aortic bifurcation or promontory of the sacrum), the sympathetic branches to the hypogastric plexus must be identified and preserved when possible. In the case discussed here, the patient's ability to have an erection should not be interfered with, because the pelvic splanchnic nerves are remote from the operating site.

66. **(B)** Oral DES was given to patients who were unable to conceive. Fortunately, this complication is unlikely to occur, because DES has been withdrawn as a drug used for this purpose.

67. **(C)** Acorpus luteum cyst is functional and uusally regresses within one menstrual cycle. If a cyst is larger than 5–6 cm, one should reevaluate the patient in 4–6 weeks before suggesting laparotomy. Dermoid cysts are benign variations of teratomas. They usually are cured by simple excision, but the opposite ovary may be involved in 10% of cases.

68. **(C)** The treatment related incidence of abnormal ejaculation observed in 0.4 mg of tamsulosin is 11% and 0.8 mg of tamsulosin is 18%.

69. **(C)** Tamsulosin has the advantage of not lowering blood pressure in men who are hypertensive at baseline over the other α-blockers.

70. **(C)** Finasteride (a 5-α-reductase inhibitor for treatment of BPH) at 5 mg has been shown to lower PSA levels by 50% after 12 months of treatment. Men who are to be treated with finasteride should have a baseline PSA measurement before starting therapy. If the PSA value does not decrease by 50%, or if there is a rise in PSA value when the patient is taking finasteride, these men should be suspected of having an occult prostate cancer.

CHAPTER 10

Vascular

Nilesh N. Balar and Mayank V. Patel

Questions

DIRECTIONS (Questions 1 through 59): Each of the numbered items in this section is followed by five answers. Select the ONE lettered answer that is BEST in each case.

1. A 56-year-old male has history of leg pain at rest. Patient also has history of severe coronary artery diseases. He cannot walk two flights of steps without getting short of breath. He underwent evaluation and was noted to have complete aortoiliac occlusive disease. He needs surgery. Which one of the following options is acceptable?

   (A) Aortobililiac bypass
   (B) Aortobifemoral bypass
   (C) Aortoiliac angioplasty and stent placement
   (D) Axillobifemoral bypass
   (E) Axilloiliac

2. A 65-year-old female on her routine examination was noted to have a pulsatile abdominal mass. She has been otherwise healthy with history of hypertension with no other history, except family history of father dying of ruptured abdominal aortic aneurysm. What are the acceptable reasons to operate on abdominal aortic aneurysms in 65-year-old female with 5-cm infrarenal aneurysm?

   (A) Presence of aneurysm
   (B) Aneurysm with intramural thrombus
   (C) Asymptomatic aneurysm 5.5 cm

   (D) Associated 2-cm iliac aneurysm
   (E) Patient with splenic artery aneurysm 1.5 cm

3. An 89-year-old male presents with asymptomatic 8-cm abdominal aneurysm. He has a recent history of myocardial infarction (MI) and is not a candidate for coronary artery bypass. What should the treatment options include?

   (A) Conservative treatment observation
   (B) Computerized axial tomography (CAT) scan to evaluate eligibility for endovascular repair
   (C) Open repair without any further workup
   (D) Axillofemoral bypass and coil embolization of aneurysm
   (E) β-blocker therapy

4. A 70-year-old male underwent an open abdominal aortic aneurysm repair for ruptured aneurysm. He was stable during the procedure. In intensive care unit he was noted to have no urine output and was also noted to have large bloody bowel movement on first postoperative day. The next step for investigation includes:

   (A) Reexploration
   (B) Arterial blood gas evaluation for acidosis
   (C) CAT scan abdomen
   (D) Sigmoidscopy/colonoscopy
   (E) Antibiotics and hydration

5. A 69-year-old man was noted to have abdominal pain in left flank with severe hypotension and pulsatile mass in abdomen. He was taken to the operating room after he coded in the emergency room. Which of the following statements regarding ruptured abdominal aortic aneurysm is TRUE?

(A) 10% of patient with ruptured aneurysm reach the Hospital.

(B) Mortality is about 10%.

(C) Aortic control is usually obtained by thoracotomy.

(D) It cannot be treated by endovascular means.

(E) Mortality following a code for ruptured AAA is 100%.

6. A 82-year-old female presented with history of loss of vision in right eye for about 15 minutes and it cleared up. She has a history of diabetes and hypertension. She had which showed old infarct on right side. Carotid duplex showed that patient had 99% carotid artery stenosis. Which one of the following statements is TRUE?

(A) 60% chance that extra cranial carotid artery stenosis is the cause of transient ischemic attack (TIA).

(B) It is always due to platelet emboli.

(C) 25% may be intracranial bleed.

(D) 0.5 to 10% may have cardiac and other causes of TIA.

(E) It is always due to thrombosis.

7. A 63-year-old male was noted to have a recent TIA. Patient was having recurrent episodes of TIA despite of being on aspirin and clopidogrel bisulfate. He does have a history of unstable angina. His workup includes magnetic resonance angiography (MRA) and carotid duplex. What are the appropriate treatment options?

(A) Carotid endarterectomy for 50% carotid stenosis on MRA

(B) Carotid endarterectomy for 60% stenosis on MRA without any treatment of unstable angina

(C) Carotid endarterectomy for 90% stenosis with coronary artery bypass graft (CABG) at the same time

(D) Start patient on heparin therapy and treat conservatively for carotid stenosis of 80%

(E) Coronary angiogram with possible coronary intervention and simultaneous carotid angiogram and angioplasty and stenting

8. A 62-year-old man had right carotid endarterectomy 7 years ago. Now he has presented with 80% stenosis on the same side. He has no symptoms from the stenosis. He has carotid artery stenosis on the opposite side of 80%. He does not have any history of TIA. What is the appropriate treatment for the patient?

(A) Medical management with aspirin

(B) Carotid artery redo surgery and patch angioplasty

(C) Angiogram and angioplasty and stenting

(D) Left carotid endarterectomy

(E) Antiocoagulation of the patient to prevent stroke

9. A 60-year-old male patient with bilateral carotid artery stenosis 90%, with history of right-sided weakness with resolution of symptoms in 15 minutes. How would you treat the patient?

(A) Right carotid endarterectomy

(B) Left carotid endarterectomy

(C) Right carotid angioplasty and stenting

(D) Start patient on aspirin

(E) Start patient on heparin

10. A 72-year-old patient is noted to have neurological deficit following elective carotid endarterectomy in recovery room. What is the most appropriate treatment at this time?

(A) Carotid duplex

(B) CAT scan of brain

(C) Angiogram of cerebral vessels

(D) Heparin drip

(E) Exploration of the same side

11. A 63-year-old man has had a cyanotic painful left fourth toe for 2 days. The dorsalis pedis and posterior tibial arteries are palpable on both sides. There is no history of cardiac or vascular disease. What is the most likely diagnosis?

   (A) Cardiac embolus
   (B) Atheroembolism
   (C) Lupus vasculitis
   (D) Digital atherosclerosis
   (E) Raynaud's syndrome

12. A 40-year-old chronic smoker presents with ulceration of the tip of the right second, third, and fourth toes. He gives a history of recurrent migratory superficial phlebitis of the feet occurring a few years ago. Physical examination findings are remarkable for absent bilateral posterior tibial and dorsalis pedis pulses with palpable popliteal pulses. What is the single most important step in management?

   (A) Multiple toe amputations
   (B) Long-term anticoagulant therapy
   (C) Immediate operative intervention
   (D) Angiography followed by bypass surgery
   (E) Cessation of smoking

13. A middle-aged man is found to have a small pulsating mass at the level of the umbilicus during a routine abdominal examination. What is the best initial test to establish the diagnosis?

   (A) Aortography
   (B) Ultrasound
   (C) Computed tomography (CT)
   (D) Magnetic resonance imaging (MRI)
   (E) Plain films of the abdomen

14. A 58-year-old woman is found to have a right carotid bruit on routine examination. She is completely asymptomatic. A carotid duplex scan and carotid arteriogram (Fig. 10–1) reveal a right carotid stenosis. Which of the following statements is true?

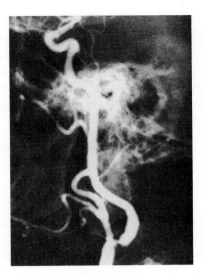

Figure 10–1.
Preoperative carotid arteriogram showing stenosis of the proximal internal carotid artery (immediately distal to the bifurcation of common carotid artery). *(Reproduced, with permission, from Doherty GM: Current Surgical Diagnosis and Treatment, 12th ed. 825. McGraw-Hill, 2006.)*

   (A) Operative treatment is indicated if the stenosis is greater than 80%, even if the patient is asymptomatic.
   (B) The incidence of stroke can be decreased by prophylactic carotid endarterectomy in patients with as little as 40% stenosis.
   (C) Aspirin is always a superior treatment to surgery regardless of the degree of stenosis.
   (D) If symptoms eventually develop, they are invariably TIAs, not stroke.
   (E) Neither surgery nor aspirin is indicated, because the patient is asymptomatic.

15. A 57-year-old male smoker is referred to you because of two episodes of right upper extremity weakness over the past 6 months, each lasting for 10–15 minutes. Findings on CT scan of the head are negative. An angiogram shows a 75% stenosis of the left carotid artery. What is the most appropriate treatment?

   (A) Antiplatelet therapy
   (B) Oral anticoagulants
   (C) Carotid endarterectomy
   (D) Carotid artery bypass to vertebral system
   (E) Surgery only if a stroke develops

16. A 24-year-old man complains of progressive intermittent claudication of the left leg. On examination, the popliteal, dorsalis pedis, and posterior tibial pulses are normal; but they disappear on dorsiflexion of the foot. What is the most likely diagnosis?

   (A) Embolic occlusion
   (B) Thromboangiitis obliterans
   (C) Atherosclerosis obliterans
   (D) Popliteal artery entrapment syndrome
   (E) Cystic degeneration of the popliteal artery

17. Four days after undergoing hysterectomy, a 30-year-old woman develops phlegmasia cerulea dolens over the right lower extremity. What is the most appropriate treatment?

   (A) Bed rest and elevation
   (B) Systemic heparinization
   (C) Venous thrombectomy
   (D) Prophylactic vena caval filter
   (E) Local urokinase infusion

18. A 21-year-old woman is referred to your office because of multiple lower extremity varicose veins. She has large varicosities in the distribution of the long saphenous vein. What is the next step in management?

   (A) A ligation and stripping operation
   (B) Ligation of both the long and short saphenous system

   (C) Sclerotherapy
   (D) Duplex evaluation along with clinical correlation as an essential initial step
   (E) Compression stockings and anticoagulation therapy

19. A 45-year-old woman undergoes cardiac catheterization through a right femoral approach. Two months later, she complains of right lower extremity swelling and notes the appearance of multiple varicosities. On examination, a bruit is heard over the right groin. What is the most likely diagnosis?

   (A) Femoral artery thrombosis
   (B) Superficial venous insufficiency
   (C) Arteriovenous (AV) fistula
   (D) Pseudoaneurysm
   (E) Deep vein insufficiency

20. A young basketball player develops an acute onset of subclavian vein thrombosis (effort thrombosis) after heavy exercise. What is the next step in management?

   (A) Active exercise of the limb
   (B) Anti-inflammatory drugs
   (C) Thrombolytic therapy
   (D) Antibiotics
   (E) First-rib resection

21. A middle-aged man undergoes a left below-knee amputation for left-foot gangrene secondary to arterial occlusive disease. Which of the following statements is true after the below-knee amputation?

   (A) There is less efficient function than after a through-knee amputation.
   (B) Stump prognosis can be judged by transcutaneous oxygen monitoring.
   (C) Poor prognosis is inevitable if Doppler fails to record a pulse at that level.
   (D) The fibula and tibia are of equal length.
   (E) The level of transection is 5 cm above the medial malleolus.

22. A 72-year-old retired banker complains of left-leg intermittent claudication while playing golf. An angiogram shows occlusion of the superficial femoral artery and reconstitution of the popliteal artery below the knee. What is the treatment of choice?

    (A) A vigorous exercise program
    (B) Endarterectomy of the superficial femoral artery
    (C) Femoropopliteal bypass with expanded polytetrofluoroethylene (PTFE) graft
    (D) In situ femoropopliteal bypass
    (E) Femoropopliteal bypass with reversed saphenous vein graft

23. A 40-year-old patient undergoes a CT scan of the abdomen for nonspecific abdominal pain. A splenic artery aneurysm is incidentally identified. What is true of the splenic artery aneurysm?

    (A) It requires splenectomy for optimal treatment.
    (B) It is more common in men.
    (C) It is caused by atherosclerosis in most cases.
    (D) It may rupture during pregnancy.
    (E) It is rarely calcified on an abdominal x-ray.

24. A 70-year-old man with a long-standing history of diabetes develops gangrene of the right second toe. What is true of his diabetic foot?

    (A) Dorsalis pedis and posterior tibial arteries are always absent.
    (B) Gangrene of the toe always requires urgent below-knee amputation.
    (C) Arterial reconstruction is invariably required.
    (D) His right femoral artery is most probably occluded or stenosed.
    (E) Trophic ulcers are sharply demarcated.

25. Eleven years after undergoing right modified radical mastectomy, a 61-year-old woman develops raised red and purple nodules over the right arm. What is the most likely diagnosis?

    (A) Lymphangitis
    (B) Lymphedema
    (C) Lymphangiosarcoma
    (D) Hyperkeratosis
    (E) Metastatic breast cancer

26. Four days after undergoing subtotal gastrectomy for stomach cancer, a 58-year-old woman complains of right leg and thigh pain, swelling and redness, and has tenderness on examination. The diagnosis of deep vein thrombosis is entertained. What is the initial test to establish the diagnosis?

    (A) Venography
    (B) Venous duplex ultrasound
    (C) Impedance plethysmography
    (D) Radio-labeled fibrinogen
    (E) Assay of fibrin/fibrinogen products

27. A middle-age woman has right leg and foot nonpitting edema associated with dermatitis and hyperpigmentation. The diagnosis of chronic venous insufficiency is made. What is the treatment of choice?

    (A) Vein stripping
    (B) Pressure-gradient stockings
    (C) Skin grafting
    (D) Perforator vein ligation
    (E) Valvuloplasty

28. A 55-year-old woman has bilateral leg edema associated with thick, darkly pigmented skin. A Trendelenburg's test is done, and results are interpreted as positive/positive. What does this patient have?

    (A) Competent varicose veins/competent perforators
    (B) Competent varicose veins/incompetent perforators
    (C) Deep vein thrombosis (DVT)
    (D) Incompetent varicose veins/competent perforators
    (E) Incompetent varicose veins/incompetent perforators

29. A middle-aged man known to have peptic ulcer disease is admitted with upper gastrointestinal (GI) bleeding. During his hospital stay, he develops DVT of the left lower extremity. What is the most appropriate management?

   (A) Anticoagulation
   (B) Observation
   (C) Thrombolytic therapy
   (D) Inferior vena cava (IVC) filter
   (E) Venous thrombectomy

30. A 70-year-old executive is complaining of three-block intermittent claudication of both legs. What is the percentage chance of his developing limb-threatening gangrene?

   (A) Less than 10%
   (B) 20%
   (C) 45%
   (D) 60%
   (E) More than 75%

31. Thirty-six hours after undergoing an abdominal aortic aneurysm repair, a 70-year-old woman develops abdominal distension associated with bloody diarrhea. What is the most likely diagnosis?

   (A) Aortoduodenal fistulas
   (B) Diverticulitis
   (C) Pseudomembranous enterocolitis
   (D) Ischemic colitis
   (E) Acute hepatic failure

32. A 65-year-old man is referred to you because of an incidental finding of a 3-cm left popliteal aneurysm (Fig. 10–2). The patient is completely asymptomatic and has normal pulses. How should the aneurysm be treated?

   (A) It should be observed.
   (B) It should be repaired because it may lead to spontaneous rupture.
   (C) It should be repaired only if it is larger than 5 cm.

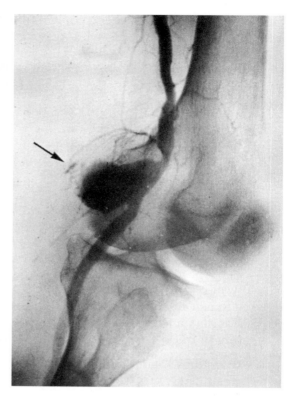

Figure 10–2.
Arteriogram showing aneurysm of the popliteal artery (arrow). *(Reproduced, with permission, from Doherty GM: Current Surgical Diagnosis and Treatment, 12th ed. 809. McGraw-Hill, 2006.)*

   (D) It should be repaired because of its tendency to either undergo thrombosis or embolize distally.
   (E) It should be repaired because of its tendency to cause nerve compression if it enlarges.

33. A 72-year-old woman falls at home after an episode of dizziness. She had been complaining of low-back pain for 3 days before the fall. In the emergency department, she is hypotensive and has cold, clammy extremities. A pulsating mass is palpable on abdominal examination. Following resuscitation, the next step in the management should involve which of the following?

   (A) Peritoneal lavage
   (B) Immediate abdominal exploration

(C) CT scan of the abdomen

(D) Abdominal aortogram

(E) Abdominal ultrasound

34. A 60-year-old man complains of dizziness, vertigo, and mild right-arm claudication. On physical examination, there is decreased pulse and blood pressure of the right upper extremity. What is the treatment of choice?

(A) Anticoagulation

(B) Repair of coarctation of the aorta

(C) Ligation of vertebral artery

(D) Carotid endarterectomy

(E) Carotid subclavian bypass

35. An 18-year-old man develops a painful, swollen leg while training for the New York Marathon. There is tenderness in the calf and ecchymosis is present. What is the most likely diagnosis?

(A) Cellulitis

(B) DVT

(C) Superficial thrombophlebitis

(D) Tear of the plantaris muscle

(E) Medical lemniscus tear

Questions 36 and 37

Four days after suffering MI, a 78-year-old woman suddenly develops severe diffuse abdominal pain. Her electrocardiogram (ECG) shows atrial fibrillation. On examination, the abdomen is soft, minimally tender, and slightly distended. Hyperactive bowel sounds are present.

36. What is the most likely diagnosis?

(A) Mesenteric embolus

(B) Nonocclusive ischemic disease

(C) Perforated peptic ulcer

(D) Congestive heart failure (CHF)

(E) Digoxin toxicity

37. The most appropriate initial examination consists of which of the following?

(A) Gastrografin upper GI series

(B) White blood cell (WBC) counts and serial abdominal examination

(C) Colonoscopy

(D) Diagnostic peritoneal lavage

(E) Angiography

38. A 28-year-old woman has new-onset hypertension and a bruit on abdominal examination. An arteriogram shows fibromuscular dysplasia (FMD) of the right renal artery. What is the best treatment option?

(A) Aortorenal saphenous vein bypass

(B) Patch angioplasty of the renal artery

(C) Percutaneous transluminal angioplasty (PTA)

(D) Transaortic renal endarterectomy

(E) Hepatorenal bypass

Questions 39 through 41

A 60-year-old man with a history of atrial fibrillation is found to have a cyanotic, cold right lower extremity.

39. The embolus is most probably originating from which of the following?

(A) An atherosclerotic plaque

(B) An abdominal aortic aneurysm

(C) Heart

(D) Lungs

(E) Paradoxical embolus

40. Which is the most common site at which an arterial embolus lodges?

(A) Aortic bifurcation

(B) Popliteal artery

(C) Tibial arteries

(D) Common femoral artery

(E) Iliac artery

41. What is the most appropriate management?

(A) Embolectomy

(B) Lumbar sympathectomy

(C) Bypass surgery

(D) Amputation

(E) Arteriography

42. An elderly patient with ischemic rest pain is found to have combined aortoiliac and femoropopliteal occlusive disease. What is the treatment of choice?

    (A) Aortofemoral bypass
    (B) Femoropopliteal bypass
    (C) Aortofemoral and femoropopliteal bypass
    (D) Lumbar sympathectomy
    (E) Vasodilator therapy

43. A 66-year-old woman has a 5.5-cm infrarenal abdominal aortic aneurysm. What is the most common manifestation of such an aneurysm?

    (A) Abdominal or back pain
    (B) Acute leak or rupture
    (C) Incidental finding on abdominal examination
    (D) Atheroembolism
    (E) Spontaneous thrombosis

44. A 72-year-old man complains of bilateral thigh and buttock claudication of several months duration. He was told by his physician that the angiogram revealed findings indicating that he has Leriche syndrome. What does this patient have?

    (A) Abdominal aortic aneurysm
    (B) Aortoiliac occlusive disease
    (C) Iliac artery aneurysm
    (D) Femoropopliteal occlusive disease
    (E) Tibial occlusive disease

45. A young woman develops a left femoral arteriovenous fistula a few months after a stab wound to the groin. Which of the following physiological changes (Nicoladoni-Branham sign) is elicited on physical examination?

    (A) Appearance of CHF when the artery proximal to the fistula is compressed
    (B) Slowing of the pulse rate when the fistula is compressed
    (C) A rise in the pulse rate when the artery distal to the fistula is compressed
    (D) A bruit heard only after the fistula is occluded
    (E) Absent dorsalis pedis after leg is elevated

46. A young patient sustains blunt trauma to his right knee that results in acute thrombosis of his popliteal artery. Which tissue is most sensitive to ischemia?

    (A) Muscle
    (B) Nerve
    (C) Skin
    (D) Fat
    (E) Bone

47. Seven years after undergoing resection of an abdominal aortic aneurysm and repair with a Dacron graft, a 65-year-old man develops an aortoenteric fistula. What would be the safest method to treat this patient?

    (A) Administration of a prolonged course of antibiotics
    (B) Removal of the Dacron graft, closure of the enteric defect, and the insertion of a new aortic graft
    (C) Closure of the enteric fistula, removal of the Dacron graft, ligation of the infrarenal aorta, and insertion of an extra-anatomic axillobifemoral bypass graft
    (D) Division of the fistula, closure of the aortic and enteric defects, and interposition of omentum in between
    (E) Closure of the enteric fistula, removal of the Dacron graft, ligation of the infrarenal aorta, and insertion of an extra-anatomic bypass at a later date

48. A 24-year-old male cyclist undergoes repair of both popliteal artery and vein following a gunshot wound to the right knee. Thirty-six hours postoperatively, there is increasing swelling of the leg and foot, and the patient complains of increasing foot pain and inability to move his toes. His pedal pulses are palpable. What is the most immediate next step that should be undertaken?

    (A) Arteriography
    (B) Leg and foot elevation
    (C) Fasciotomy
    (D) Venography
    (E) Immediate reexploration of the popliteal space

49. A homeless elderly man is brought to the emergency department after sustaining frostbite to both feet. What is the most appropriate immediate management?

    (A) Slow rewarming at room temperature

    (B) Amputation of the gangrenous toes

    (C) Rapid rewarming with warm water

    (D) Rapid rewarming with hot water or dry heat

    (E) Thorough debridement of blisters and devitalized tissue

50. A 55-year-old woman who comes from a high-altitude location is diagnosed as having a carotid body tumor (Fig. 10–3). What is true of these tumors?

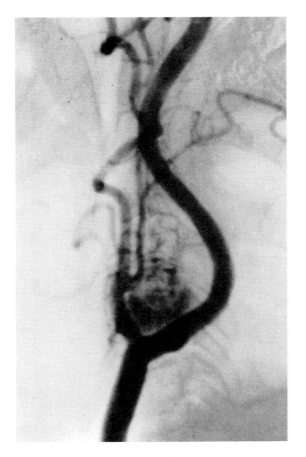

Figure 10–3.
Carotid body tumor. *(Reproduced, with permission, from Doherty GM: Current Surgical Diagnosis and Treatment, 12th ed. 819. McGraw-Hill, 2006.)*

    (A) They most frequently present as a painless neck mass.

    (B) They arise from endothelial cells.

    (C) They are usually hypovascular.

    (D) They frequently manifest with a stroke.

    (E) They are usually treated by embolization.

51. A middle-aged man complains of short-distance claudication in the right thigh. The angiogram shows a right common iliac artery stenosis of 90% over a short segment. What is the treatment of choice?

    (A) Aortofemoral bypass

    (B) Left-to-right fermorofemoral bypass

    (C) Iliofemoral bypass

    (D) PTA and stent placement

    (E) Axillofemoral bypass

52. A 65-year-old man with hypertension and a blood pressure of 190/105 mm Hg has unilateral renal artery stenosis. What is the best diagnostic test to determine the physiologic significance of the lesion?

    (A) Aortography

    (B) Renal scan

    (C) Renal ultrasound

    (D) Renal vein renin assay

    (E) Rapid-sequence intravenous pyelogram

53. A young college student injures his left knee while playing football and is unable to bear weight. The provisional x-ray report indicates that there are no fractures seen. He is discharged home but presents the next morning to the emergency department with a severely swollen, painful left knee and severe pain in the foot. On examination, the foot is pale, cold, and pulseless. What is the most likely diagnosis?

    (A) Traumatic deep vein thrombosis

    (B) Gastrocnemius muscle tear

    (C) Traumatic arteriovenous fistula

    (D) Posterior knee dislocation with thrombosed popliteal artery

    (E) Traumatic sciatic neuropathy

54. An elderly patient complains of recurrent episodes of amaurosis fugax. This is attributable to microembolization of which of the following?

    (A) Facial artery
    (B) Retinal artery
    (C) Occipital artery
    (D) Posterior auricular artery
    (E) Superficial temporal artery

55. A 65-year-old woman television technician undergoes femoral embolectomy and leg fasciotomy. Following surgery, she is noted to have oliguria, and her urine is red. What is the most probable diagnosis?

    (A) Hematuria secondary to heparin
    (B) Embolus of the renal artery
    (C) Myoglobinuria
    (D) Retroperitoneal hematoma
    (E) Hemoglobinuria

56. A 24-year-old woman on oral contraceptive pills develops an episode of deep vein thrombosis that is adequately treated with anticoagulation. She is at increased risk of developing which of the following?

    (A) Recurrent foot infections
    (B) Claudication
    (C) Pulmonary embolism
    (D) Postphlebetic syndrome
    (E) Superficial varicose veins

57. A 72-year-old businessman undergoes a femoral-to-posterior tibial *in situ* bypass graft for a nonhealing foot ulcer. During routine follow-up examination 4 years later, the graft is found to be occluded. The cause of his graft failure is most probably secondary to which of the following?

    (A) Progression of atherosclerosis
    (B) Technical error
    (C) Retained valve in the conduit
    (D) Venous aneurysm
    (E) Intimal hyperplasia

58. A 60-year-old woman has an asymptomatic right carotid bruit. A carotid duplex scan shows no evidence of significant carotid bifurcation disease but reveals reversal of flow in the right vertebral artery. What is the most likely diagnosis?

    (A) Stenosis of the origin of the common carotid artery
    (B) Stenosis of the vertebral artery
    (C) Stenosis of the subclavian artery
    (D) Stenosis of the external carotid artery
    (E) Stenosis of the intracranial portion of the internal carotid artery

59. A newborn girl with family history of lymphedema is noted to have bilateral lower extremity swelling. What is the diagnosis?

    (A) Secondary lymphedema
    (B) Lymphedema praecox
    (C) Milroy disease
    (D) Lymphedema tarda
    (E) Meigs's syndrome

Answers and Explanations

1. **(D)** The treatment goal in these patients is to reestablish blood flow to the lower extremity. The treatment is based on the findings at angiogram. All the treatment options are valid and are used in treatment of the aortooclusive disease. Patients with short-segment (TASCA) stenosis in common iliac artery are treated with angioplasty and/or stent placement and the patency results are expected to be comparable to surgery. In patients with long-segment stenosis and good risk patient treatment options would include aortobifemoral bypass. These procedures are long lasting. The long-term patency rates are reported to be 65–90%. Axillobifemoral bypass is utilized in patients with high risk and poor general condition. The patency rates for this group vary between 50–85% in 5 years. The patient described would be an ideal candidate for axillobifemoral bypass.

2. **(C)** The current indication for repair of abdominal aortic aneurysm in female includes aneurysm size 5 cm in acceptable risk patient. A United Kingdom small aneurysm study has increased the size that could be observed to 5.5 cm in male while in female it is acceptable to treat aneurysm at 5 cm size for acceptable risk. Any aneurysm with associated complication should be treated; just the presence of intramural thrombus does not justify repair. Asymptomatic 5.5-cm aneurysm should be treated in all patients, male or female, at acceptable cardiac risk. Patients with 2-cm aneurysm of iliac artery without any symptoms and complications should be observed; as the risk of surgery is higher than risk of observation till they reach to 4 cm. In patients, not in child-bearing age, 1.5-cm splenic aneurysm could be observed.

3. **(B)** An 8-cm aneurysm carries significant mortality which exceeds 50% in 1 year from aneurysm related death if observation or medical management is chosen as treatment option. It would be appropriate, if the neck size is greater than 1.5 cm and diameter is less than 26 mm, without any significant thrombus or calcification in the neck. This patient does well at least on mid term follow-up. They have lower perioperative morbidity compared to traditional open repair. Open repair with given cardiac history would carry high morbidity and morotality. β-blocker therapy would be indicated for his cardiac condition but is not a standard therapy for aneurysm.

4. **(D)** Mortality associated with aortic aneurysm is usually around 0–3%. A ruptured AAA carries mortality in range of 60–80% depending on presentation. Risk of large-bowel ischemia with ruptured AAA is about 10%. The first investigation with patients where colonic ischemia is suspected is to perform sigmoidoscopy. All other investigations may be done but none of them would be the primary investigation for the suspected pathology.

5. **(E)** Ruptured AAA carries a mortality of 40–50%. It is true that only 50% of all ruptured AAA reaches the hospital. Free peritoneal rupture carries a very high mortality. Thoracotomy is not the standard approach for proximal aortic control. Ruptured AAA can be treated with endovascular grafts. Preoperative hypotension is a good predictor of poor outcome but cardiac arrest is associated with 100% mortality in most of the studies.

6. **(A)** Neurological events are associated with extracranial carotid artery in about 60%. Fourty percent may have extracranial/intracranial cause for neurological events, which includes cardiac emboli, arch of aorta as source of emboli; intracranial bleed may be more than just a TIA. It is not always that platelet emboli are the cause of TIA, it could be due to atheroma. It is not always attributed to thrombus.

7. **(D)** Asymptomatic carotid artery stenosis is only treated surgically if it is greater than 70% stenosis. The risk reduction with surgical treatment is favorable with 70% stenosis when compared to nonoperative treatment. Any symptomatic stenosis is an indication for surgical intervention including ulcerated plaque. Any amount of stenosis with unstable angina would need appropriate workup for cardiac risk prior to carotid intervention. Carotid endarterectomy and CABG are viable options if they are left main disease and have undergone coronary angiogram. In this patient the most appropriate treatment is option to perform coronary angiogram and possible carotid stenting if feasible. Role of anticoagulation to prevent recurrent TIA is not well established. Aspirin and clopidogrel bisulfate are appropriate options for TIA.

8. **(D)** Recurrent stenosis is secondary to intimal hyperplasia but it occurs in first two years. If more than two years, it is progression of disease and it does not carry high risk for embolization, so it is reasonable to observe it. It is also a surgery which carries higher stroke rate and morbidity with nerve injury which is in range of 7%. Patient is treated with antiplatelet therapy which includes aspirin and clopidogrel bisulfate. Anticoagulation with warfarin is not a standard therapy. It is appropriate to treat the opposite side with 80% carotid stenosis. Angiogram and angioplasty is an option but if the stenosis is significant and symptomatic. Priority in this case would be to treat the opposite side.

9. **(B)** The treatment for symptomatic carotid artery stenosis greater than 70% is carotid endarterectomy. Since patient has left cerebral symptoms, it would be appropriate to treat that side first. Patient would need bilateral carotid endarterectomy but symptomatic side would be the first one to be operated. Heparin has no significant role in preventing stroke. Aspirin is a part of therapy but would not constitute a primary modality for treatment.

10. **(E)** In recovery room, the immediate approach would be to explore the patient. The cause for immediate stroke is usually technical and is most likely reversible if treated early on. All investigations are valid options once the technical cause is addressed and it would not be a primary option.

11. **(B)** All the listed conditions may result in isolated digital ischemia. In this age group, atheroembolism is the most likely diagnosis in a man. The atheroma is derived from an occult aortic aneurysm or a proximal ulcerative atherosclerotic lesion. This plaque or ulcer can be any part of the vascular tree proximal to the ischemic toe. Cardiac emboli also are common in this age group but are a less likely cause in the absence of previous MI, arrhythmia, or valvular disease.

12. **(E)** This patient suffers from thromboangiitis obliterans (Buerger's disease), a disease found most frequently in white men between 20 and 40 years of age. It is a form of panvasculitis involving the artery, vein, and nerve. Heavy tobacco smoking is strongly associated with this disease. Early in the course of the disease, there is involvement of the superficial veins, producing recurrent migratory superficial phlebitis. The distribution of arterial involvement is usually segmental, involving the peripheral arteries. In the lower extremities, the disease occurs generally beyond the popliteal arteries and distal to the forearm in the upper extremities. As long as ulceration or gangrene is confined to a digit, amputation should be postponed as long as possible unless rest pain or infection cannot be otherwise controlled. Bypass surgery is rarely indicated, and long-term anticoagulation has not been of much benefit. The most important aspect of treatment is cessation of smoking, which can halt progression of the disease.

13. **(B)** Although aortography, CT, and MRI can all establish the diagnosis of abdominal aortic aneurysm, ultrasound remains the best screening test. It is the preferred method for making the initial diagnosis, because it is reliable, inexpensive, and noninvasive. Aortography is used infrequently because of the small but definite risk it entails and because diagnosis can be made by other means. Once the aneurysm meets the criteria for repair, then a CT scan is done preoperatively to establish the true size and to delineate the aneurysm more accurately. Plain films of the abdomen are inaccurate in establishing the diagnosis.

14. **(A)** Operative treatment is indicated if the diameter of the stenosis is greater than 60%, even if the patient is asymptomatic. The value of prophylactic carotid endarterectomy, for hemodynamically significant carotid stenosis, decreases the incidence of subsequent cerebral ischemic events if performed with morbidity and mortality rates under 4%. Several studies including asymptomatic carotid artery surgery (ACAS) have shown that surgical treatment is superior to medical management if the stenosis is 60% or greater. The ACAS trial has shown the benefits of surgical treatment over medical management if the stenosis is greater than 60%. However, there are no data to support the use of carotid endarterectomy in asymptomatic patients with stenosis of less than 60%. If ischemic events eventually develop, stroke can be the presenting symptom.

15. **(C)** This patient is experiencing recurrent left hemispheric TIA with a hemodynamically significant stenosis of the left carotid artery. This is clearly an indication for surgery because operative management is superior to aspirin in symptomatic carotid bifurcation disease with stenosis greater than 70%. Oral anticoagulants may decrease the incidence of TIAs but not of completed strokes, and they are associated with a considerable risk of hemorrhage. Carotid endarterectomy, and not carotid artery bypass, is the surgical procedure of choice. Surgical treatment must be performed before and not after major neurologic deficits are produced from cerebral infarction.

16. **(D)** Popliteal artery entrapment syndrome consists of intermittent claudication caused by an abnormal relation of that artery to the muscles, usually the medial head of the gastrocnemius muscle. As a consequence of developmental abnormalities, the popliteal artery may be compressed by the medial head of the gastrocnemius muscle, resulting in ischemia of the leg at an unusually early age. On examination, the pulses may be diminished or absent, but they may also be normal and be made to disappear on dorsiflexion of the foot. Angiography is essential to establish the diagnosis.

17. **(C)** Phlegmasia cerulae (blue) dolens, indicates that major venous obstruction has occurred. The standard treatment for postoperative thrombosis includes bed rest and anticoagulation. Venous thrombectomy may be indicated when impending gangrene is noted. Vena caval filters are inserted in patients with established pulmonary emboli, but they may be considered as a prophylactic measure when iliofemoral thrombosis is massive. They are also inserted as an adjunct to venous thrombectomy along with creation of an arteriovenous fistula to prevent the venous system from rethrombosing. Thrombolysis of major venous thrombi requires placement of a multihole pigtail catheter inside the thrombus and administration of tPA, including systemic heparinization and is therefore contraindicated postoperatively.

18. **(D)** A through clinical evaluation followed by a venous duplex examination are the two most important steps in managing varicose vein of the lower extremity. An asymptomatic patient without complications of phlebitis, ulceration, or hemorrhage should be treated with compression stocking. Duplex evaluation will help map the valvular incompetence of the superficial and deep system including the perforators that guide the extent of the initial surgical intervention, and also investigate if these are primary or secondary varicosities. Sclerotherapy is an alternative to surgery but in the presence of saphenofemoral, saphenopopliteal, or perforator reflux is associated with a high incidence of recurrence and complications.

19. **(C)** A traumatic AV fistula results from a penetrating injury to adjacent artery and vein, permitting blood flow from the injured artery into the vein. The iatrogenic injury in this case occurred during cardiac catheterization. Femoral artery thrombosis results in signs of limb ischemia. A bruit is usually not heard with venous insufficiency. Traumatic pseudoaneurysm presents as an enlarging pulsating mass. Once the diagnosis of AV fistula is made, an angiogram is performed, and surgical repair (division of the fistula and reconstruction of the artery and preferably of the injured vein as well) is carried out.

20. **(C)** Effort thrombosis, also called Paget-von Schroetter syndrome, is the development of thrombosis of the axillary-subclavian vein as a result of injury or compression. It occurs primarily in young athletes and is disabling. When these patients are seen early, thrombolytic therapy is the first step in management and is followed by a venogram to detect correctable lesions. If effort thrombosis is associated with thoracic outlet syndrome, then thrombolytic therapy should be followed by cervical rib resection. If the condition is chronic, thrombolytic therapy might not be successful; these patients usually respond to limb elevation and anticoagulation.

21. **(B)** Stump prognosis can be judged by transcutaneous oxygen monitoring. Doppler is not fully reliable to select the level of transection, because it cannot calculate the quantity of vascular flow. Transcutaneous oxygen (PO_2 >40 mm Hg) offers a fairly accurate prediction of a favorable result; although, Doppler fails to confirm a patient pulse at the level of transection. On the other hand, a duplex evaluation with blood flow of more than 50 cm/s is also a fairly accurate predictor for stump prognosis. The level of transection is 13–15 cm below the level of the medial condyle of the tibia.

22. **(A)** If claudication is the only symptom, elective vascular reconstruction is considered only if claudication is disabling and interferes with day-to-day activity. Because the risk of gangrene, occurring in a patient who has only claudication,

is small, this alone does not constitute a clear-cut indication for operation. Vigorous exercise programs have resulted in marked improvement in claudicants. Revascularization surgery is usually reserved for rest pain or tissue loss (nonhealing ulcer, gangrene). Addition of a phosphodiastraze inhibitor, cilostazol (pletal), or pentoxiphyline (trental) can help increase the claudication distance. It should also be kept in mind that an angiogram is not indicated for claudication. An initial evaluation with noninvasive vascular studies is the investigation of choice. Angiogram is only requested if the decision is made to intervene surgically.

23. **(D)** Splenic artery aneurysms are rare and are most frequently caused by medial necrosis. Small asymptomatic aneurysms caused by atherosclerosis are more commonly incidental findings at autopsy. Larger (>3 cm) aneurysms predominate in women and characteristically may rupture during late pregnancy. Rupture may be preceded by an initial warning bleed into the retroperitoneum, with massive bleeding following after 1 or 2 days.

24. **(E)** Patients with a diabetic foot may have localized arterial occlusion involving the popliteal artery and its branches, usually sparing the femoral artery. Although patients have gangrene of the toes, there may be a palpable pulse in the foot. In the presence of localized disease, trophic ulcers and even gangrene of the toes may respond to local foot care, and major vascular reconstruction or amputations are not required. The trophic ulcers have punched sides. Patients may not realize the gravity of localized gangrene with spreading cellulitis, which develops because of the neurotropic nature of the lesions with the absence of pain sensation.

25. **(C)** Lymphangiosarcoma is a rare complication of long-standing lymphedema, most frequently described in a patient who has previously undergone radical mastectomy (Stewart-Treves syndrome). It usually presents as blue, red, or purple nodules with satellite lesions. Early metastasis, mainly to the lung, may develop if it is not recognized early and widely excised. Lymphedema is a complication of radical mastectomy and

presents as diffuse swelling and nonpitting edema of the limb. Lymphangitis and hyperkeratosis are complications of lymphedema.

26. **(B)** The most accurate method of confirming the diagnosis of venous thrombosis is the injection of contrast material to visualize the venous system (venography). However, this method is invasive and time-consuming and must be done in the radiology suite. Venous duplex ultrasound is noninvasive, can be done bedside, and has a sensitivity and specificity of 96 and 100%, respectively. The other methods listed are used less often in certain selected patients.

27. **(B)** The mainstay of treatment of chronic venous insufficiency and its complication, venous stasis ulceration, is conservative management. Elastic stocking support, frequent elevation of the legs, and avoidance of prolonged sitting and standing is used for venous insufficiency in the absence of ulceration. If venous stasis ulcers develop, then paste boots (e.g., Unna's boots) are used along with appropriate bed rest and foot elevation until the ulcer heals. Patients whose ulcers fail to heal after such conservative management may need perforator vein ligation. Skin grafting should be considered for chronic stasis ulcers that are large, and perforator incompetance has been treated. Venous reconstruction procedures, including valvuloplasty, can be useful for a selected group of patients, especially those with venous claudication to less than half a block, that have been treated with all the procedures above, including stripping and ligation. Unlike previous opinions, superficial venous stripping and ligation is not always contraindicated in the presence of chronic venous insufficiency and even previous history of deep vein thrombosis.

28. **(E)** The Trendelenburg's test is a two-part test used to access the competency of the superficial and perforating veins. The legs are elevated to evacuate the veins, and pressure is applied to the saphenofemoral junction either by hand or tourniquet. The four possible results are: (a) negative/negative response if there is gradual filling of veins from below and continued slow filling after release of pressure, indicating absence of incompetent superficial and perforating veins; (b) negative/positive response if there is gradual filling of veins from below while there is rapid retrograde filling after release of pressure, indicating incompetent superficial veins only; (c) positive/negative response if there is rapid initial filling of the veins from below while only continued slow filling after the release of pressure, indicating incompetent perforators only; and (d) positive/positive response if there is rapid filling of the saphenous vein before and after release of pressure, indicating incompetent superficial and perforating veins.

29. **(D)** The main treatment of DVT is adequate anticoagulation. However, if pulmonary embolism develops during anticoagulant therapy or if there is contraindication to anticoagulation, the insertion of an IVC filter is indicated either to prevent occurrence of or to offer prophylaxis against recurrence of pulmonary embolism (Fig. 10–4). Observation alone leaves the patient unprotected against pulmonary embolism, and operative thrombectomy is reserved for limb salvage in the presence of impending venous gangrene. Obviously, if anticoagulation is contraindicated (as in the patient presented), thrombolytic therapy cannot be used.

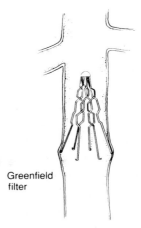

Greenfield filter

Figure 10–4.
Surgical prevention of pulmonary embolism. Large emboli can be trapped by partial interruption of the IVC (Greenfield filter). *(Reproduced, with permission, from Way LW: Current Surgery Diagnosis & Treatment, 10th ed. Appleton & Lange, 1994.)*

30. **(A)** The relatively benign course of intermittent claudication has been well established. The risk of gangrene developing within 5 years in an extremity with claudication as the only symptom is only about 5%. The patient must be encouraged to stop smoking, to exercise, and be placed on a diet that lowers cholesterol.

31. **(D)** The occurrence of bowel movements during the first 24–72 hours after repair of an abdominal aortic aneurysm (especially if the hemoccult test is positive), should raise suspicion for ischemic colitis. It may develop as a result of interruption of flow to the inferior mesenteric artery with inadequate collateral circulation from either the superior mesenteric artery or the iliac arteries. Aortoduodenal fistula is a late complication of aneurysm repair. Pseudomembranous enterocolitis occurs late in the postoperative course.

32. **(D)** Popliteal aneurysms are usually arteriosclerotic and are bilateral in at least 50% of cases. Any popliteal aneurysm twice the size of the normal artery is an indication for surgical repair. Although often asymptomatic and small, they should be treated surgically because of their propensity to produce limb-threatening ischemia related to thrombosis or embolism. Spontaneous rupture and/or nerve compression are rare complications of a popliteal aneurysm. The ideal repair consists of ligation of the aneurysm, including its branches and a bypass to the open distal vessels.

33. **(B)** The presence of acute vascular collapse with history of abdominal or flank pain and associated pulsating abdominal mass is characteristic of a ruptured abdominal aneurysm. Operation should be performed as quickly as possible, because the first priority is to control the hemorrhage. No time should be lost in obtaining diagnostic studies, because these patients often crash in the radiology suite. These patients should not be resuscitated aggressively, because an increase in systolic pressure will only cause more intra-abdominal hemorrhage.

34. **(E)** The clinical picture presented is that of a subclavian artery stenosis resulting in subclavian steal syndrome, represented by vertebrobasilar symptoms and extremity ischemia. The symptoms are due to a decrease of posterior circulation (vertebral artery) blood flow. Claudication occurs more commonly than ischemic findings. Most patients have no triggering events, and the symptoms are not readily reproducible. Carotid subclavian bypass restores the circulation beyond the stenotic area and corrects the steal syndrome. Ligation of the vertebral artery will correct the steal syndrome but will not improve the circulation of the arm. Anticoagulation has no role in the treatment of this entity. Other treatment options include subclavian artery transposition, axilloaxillary bypass, and subclavian artery angioplasty. Coarctation of the aorta results in pulse and pressure difference between the upper and lower extremities.

35. **(D)** Spontaneous thrombophlebitis in this age group is unlikely. Plantaris or gastrocnemius tear may occur during physical exertion involving running or walking, causing a sharp pain in this region. After resolution of a hematoma in this region, it may be difficult to exclude cellulitis if there is any question that the integrity of the skin has been damaged. In superficial thrombophlebitis, there is tenderness along the distribution of the long or short saphenous veins. A tear of the medial lemniscus of the knee joint is detected by tenderness over the medical aspect of the knee joint during flexion and internal rotation of the knee joint (McMurray sign).

36. **(A)** Patients with atrial fibrillation are more likely to develop emboli to different sites throughout the body. Nonocclusive ischemic disease is characterized by spasm of the major mesenteric arterial vessels, with a characteristic beading effect. Early recognition may result in improvement with direct intra-arterial infusion of papaverine (which causes vasodilation), thus avoiding operative intervention.

37. **(E)** Clinical findings of peritoneal irritation and leukocytosis in patients with suspected visceral ischemia indicate necrosis of ischemic bowel. Immediate arteriography is required to establish the diagnosis and initiate treatment to restore circulation before massive bowel infarction,

acidosis, and possible perforation occur. The most likely diagnosis is a mesenteric embolus arising from the heart, especially in the presence of atrial fibrillation. The catheter should be left in place to allow papaverine infusion to an area of borderline ischemic bowel.

38. **(C)** Among all causes of renovascular hypertension, FMD responds best to angioplasty. Intermediate results of PTA for FMD are similar to those of bypass. PTA has lower morbidity, causes less discomfort, and is less expensive. Recurrence can be treated by repeated PTA.

39. **(C)** The heart is the origin of about 90% of lower extremity emboli. The causes are usually mitral stenosis, atrial fibrillation, or MI. A rare source of left atrial emboli is a left atrial myxoma. The remaining 10% arise from ulcerated plaques in the aorta or peripheral arteries. Paradoxical emboli arising from the venous system may reach the arterial circulation through a patent foramen ovale.

40. **(D)** Arterial emboli usually lodge proximal to bifurcations, the most common site being the common femoral artery.

41. **(A)** Once the diagnosis is made clinically, heparin is administered intravenously to prevent the development of thrombi distal to the embolus. Then embolectomy can be done in most instances under local anesthesia. Arteriography to confirm what is already clinically apparent only delays the needed surgical procedure. If there is a doubt, duplex evaluation will help confirm the diagnosis. Lumbar sympathectomy locks are of dubious value. In patients who have known occlusive disease, absent pulses in the contralateral extremity, absence of clinical features of hyperacute ischemia would be best managed by an angiogram and thrombolytic infusion.

42. **(A)** Patients with combined segmental occlusive disease require correction of proximal hemodynamically significant disease before distal (infrainguinal) bypass. Only about 20% of patients undergoing aortofemoral reconstruction in the presence of superficial femoral artery occlusion will subsequently require femoropopliteal bypass. Combined procedures should be reserved for patients with severe life-threatening ischemia. Lumbar sympathectomy and vasodilator therapy are ineffective in treating severe arterial occlusive disease.

43. **(C)** Most patients are unaware of their abdominal aneurysm until it is incidentally discovered by their physician. The importance of careful deep palpation of the abdomen cannot be overemphasized. On occasion, these aneurysms may expand, causing abdominal or back pain, and may even leak or rupture, mimicking other acute intra-abdominal conditions. Signs and symptoms of acute ischemia in the lower extremities are rare and usually follow thrombosis or embolization from an abdominal aneurysm.

44. **(B)** Leriche syndrome consists of the manifestations of aortoiliac occlusive disease and includes thigh and buttock claudication, atrophy of the leg muscles, diminished femoral pulses, and impotence in men.

45. **(B)** The Nicoladoni-Branham sign can be elicited in some patients with an AV fistula. Occlusion of the fistula or the artery proximal to the fistula may result in slowing of the heart rate. By this compression, the peripheral resistance is increased, venous return is decreased, and the pulse rate falls.

46. **(B)** Peripheral nerve endings are the tissues most sensitive to anoxia in the extremity. Therefore, paralysis and paresthesia are most important when evaluating an extremity with acute arterial occlusion. The second most sensitive tissue is the muscle. This is why an extremity with paralysis and paresthesia will develop gangrene if circulation is not restored. Gangrene is less likely to occur if signs of ischemia are present, but motor and sensory functions are intact.

47. **(E)** The use of an extra-anatomic bypass (axillobifemoral) is indicated in the presence of "hostile" abdomen (infection, dense and severe adhesions, tumors) or if the patient is too sick to undergo an abdominal operation. If a previously placed graft is contaminated (infection,

aortoenteric fistula), the graft must be removed, and the enteric defect must be closed. Although some surgeons advocate removing the infected graft and replacing it *in situ* with a new graft, the safest approach remains the extra-anatomic route to restore circulation to the lower extremities (axillobifemoral bypass).

48. **(C)** Compartment syndrome can occur following repair of vascular injuries, especially if ischemia time is more than 6 hours or if there have been substantial periods of shock. Other instances include the combination of arterial and venous injury and the presence of concomitant soft-tissue crush injury or bone fracture. Compartment swelling and tenderness, pain disproportionate to the physical findings, paresthesia, and weakness are all clinical signs of compartment syndrome and require urgent surgical decompression. A palpable pulse does not rule out the presence of a compartment syndrome, because compartment pressures are high, even before loss of a palpable pulse.

49. **(C)** Rapid warming of the injured tissue is the most important aspect of treatment. The frozen tissue should be placed in warm water, with a temperature in the range of 408–448°C. Dry heat or hot water carries the risk of thermal injury because of decreased sensation in the injured part. Opening of blisters and debridement of devitalized tissue are contraindicated. Demarcation of gangrenous areas should be carefully observed, often for several weeks, before amputation is performed. The extremity should be elevated, tetanus prophylaxis should be administered as indicated, and antibiotics should be given in the presence of open wounds.

50. **(A)** Carotid body tumors are usually 3–4 mm in size and are located at the carotid bifurcation. They arise from nests of chemoreceptor cells of neuroectodermal origin (carotid body). In normal individuals, the carotid body responds to a fall in PO_2 and pH and to a rise in PCO_2 and temperature to cause an increase in cardiac contraction, heart rate, and respiratory rate. Carotid body tumors are uncommon, slow growing, and highly vascular. Although large tumors may cause compression of the vagus or hypoglossal nerves, most tumors present as a palpable painless mass at the carotid bifurcation. The treatment is definitely excision whenever possible.

51. **(D)** PTA is technically successful in approximately 90% of iliac lesions with good patency rates. It is more successful for single short stenoses rather than multiple long stenosis or occlusions. The advantages of PTA is that it is less invasive than surgery, has a lower initial cost, has a shorter hospital stay, and lower morbidity, enables an earlier return to full activity, and the procedure can be repeated without an increase in morbidity or a decrease in clinical result. It is particularly useful for patients who are at high operative risks. The ideal procedure would be and angioplasty and stent placement.

52. **(D)** Aortography and renal ultrasound can detect the presence of renal artery stenosis, but they do not determine the functional significance of the lesion. IVP is not a sensitive enough test to detect the presence of renal artery stenosis. A renal scan can show decreased flow (uptake) or decreased function of the affected kidney, but it, too, lacks sensitivity. The assessment of renal vein renin levels is a good diagnostic test to determine the physiologic significance of renal artery stenosis. It indicates whether the stenosis is significant enough to decrease the glomerular filtration rate and cause the release of renin. In addition, the opposite kidney should have suppression of renin secretion.

53. **(D)** Normal radiographic findings in the presence of severe knee trauma should raise suspicion for posterior dislocation of the knee, which is often associated with popliteal artery thrombosis. A careful vascular examination should, therefore, be made in such a situation. The presence of pain, pallor, and pulselessness (three of the five *p*'s) is indicative of severe ischemia. This patient should undergo urgent exploration for vascular repair. The other options are unlikely to cause the signs and symptoms presented.

54. **(B)** Amaurosis fugax, one type of TIA, is a manifestation of carotid bifurcation atherosclerotic disease. It is manifested by unilateral blindness, being described by the patient as a window

shade across the eye, lasting for minutes or hours. It is caused by microemboli from a carotid lesion lodging in the retinal artery, the first intracerebral branch of the internal carotid artery.

55. **(C)** Patients with sudden severe ischemia are prone to "ischemia-reperfusion" syndrome. With revascularization, there is sudden release of the accumulated products of ischemia into the circulation; namely, potassium, lactic acid, myoglobin, and cellular enzymes. Hyperkalemia, metabolic acidosis, and myoglobinuria (red urine, clear plasma) are the key features of the syndrome. Renal tubular acidosis results in myoglobin deposition in the renal tubules. Anticipation and early recognition require the induction of diuresis with mannitol, alkalinization of the urine to avoid precipitation of myoglobin in the renal tubules, and correction of hyperkalemia.

56. **(D)** Despite receiving optimal treatment for DVT, approximately 50% of the patients will develop the post-thrombotic syndrome. The recanalization of the deep veins will result in deformity and subsequently incompetence of the affected venous valves. Although patients with DVT can develop infections secondary to edema, these are usually located about the ankle and resolve with adequate treatment. Patients adequately treated for DVT are not at increased risk of developing pulmonary embolus. Neither the arterial circulation nor the superficial venous system are affected by the development of DVT. Young patients with iliofemoral thrombosis are best managed by thrombolytic infusion, which has been shown to preserve valvular function and decrease the incidence of postphlebitic syndrome.

57. **(A)** The causes of graft failure can be divided into early and late. Although early failure of vein grafts is usually attributed to either technical error or inadequate outflow tract, late failure is usually related to progressive proximal or distal atherosclerotic disease. Other less common causes of late graft failures include—local stenotic areas from trauma or endothelial damage, valve stenosis from fibrosis, and venous aneurysms and subsequent thrombosis. Intimal hyperplasia is a rare cause of late failure.

58. **(C)** Occlusion or stenosis of the subclavian artery proximal to the origin of the vertebral artery results in the "subclavian steal" syndrome. In response to decreased pressure in the distal subclavian artery, especially in instances in which increased perfusion is needed, there is reversal of flow in the vertebral artery. The clinical picture is that of vertebrobasilar symptoms in association with upper extremity exercise. Although this phenomenon is sometimes seen on duplex scanning or angiography, evolution into a clinical syndrome is relatively rare. The other mentioned options do not result in retrograde flow in the vertebral artery.

59. **(C)** Lymphedema is classified by etiology—primary versus secondary. Primary lymphedema is divided into congenital, praecox, and tarda, depending on the age of onset. The diagnosis of Milroy disease is reserved for patients with familial lymphedema in which clinical factors are present at birth or noticed soon thereafter. Lymphedema is classified as praecox if the age of onset is between 1 and 35 years. Meigs' disease is the familial form of primary lymphedema praecox. If the onset of primary lymphedema is after 35 years of age, it is called lymphedema tarda. Secondary lymphedema usually results from a disease process that causes obstruction of the lymphatic system.

CHAPTER 11

Neurosurgery

Kamran Tabaddor, MD

Questions

DIRECTIONS (Questions 1 through 58): Each of the numbered items in this section is followed by five answers. Select the ONE lettered answer that is BEST in each case.

1. A 43-year-old man experiences lower back pain after lifting a heavy object off the ground. The following morning, he notices that the pain has begun to radiate down the posterolateral aspect of the right leg and across the top of the foot to the big toe. The pain is severe, electric in quality, associated with paresthesia over the same distribution, and made worse by coughing. On examination, it is found that he has an area of diminished sensation to pinprick over the dorsum of the right foot and mild weakness in his right extensor hallucis longus muscle. The deep tendon reflexes are all intact. What is the most likely diagnosis?

   (A) Lumbar spinal fracture with compression of the cauda equina
   (B) Herniated lumbar disk on the right at the level of L4–L5
   (C) Herniated lumbar disk on the left at the level of L4–L5
   (D) Herniated lumbar disk on the right at the level of S1–S2
   (E) Intermittent claudication

2. A 48-year-old woman has a lower back pain and hypoesthesia in the left S1 dermatomal distribution (left calf and lateral left foot). What is the most likely cause?

   (A) A lesion at the right L4–L5 interspace
   (B) Pathology where the nerve exits the spinal canal immediately above the pedicle of S3 vertebra
   (C) A herniated nucleus pulposus
   (D) Compression by the L5 lamina
   (E) A lesion outside the vertebral column

3. A 35-year-old secretary complains of severe pain in the neck that radiates down the right arm. The pain is electric in quality and affects specifically the radial aspect of the right forearm and the thumb. She also describes numbness and paresthesia over the same distribution. On physical examination, she is found to have an area of diminished sensation to pinprick over the right wrist and thumb. The right biceps tendon reflex is diminished, but there is no loss of muscle strength. She has right C5–C6 disk compression and radiculopathy affecting which of the following?

   (A) The right C4 root
   (B) The right C4 mixed spinal nerve
   (C) The right C4 anterior primary rami
   (D) The right C6 root
   (E) The right C6 spinal ganglion

Questions 4 and 5

A 47-year-old man presents to the emergency department after falling from his bicycle. He claims that his neck was suddenly and violently hyperflexed. Although he is currently complaining of neck pain, his chief complaint is weakness of the arms. On examination, he is found to have profound symmetric weakness of both hands and wrists. His biceps and triceps are moderately weak. The lower extremities are only minimally weak, and he is able to ambulate, albeit with some difficulty. His sensation to all modalities is within normal limits. Plain radiographs of his neck reveal no fracture or dislocation, but there is evidence of severe spondylosis with osteophytes narrowing the neural canal at C3–C4, C4–C5, and C5–C6.

4. What is the most likely mechanism of injury?

   (A) Brachial plexus injury
   (B) Epidural hematoma
   (C) Contusion of the spinal cord
   (D) External carotid artery occlusion
   (E) Internal jugular vein occlusion

5. What is this pattern of motor findings that results from this injury termed?

   (A) Central cord syndrome
   (B) Cervical radiculopathy
   (C) Cauda equina syndrome
   (D) Lhermitte sign
   (E) Posterior cord syndrome

Questions 6 and 7

A 57-year-old woman is referred to you for evaluation of difficulty with ambulation. Her chief complaint is weakness of her left leg that has been slowly progressive over the last 6 months. On neurologic examination, her mental status and cranial nerve findings are within normal limits. She has marked (grade 4–5) weakness of both her left leg and arm. On her left side, she has diminished sensation to light touch and vibration below the C5 dermatome. Sensation to pinprick and temperature are severely diminished on the right side below approximately the C8 dermatome. Her deep tendon reflexes and muscle tone are increased on the left.

6. This pattern of neurologic deficits is which of the following?

   (A) Spondylolisthesis
   (B) Brown-Sequard syndrome
   (C) Central cord syndrome
   (D) Guillain-Barré syndrome
   (E) Poliomyelitis

7. This pattern of neurologic deficits is explained by injury to the spinal cord with damage to which of the following?

   (A) Anterior horn cells
   (B) Peripheral neuropathy
   (C) Central cord
   (D) Right half (right hemicord)
   (E) Left half (left hemicord)

8. A 73-year-old man presents for evaluation of weakness in his lower extremities and recurrent falls. On further questioning, the patient admits to having frequent spasms affecting both of his lower extremities. He also claims that his legs occasionally feel as if ants were crawling all over them. On neurological examination, he is found to have a slightly unstable gait and with minimal flexion of the knees. His strength is slightly but symmetrically diminished in both lower extremities and both triceps muscles. There is decreased sensation to vibration and light touch below approximately the level of the nipples bilaterally. In both lower extremities, muscle tone is markedly increased, and deep tendon reflexes are hyperactive. Babinski's reflex is present bilaterally. What is the most likely diagnosis?

   (A) A thoracic spinal cord compression
   (B) A thoracic radiculopathy
   (C) A cervical myelopathy
   (D) Cerebellar tumor
   (E) Intracranial aneurysm

9. An 87-year-old woman is referred to you for evaluation of lower back pain. It is exacerbated by walking or prolonged standing and occasionally made better by bending over. Physical examination reveals a thin, elderly woman who walks with a cane with her lower back moderately flexed. Motor power in her lower

extremities is normal, but she has impaired sensation to light touch and vibration below the L4 dermatome bilaterally. Deep tendon reflexes are normal in her upper extremities but absent in both lower extremities. You refer her for magnetic resonance imaging (MRI) of the lumbosacral spine. What will be the most likely finding on this study?

(A) Lumbar spinal stenosis
(B) A fracture of the odontoid process
(C) A herniated L3–L4 disk causing unilateral compression of the L4 root
(D) Spinal cord compression at the level of L1 vertebra level
(E) Spinal cord compression at the T1 vertebra level

10. A 33-year-old man is brought to the emergency department after being involved in a major motor vehicle accident. He is unable to move his legs and complains of severe pain in his mid to lower back. On physical examination, he is found to have exquisite tenderness over some of the bony prominence of his lower back, but no gross physical deformity can be appreciated. On neurologic examination, flaccid paralysis of both lower extremities and complete anesthesia to all sensory modalities below approximately the L3 dermatome are noted. Catheterization of his bladder yields approximately 700 mL of urine. Plain radiographs of the spine reveal compression fracture in the body of L3 with greater than 50% of loss in its height. A computed tomography (CT) scan through this area reveals a burst fracture of the body of L3. There are large fragments of bone driven dorsally with an 80% canal compromise. What is the cause of weakness?

(A) Compression of the conus medullaris
(B) Compression of the spinal cord at the level of L3
(C) Compression of the cauda equina
(D) Rupture of the anterior spinal ligament
(E) Associated epidural hemorrhage

Questions 11 and 12

A 17-year-old boy suffers a hyperextension injury of his neck when he jumps headfirst into a shallow pool. He does not lose consciousness. He arrives at the emergency department holding his neck stiffly and complaining of severe neck pain. He says the pain is particularly severe whenever he tries to move his head. He says he has no neurologic symptoms such as weakness, numbness, or paresthesia. On physical examination, he is found to have no areas of ecchymosis or deformity on the cervical spine. He has exquisite pain on deep palpation of the bony prominence of the mid-cervical spine. There are no neurological signs. Routine plain radiographs (anteroposterior [AP], lateral, open-mouth view) of the cervical spine in the neutral position show no fracture or subluxation of the bony elements. There is, however, thickening of the pretracheal space ventral to the body of C6, suggesting soft-tissue swelling.

11. What would the next step in management involve?

(A) Analgesics alone
(B) A hard cervical collar
(C) Internal fixation of the cervical vertebra
(D) Burr holes and traction
(E) Plaster cast to face, neck, and thorax

12. What would be the most appropriate radiologic examination?

(A) Plain lateral radiographs in flexion and extension to rule out occult ligamentous tear and instability of the cervical spine
(B) A CT scan of the cervical spine to rule out the possibility of a bony fracture not seen on plain radiographs
(C) Lateral tomogram of the cervical spine to rule out the possibility of an occult fracture
(D) Angiography
(E) Ultrasound of the neck

Questions 13 and 14

A 63-year-old woman with a history of local inoperable breast cancer is referred to you for the evaluation of new-onset diplopia. Upon questioning, she admits that diplopia occurs mostly when she attempts to look at objects in the distance and when she attempts to look toward the left side. In addition, she reports having severe headaches and an electric-type discomfort affecting her right deltoid region for approximately 3 weeks. On neurologic examination, she is found to have left abducens (sixth) nerve palsy; the rest of her cranial nerves are intact. She also has mild weakness of the right deltoid and a diminished biceps tendon jerk on the same side. Findings on an MRI of the brain with intravenous contrast are unremarkable.

13. In this patient, what would be the most likely site where metastasis occurs?

    (A) Brain
    (B) Orbital cavity
    (C) Meninges
    (D) Cerebellum
    (E) Optic chiasm

14. What would the next step in management involve?

    (A) An MRI of the cervical spine to rule out metastatic deposits within the cervical roots
    (B) A CT scan of the brain with intravenous contrast
    (C) A lumbar puncture to measure opening pressure and obtain cerebrospinal fluid (CSF) for cytologic analysis
    (D) Repeated breast biopsy
    (E) No further tests until further symptoms develop

15. A 57-year-old woman presents to the emergency department with new-onset seizures. She was witnessed by her husband to have a generalized seizure lasting approximately 1 minute. She has smoked 1 pack of cigarettes a day for over 40 years. In the past 3 months, she has lost 25 lb in weight. On examination, she appears thin and nervous but findings on her neurologic examination are otherwise essentially within

normal limits. Plain radiographs of the chest obtained in the emergency department show a 4-cm nodule in the upper lobe of her right lung. To exclude cerebral metastasis as a cause of her seizure, what should the next test requested be?

    (A) An electroencephalogram (EEG)
    (B) A CT scan of the brain with intravenous contrast
    (C) A spinal tap to measure opening pressure and obtain CSF for cytology
    (D) An MRI of the brain with intravenous contrast
    (E) Doppler ultrasound

Questions 16 and 17

A 58-year-old woman is admitted from the emergency department with a history of approximately 2 weeks of headache. She has a history of breast cancer. Her headache is severe, particularly in the mornings when she wakes up. It is accompanied by occasional vomiting. She says she experiences no focal weakness, numbness, or paresthesia. On physical examination, she is found to have a mild weakness of her left arm. An MRI of the brain with intravenous contrast reveals the presence of a neoplasm in the right motor cortex that is considered responsible for her weakness.

16. If the MRI shows multiple brain metastasis, what should be the treatment required in addition to corticosteroids?

    (A) Whole-brain radiotherapy
    (B) Craniotomy to resect the lesion responsible for her left arm weakness
    (C) Chemotherapy
    (D) Placement of an Ommaya reservoir for use in treatment by intrathecal chemotherapy
    (E) No further treatment

17. If the MRI shows a single brain metastasis, what should be the next step in management?

    (A) Whole-brain radiotherapy
    (B) Craniotomy to resect the lesion responsible for her left arm weakness
    (C) Chemotherapy

(D) Placement of an Ommaya reservoir for use in treatment by intrathecal chemotherapy

(E) No further treatment

18. A 63-year-old woman presents with a several-week history of headaches and difficulties with speech. A sister who lives with her claims that her language "has recently not been making much sense" and that she is a bit confused. Her condition seems to be deteriorating. On neurologic examination, she has a moderately severe aphasia, with difficulty understanding language and following commands, and she makes frequent paraphasic errors when she speaks. There are no other motor or sensory deficits. An MRI with intravenous contrast reveals the presence of a ring-enhancing mass lesion within the substance of the left temporal lobe. The lesion is approximately 3 cm in greatest diameter, poorly demarcated from the surrounding brain, and surrounded by a moderate amount of cerebral edema. Findings on routine admission tests, including a chest x-ray and serum chemistry, are unremarkable. What is the most likely diagnosis?

(A) Low-grade cerebral astrocytoma

(B) Glioblastoma multiforme

(C) Metastasis to the brain from an occult primary cancer

(D) Meningioma

(E) Glomus tumor

19. A 64-year-old man presents with headache and left-sided upper extremity weakness. The MRI findings suggest that this is a glioblastoma multiforme. This is because the tumor exhibits which of the following?

(A) It is regular in shape.

(B) It is well demarcated from surrounding brain tissue.

(C) It shows a ring pattern of enhancement with intravenous contrast and has a nonenhancing necrotic center.

(D) It shows an absence of surrounding white-matter edema.

(E) It arises from the carotid body.

20. A 63-year-old woman presents for workup to determine the reason for a gradual hearing loss over approximately 5 years and intermittent tinnitus over the last several months. Findings on physical and neurologic examination are entirely within normal limits, except for the presence of sensorineural hearing loss in the left ear. She has no cranial nerve deficits. An MRI of the brain with gadolinium reveals the presence of an extra-axial tumor in the region of the left cerebella-pontine angle. What is the most likely diagnosis?

(A) Epidermoid tumor (cholesteatoma)

(B) Glioblastoma multiforme

(C) Meningioma

(D) Acoustic neuroma

(E) Glomus tumor

Questions 21 and 22

A 4-year-old boy is brought to the emergency department with the complaint of approximately 2 weeks of headache and vomiting. He was seen in the emergency department 1 week earlier with the same complaints. At that time, his parents were told that the probable cause was a gastrointestinal virus, and the boy was sent home. His symptoms have not improved. On general examination, the child appears somewhat dehydrated and has a dry mouth and sunken eyes. His examination findings are also remarkable for the presence of bilateral papilledema and marked nystagmus. An MRI with intravenous contrast is obtained that reveals the presence of a 2-cm mass in the posterior fossa. The mass is entirely within the fourth ventricle and appears to be arising from the vermis of the cerebellum. It enhances uniformly with contrast. The lateral and third ventricles are moderately dilated with hydrocephalus.

21. What is the most likely diagnosis?

(A) Acoustic neuroma

(B) Craniopharyngioma

(C) Medulloblastoma

(D) Brain metastasis

(E) Polycystic cerebellar astrocytoma

22. If at craniotomy the tumor found is not that listed in question 21 and the pathologist reports that it is a benign lesion, what is that lesion?

(A) Ependymoma

(B) Choroid plexus papilloma

(C) Polycystic (cystic) cerebellar astrocytoma

(D) Teratoma

(E) Dermoid cyst

Questions 23 and 24

A 5-year-old girl undergoes debulking of medulloblastoma. She undergoes a repeat MRI of the brain with intravenous contrast, which shows a small amount of enhancement consistent with limited residual tumor. She is given a full course of radiotherapy to the posterior fossa and does very well for 6 weeks, until she experiences difficulty in walking. Physical examination at this time indicates moderate weakness of both lower extremities (particularly on the right side) but strength in her upper extremities and cranial nerves are normal. Her sensation to light touch and vibration are intact, but she has diminished sensation to pinprick throughout her left leg.

23. What should be the next step in management?

(A) Repeat the MRI of the brain to rule out an early recurrence

(B) Obtain a single-photon-emission CT (SPECT) scan of the brain to rule out the possibility of radiation-induced toxicity

(C) Begin treatment with chemotherapy for the residual tumor within the brain

(D) Obtain an MRI or myelogram of the entire spinal axis to rule out the possibility of "drop metastasis" from the medulloblastoma

(E) Obtain an ultrasound of the lumbar spine

24. What should treatment of this girl involve?

(A) Removal of recurrent medulloblastoma and neck dissection

(B) Ventriculoperitoneal shunt

(C) Repeat irradiation to the posterior cranial fossa

(D) Complete craniospinal irradiation with local boosts to the areas where tumor nodules are detected

(E) Cortisone alone

25. A 35-year-old man is brought to the hospital unconscious after being resuscitated in an ambulance from the site of a motor vehicle accident. No other history or information is available. On general inspection, he is found to have multiple bruises over his body and has a massively swollen left thigh. His vital signs are stable with a heart rate of 100 beats per minute (bpm) and a blood pressure of 150/75 mm Hg. He is obtunded and does not follow commands or open his eyes. He withdraws his left arm and leg from painful stimuli, but not his right. His left pupil is 3 mm in diameter, and it is sluggishly reactive to light, while his right is 5 mm in diameter and fixed. Corneal reflexes are present bilaterally. His pulse rate is 120 bpm and respiration rate is 40 breaths per minute. To avoid injury to his spinal cord by an unstable cervical spine, an order is issued to not perform testing of his doll's eye reflex. Intracranial hemorrhage causing increased intracranial pressure (ICP) is suspected, along with a right uncal herniation. What is the next step in management?

(A) Intubation of his airway for hyperventilation and administration of intravenous mannitol

(B) Immediate CT scanning of the brain to confirm the presence of the suspected intracranial hemorrhage

(C) Intubation of his airway for hyperventilation and intravenous administration of corticosteroids

(D) Immediately evacuation of the suspected intracranial hematoma

(E) Controlled hypoventilation

26. In the management of a 64-year-old woman struck by a car, mannitol is given to do which of the following?

(A) Increase CSF formation

(B) Increase the respiratory rate

(C) Increase the pulse rate

(D) Replace extensive fluid loss

(E) Lower raised ICP

27. A 17-year-old boy is brought to the emergency department after he was assaulted. Witnesses claim that he was hit on the head with a lead pipe, after which he was unconscious for several minutes. No seizure activity was witnessed. On arrival, he complains of a headache, particularly severe at the point where he was hit in the right frontoparietal region. On examination, he is found to have swelling and ecchymosis over this region. He is awake, alert, and fully oriented. A complete neurologic examination reveals no deficit. Plain radiographs of the skull show a linear, nondepressed skull fracture in the frontoparietal skull that crosses the groove of the medial meningeal artery. During the following hour, he becomes sleepier and begins to vomit. A repeat neurologic examination at that time reveals him to be lethargic but without weakness, numbness, paresthesia, or other focal deficit. What is the most likely cause of the neurologic deterioration?

(A) Diffuse axonal injury (DAI)

(B) Todd's phenomenon

(C) Subdural hematoma

(D) Epidural hematoma

(E) Trigeminal ganglion hematoma

28. Following a sudden impact in an accident, the 34-year-old race car driver becomes unconscious and is admitted to the hospital. A CT scan is performed, and a right space-occupying lesion is noted (Fig. 11–1). What is the most likely diagnosis?

(A) Corpus callosum injury

(B) Pituitary apoplexia

(C) Acute subdural hematoma

(D) Acute epidural hematoma

(E) Chronic subdural hematoma

29. A 44-year-old woman was brought to the emergency department after she was involved in a

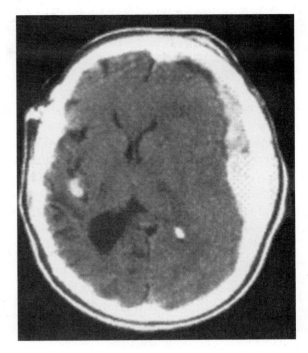

Figure 11–1.
(Reproduced, with permission, from Doherty GM: Current Surgical Diagnosis and Treatment, 12th ed. 876. McGraw-Hill, 2006.)

high-speed motor vehicle accident. She was extracted from the wreckage by paramedics. She was intubated at the site and rushed to the emergency department. On arrival, her blood pressure was 160/80 mm Hg and heart rate was 100 bpm, and exam showed evidence of decerebrate rigidity. A CT scan of the head revealed small punctate hemorrhages in the corpus callosum and the midbrain tegmentum, but there was no mass effect on adjacent structures. The size of the ventricles was normal. This grave clinical presentation and these CT findings are most consistent with the diagnosis of which of the following?

(A) DAI

(B) Cerebral contusion

(C) Cerebral concussion

(D) Traumatic subarachnoid hemorrhage (SAH)

(E) Petrous temporal lobe fracture

30. A 43-year-old man presents to the emergency department after falling down a flight of stairs and landing on his head. He did not lose consciousness. He complains of severe headache, marked decreased acuity in hearing in the left ear, and a "runny nose" since the fall. On physical examination, he is found to have a left-sided Battle's sign (an ecchymosis in the area of the left mastoid process) and hemotympanum. He has a constant dripping of a clear, watery fluid through his nose. Findings on his neurologic examination, other than the hearing loss, are completely normal. X-ray studies will reveal which of the following?

   (A) A fracture of the cribriform plate with a CSF leak into the paranasal sinuses
   (B) A skull-base fracture with a mucocele
   (C) A temporal bone fracture with paradoxical rhinorrhea
   (D) Occipital bone fracture
   (E) Fracture of the maxillary antrum and greater wing of the sphenoid

31. A 52-year-old painter injured his lower back 3 weeks ago when he fell off a ladder. He presents for evaluation of abnormal findings on plain radiographs of his lumbar spine. His pain has subsided, and he is now asymptomatic. Physical examination reveals a dense tuft of hair in his lumbosacral region that has been present for as long as he can remember. There is no tenderness or palpable abnormality in his spine. Findings on his neurologic examination are unremarkable. The radiographs mentioned show absence of the spinous processes and laminae at the levels of L5 and S1, with their corresponding pedicle displaced and angled laterally. What is the diagnosis?

   (A) An L5–S1 spondylolisthesis
   (B) A burst fracture of L5 and S1
   (C) Spina bifida
   (D) Spinal stenosis
   (E) Fracture of the vertebral bodies and nucleus pulposus

32. In the investigation of chronic back pain, a 72-year-old man is found on radiologic examination to have congenital spondylolisthesis.

The pathology is based upon disruption between two adjacent vertebra at which site?

   (A) Bodies and disks
   (B) Spinous process
   (C) Transverse process
   (D) Articular process(pars interarticularis)
   (E) Pedicle

33. A baby is born with a 2.5- × 2.0-cm myelomeningocele in the mid to lower lumbar region. Just hours after birth, he is rushed to the operating room (OR) for repair of this defect. Approximately 48 hours later, the baby is doing well, but it is noted that his head circumference has increased by 2 cm. On examination, the fontanelle is found to be slightly bulging and tense. On neurologic examination, the baby is awake but is found to have no spontaneous sensory or motor function below approximately the L3 dermatome. An ultrasound of the brain is obtained through the open fontanelle. This study shows an enlarged ventricular system, consistent with the presence of hydrocephalus. What is the related abnormality responsible for the hydrocephalus?

   (A) A fourth-ventricle ependymoma
   (B) Stenosis of the aqueduct of Sylvius
   (C) Amelia (failure of limbs to develop)
   (D) Arnold-Chiari malformation
   (E) Nasopharyngeal hamartoma

34. A 4-month-old infant has undergone surgical treatment for meningomyeloencephalocele. A CT tomogram of head was made immediately after birth (see Fig. 11–2). At birth, an operation was carried out in the posterior cranial fossa to partially replace brain cerebellar contents to an intracranial position. In investigations for progressive hydrocephalus, it is noted that there is herniation of the cerebellar tonsils through the foramen magnum, and a diagnosis of Arnold-Chiari syndrome is established. This syndrome may also include which of the following?

   (A) Fusion of the frontal lobes
   (B) Fusion of the temporal, parietal, and occipital lobes

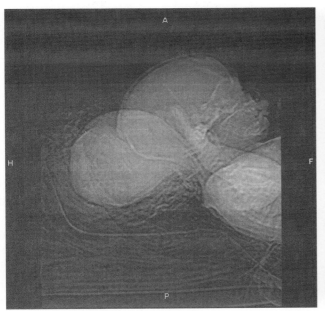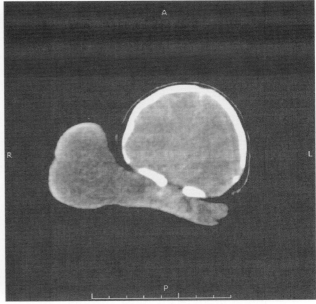

Figure 11–2.
Tomogram from CT head taken 4 months previously (immediately after birth). Opening in the posterior cranial fossa showing brain and meninges protruding into sac (axial view).

(C) Abnormal elongation of the medulla and lower cranial nerves

(D) Partial or complete absence of the pituitary gland

(E) Hypertrophy of cerebral lobes

35. During a regular visit to the pediatrician 1 week after birth, an infant's size and head circumference are recorded as being in the seventy-fifth percentile. Repeat measurement 1 month later still shows the size of the baby at the seventy-fifth percentile, but the baby's head circumference is now at the ninty-fifth percentile. The pediatrician notices that the baby's anterior fontanelle is tense and that the skull sutures are open. He obtains an MRI of the brain with intravenous contrast. This study shows the presence of greatly dilated lateral and third ventricles. The aqueduct of Sylvius cannot be easily visualized. The fourth ventricle is small. There are no lesions within the subarachnoid space or cerebral parenchyma. The appearance of the MRI is consistent with which of the following?

(A) Noncommunicating hydrocephalus

(B) Communicating hydrocephalus

(C) Normal-pressure hydrocephalus

(D) Arnold-Chiari malformation with herniation of the cerebellum into the foramen magnum

(E) Anencephalus

36. A 64-year-old woman complains of gait imbalance, headache and deterioration of mental status over the past several months. Her vision is normal. A CT scan reveals hydrocephalus, but the lumbar puncture pressure is unexpectedly low. What does she have?

(A) Meningitis

(B) Normal-pressure hydrocephalus

(C) Sigmoid sinus thrombosis

(D) *Echinococcus*

(E) Glioblastoma multiforme

37. A 23-year-old woman complains of progressive loss of vision and papilledema. Investigations show normal findings on CT scan. A lumbar puncture shows marked elevation of pressure. What is the most likely diagnosis?

    (A) Pseudotumor cerebri
    (B) Corpus cavernous thrombosis
    (C) Cavernous sinus thrombosis
    (D) Retinoblastoma
    (E) Chordoma

38. During her eighth month of pregnancy, a 29-year-old woman is noted to have hydramnios. Further testing shows anencephalus. In this case hydramnios is caused by which of the following?

    (A) Impairment of the fetus's swallowing mechanism
    (B) Tumor of the fetus's brain
    (C) A secretory peptide from the placenta
    (D) Excess antidiuretic hormone (ADH) from the fetus
    (E) Renal agenesis

39. A 28-year-old man presents with a history of chronic headache. The headache is intermittent, severe, poorly localized, and most often present when he arises in the morning. He suffered a severe blow to the head and sustained a skull fracture at the age of 15. Findings on his physical and neurologic examinations are within normal limits. An MRI of the brain with gadolinium reveals the presence of a large, nonenhancing extra-axial cyst in the region of the right temporal tip. This most likely represents which of the following?

    (A) An arachnoid cyst
    (B) A cystic astrocytoma
    (C) Rathke's cleft cyst
    (D) A Dandy-Walker cyst (failure of proper formation of the foramina of Lushka and Magendie)
    (E) Polycystic disease

40. A 15-year-old boy complains of right-sided weakness and gait impairment. A CT scan shows a large, nonenhancing cyst in the posterior cranial fossa, with an enhancing tumor nodule in the left cerebellum. What is the most likely diagnosis?

    (A) An arachnoid cyst
    (B) A cystic astrocytoma
    (C) Rathke's cleft cyst
    (D) Glioblastoma multiforme
    (E) A large sebaceous cyst

41. A 56-year-old woman presents with a history of several months of pain involving both hands. She describes the pain as electric and severe. It is localized to the palmar aspect of the first three digits of each hand and associated with numbness. The pain is particularly severe in the morning when she wakes up. She reports no weakness of the hands, but she says that sometimes objects fall off her hand because she cannot feel them. Physical examination reveals atrophy and weakness in the muscles of the thenar eminence bilaterally. She also has numbness in the distribution of the median nerve within the hands. Phalen test is positive. Which is the best test to confirm the clinical diagnosis?

    (A) An MRI of the hand to visualize an enlarged carpal ligament
    (B) An EMG and nerve-conduction study
    (C) MRI of the cervical spine to rule out radiculopathy
    (D) An x-ray of the hand
    (E) Physical examination

Questions 42–44

A 28-year-old police officer is brought to the emergency room (ER) by ambulance following a gunshot to the head. Emergency medical services (EMS) reports that he was found unresponsive at the site of the shooting and was immersed in a pool of blood. There were no witnesses. On arrival to the emergency department, he is noted to have a bullet entry wound on the right frontal region without any exit wound. His blood pressure is 80/35 mm Hg, pulse rate 150 bpm, and on examination, he does not open his eyes or follow commands. He is unresponsive to deep painful stimuli such as testing by sternal rub. His pupils are dilated approximately 4 mm bilaterally, but sluggishly reactive. He is aggressively resuscitated with colloid and blood products. The blood pressure is now 140/75 mm Hg. There is improvement in his neurologic examination—1 hour after admission, he withdraws his limbs from painful stimuli. A CT scan shows a small-skull defect in the right frontal region, representing the bullet entry site. The bullet is lodged within the cerebral parenchyma, approximately 2 cm from the surface of the brain, and there is a trail of bone fragments along the bullet path. The bullet has not crossed the midline. There is a $2 \times 2 \times 2.5$-cm hematoma within the substance of the right frontal lobe with surrounding edema and subfalcian herniation.

42. Which item is *least* likely to be useful as a prognostic marker for subsequent recovery?

   (A) Neurologic examination upon presentation and early response
   (B) The fact that the bullet did not cross the midline
   (C) The presence of an intracerebral hematoma
   (D) The presence of edema with subfalcian herniation
   (E) Bullet crosses the midcoronal plane

43. What is the next step in management?

   (A) Administration of mannitol (1 g/kg) through a rapid IV infusion followed by the placement of an intracranial pressure monitor
   (B) Administration of mannitol (1 g/kg) through a rapid IV infusion followed by urgent craniotomy
   (C) Administration of mannitol (1 g/kg) through a rapid IV infusion followed by the placement of burr holes for emergent decompression of raised intracranial pressure
   (D) No treatment should be administered, because the patient's prognosis is poor, and he is unlikely to survive
   (E) Steroids and antibiotics alone

44. Intraoperative management of this patient should be avoidance of which of the following?

   (A) Placement of an intracranial pressure monitor
   (B) Performance of a wide craniotomy for evacuation of the intraparenchymal hematoma
   (C) Extensive debridement of all bullet and bone fragments
   (D) Reconstruction of the cranial defect caused by the bullet
   (E) Removal of necrotic brain material

Questions 45 and 46

A 54-year-old-man comes to the emergency department complaining of a severe headache for several hours. He describes this headache as the worst of his life. It started suddenly "like a firecracker had gone off" inside his head. He has had no loss of consciousness but has had several episodes of vomiting. General physical examination reveals a patient who is in severe distress due to the headache. His blood pressure is 180/70 mm Hg, and his pulse racing at 120 bpm. He is afebrile. He has photophobia and gross neck rigidity. Neurologically, he is fully alert and oriented. He has a normal motor and sensory examination. His left pupil is 2 mm and briskly reactive to light; his right is 4.5 mm and fixed to both light and accommodation.

45. What is the most likely diagnosis?

   (A) Acute bacterial meningitis
   (B) Incipient uncal herniation due to an expanding lesion in the right temporal lobe
   (C) Acute SAH from an anterior communicating artery aneurysm
   (D) Acute SAH from a right posterior communicating aneurysm
   (E) Cavernous sinus thrombosis

46. What is the most appropriate test to establish the diagnosis?

(A) MRI of the brain with and without gadolinium
(B) CT scan of the brain without contrast
(C) A lumbar puncture
(D) An electroencephalogram
(E) Optometry

47. A 43-year-old man is treated with pyridostigmine for facial, ocular, and pharyngeal weakness due to myasthenia gravis. Which statement is true of pyridostigmine?

(A) It is unrelated to neostigmine.
(B) It has far more side effects than neostigmine.
(C) Pyridostigmine and neostigmine reverse depolarizing neuromuscular blockade.
(D) It causes greater muscarinic effect than neostigmine.
(E) It is an anticholinesterase agent.

48. During anesthesia using a narcotic, thiopental, and N_2O, the respiratory response to a rising end-respiratory CO_2 tension is which of the following?

(A) Depressed only by the narcotic
(B) Depressed only by thiopental
(C) Depressed progressively by the addition of each agent
(D) Depressed by the narcotic and thiopental, then elevated by N_2O
(E) Unchanged from control response

49. A plastic surgeon is performing a minor procedure on the face of an 18-year-old woman. She has a seizure that is attributed to the local anesthetic agent. Convulsion following an overdose of local anesthesia is best treated by which of the following?

(A) Droperidol
(B) Hydroxyzine (Vistaril)
(C) Diazepam (Valium)
(D) Fentanyl ketamine

Questions 50 and 51

50. A 17-year-old male presents with 3-month history of headache, weight gain, decreased concentration, polyuria, and polydypsia. His headaches are mostly in morning and involves the frontal region. On examination he was found to have bitemporal visual field defect and no facial hair. MRI scan revealed a suprasellar partially calcified cystic lesion with displacement of optic chiasm. The most likely pathology is:

(A) Giant aneurysm of carotid artery
(B) Pituitary macroadenoma
(C) Glioblastoma multiforme
(D) Craniopharyngioma
(E) Testicular metastasis

51. He underwent a craniotomy for resection of his lesion. Twelve hours postoperatively, he developed diuresis of over 500 mL/h. The diagnosis of (DI) was entertained. What laboratory findings are most consistent with the clinical impression?

(A) Urine specific gravity of over 1010
(B) Serum sodium of less than 135
(C) Decreased both serum and urine osmolality
(D) Increased serum osmolality and decreased urine osmolality
(E) Increased both serum and urine osmolality

Questions 52 and 53

52. A 55-year-old female presents with 3-years history of severe lancinating pain extending from left ear to her maxillary area. Pain is triggered by chewing and brushing teeth. She was treated by otolaryngologist for sinus infection a year ago and undergone multiple dental work and teeth extraction with transient or no improvement. The most likely diagnosis is:

(A) Maxillary sinusitis
(B) Trigeminal neurolgia
(C) Maxillary osteomyelitis
(D) Gradenigo's syndrome
(E) Otitis media

53. Which one of the following medications is not indicated in treatment of this condition?

(A) Carbamezapin
(B) Cefatin
(C) Phenytoin
(D) Gabapentin
(E) Baclofen

Questions 54 through 56

54. A 45-year-old woman was brought to emergency department for sudden onset of severe headache associated with photophobia, nausea, and transient loss of consciousness. On examination, she is awake and alert with normal cranial nerve function. She also exhibits normal muscle strength and sensation.Her past medical history is significant for sickle cell disease (SCD) and hypertension. CT scan confirms the diagnosis of SAH without any intraparenchymal abnormality.What is the least likely cause of SAH?

(A) Aneurysmal bleed
(B) Sickle cell angiopathy
(C) Arteriovenous malformation (AVM)
(D) Hemorrhagic meningioma
(E) Blood dyscrasia

55. What is the most definitive diagnostic test in this condition?

(A) CT angiography
(B) Magnetic resonance angiography (MRA)
(C) Cerebral angiogram
(D) MR spectroscopy
(E) Positron emission tomography (PET) scan

56. What is the most likely complication of angiography in this patient?

(A) Cerebral stroke
(B) Aneurysmal rupture
(C) Increased intracranial pressure
(D) Vascular wall damage
(E) Sickle cell crisis

Questions 57 and 58

57. A 69-year-old well-controlled, hypertensive man was seen in ER with 3-month history of mild headache and sudden onset of hemiparesis. On examination, he exhibit mild dysphasia and lethargy. His cognitive function testing indicates moderate diminution of his recent memory and executive function. His hemiparesis is more dense in arm and leg and is mild in his face.CT scan without contrast demonstrates a 3-cm irregular hemorrhage surrounded by marked edema and mass effect in frontal-temporal region. The most likely cause of bleed is?

(A) Amyloid angiopathy
(B) Hypertensive hemorrhage
(C) Hemorrhagic neoplasm
(D) Arterial-venous malformation
(E) Coagulopathy

58. What is the next diagnostic test that should be ordered?

(A) EEG
(B) Cerebral angiography
(C) MRI with contrast
(D) Spinal tap to determine the ICP
(E) Transcranial Doppler

Answers and Explanations

1. **(B)** The patient has a right-sided L5 radiculopathy, most likely resulting from a disk herniation at the right L4–L5 interspace. The key to this diagnosis is in understanding the dermatomal anatomy of the lower extremity. The L5 dermatomal distribution involves the lateral calf and the dorsomedial aspect of the foot. The dermatome also typically includes the big toe.

2. **(C)** Thoracic, lumbar, and sacral nerves exit off the spinal canal immediately below the pedicle of the corresponding numbered vertebra. The left S1 root, for example, passes immediately dorsal to the L5–S1 disk, where it can be susceptible to compression by a herniated nucleus pulposus. The root then swings laterally to exit immediately caudal to the left L5 pedicle. For a correlation between level of disk herniation and the root affected, see the table below.

Level of Herniation	Root Affected
L1–L2	L2
L2–L3	L3
L3–L4	L4
L4–L5	L5
L5–S1	S1

3. **(D)** This patient has radiculopathy of her right C6 root. To make this diagnosis, it is essential to understand the dermatomal anatomy of the upper extremity. The C6 dermatome includes the radial aspect of the distal forearm and hand. The C4 dermatomes include the deltoid region. The biceps tendon jerk is mediated by the C5 and C6 roots.

4. **(C)** The mechanism of injury was a contusion to the cervical spinal cord. This probably occurred when the violent hyperflexion of the neck caused the cervical cord to bump against the osteophytic ridges of the spine. The typical clinical picture of a spinal cord contusion is a central cord syndrome.

5. **(A)** The central spinal cord syndrome describes the following pattern of weakness: (a) weakness in upper extremity is greater than weakness in lower extremity; (b) weakness in distal muscles is greater than weakness in proximal muscles and limb girdle. This results from the distribution of motor fibers within the corticospinal tracts of the cervical cord. Fibers supplying the upper extremity and more proximal muscles are more centrally located and, thus, more susceptible to dysfunction from a central injury. Within the spinal cord, sensory fibers are more peripherally located and, thus, less frequently affected. Sensory deficits, when present, are often variable and inconsistent. A Lhermitte's sign or syndrome also results from stenosis of the cervical canal, causing compression of the spinal cord. The patient develops severe numbness and paresthesia of the upper extremities as the result of sustained hyperextension of the neck.

6. **(B)** Brown-Sequard syndrome (Fig. 11–3) describe (a) weakness of muscle *ipsilaterally* below the spinal cord lesion, (b) impaired sensation to light touch and vibration *ipsilaterally* below the spinal cord lesion; and (c) impaired sensation to pain and temperature *contralaterally* below the spinal cord lesion.

7. **(E)** The motor deficit is on the left ipsilateral side. Brown-Sequard syndrome is caused by unilateral injury or dysfunction following

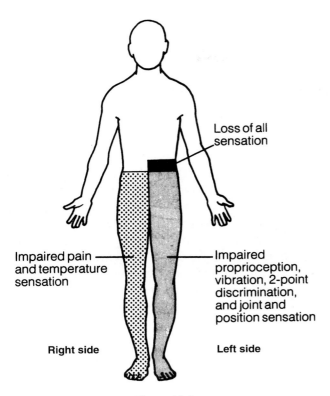

Figure 11–3.
Brown-Sequard syndrome. The lesion depicted here is at a lower spinal cord level than that described in the text. *(Reproduced, with permission, from Lindner HH: Clinical Anatomy. Appleton & Lange, 1989.)*

Loss of all sensation

Impaired pain and temperature sensation

Impaired proprioception, vibration, 2-point discrimination, and joint and position sensation

Right side

Left side

hemisections of the spinal cord. In the human nervous system, motor and sensory functions on one side of the body are under the direct control of the opposite side of the brain. All major motor and sensory tracts decussate. The decussation of the various tracts occurs at different levels of the neuraxis.

8.   **(C)** On subsequent MRI of the cervicothoracic spine, this patient is found to have severe spondylosis at multiple levels of the spine. There is spinal cord compression by a large osteophyte at the level of C6–C7. The patient has all the signs and symptoms of cervical spinal cord dysfunction. The weakness affecting the triceps muscles in addition to the lower extremities indicates that the lesion is above the level of the thoracic cord. Absence of similar symptoms on the face as well as the absence of cranial nerve abnormalities indicate that the lesion is not intracranial. The diffuseness of the symptoms as well as the fact that they are associated with increased reflexes and tone

indicate that the problem lies within the CNS (upper motor neuron) rather than the peripheral nervous system (lower motor neuron).

9.   **(A)** The clinical presentation indicates a lower motor neuron lesion. The clinical diagnosis is neurologic claudication secondary to lumbar spinal stenosis, which is commonly seen in elderly persons in whom (as a consequence of wear and tear over the years) bony structures of the lumbar spine hypertrophy and develop osteophytes. These bony changes, in turn, lead to stenosis of the spinal canal and intervertebral foramina. Thus, the result is compression and dysfunction of multiple lumbosacral nerve roots bilaterally. Bending over opens the lumbar canal and relieves the stenosis.

10.   **(C)** This patient has suffered a traumatic fracture of L3 in which bony fragments were displaced dorsally to compress the cauda equina at that level. It is important to remember that the spinal cord does not extend along the entire length of the spine. The conus medullaris, the most caudal tip of the spinal cord, ends in 98% of people at or above L2 vertebrae. Thus, it is highly unlikely for an L3 fracture to cause compression of the spinal cord or conus medullaris.

11.   **(B)** The most appropriate step is to place him in a hard cervical collar to protect his neck and obtain plain lateral radiographs in flexion and extension. In this boy, the continuous neck pain and the prevertebral swelling on the plain radiographs are strongly suggestive of an injury to the ligamentous structures of the cervical spine. A severe ligamentous tear can lead to instability of the spine from excessive movement between adjacent vertebrae. Ligamentous injury must be ruled out by obtaining lateral radiographs in flexion and extension to demonstrate any excessive movement between adjacent vertebrae. This excessive movement, if missed, can result in compression of the cervical spinal cord and a serious neurologic deficit. These studies require supervision by appropriate specialist consultants.

12.   **(A)** A CT scan of the cervical spine is more sensitive for fractures of the spine than are plain

radiographs. Because CT images are in the axial plane, only one vertebral body can be seen at a time. This makes CT scanning entirely inadequate to rule out all but large subluxation resulting from the most major ligamentous disruptions. Sagittal MRI of the cervical spine in this case may show swelling or hematoma within the soft tissues of the spine. MRI, however, is poor in demonstrating bony anatomy and detail. Furthermore, without flexion and extension of the neck, an MRI of the cervical spine is no better in showing bony instability than plain radiographs in the neutral position.

13. **(C)** Meningeal carcinomatosis results when malignant cells gain access to the CSF and are able to disseminate within it. Cells most commonly adhere to and affect the neural structures traversing the CSF, such as cranial nerves and peripheral nerve roots. Cells cause dysfunction at multiple sites of the CNS. This patient has a left abducens nerve palsy and a right C5 radiculopathy, making the diagnosis of meningeal carcinomatosis highly likely.

14. **(C)** In the presence of meningeal carcinomatosis (also called carcinomatous meningitis), the lumbar puncture CSF examination may reveal elevated protein and positive cytology. The sensitivity of MRI to detect small tumor deposits within the intracranial compartment is much greater than that of a CT scan. Thus, a CT scan is unlikely to be helpful in this clinical scenario.

15. **(D)** An adult with new onset seizures is considered to have a brain tumor until proved otherwise. The best test available to detect metastatic deposits in the brain is the MRI with intravenous contrast. MRI is exquisitely sensitive in diagnosing brain metastasis, sometimes detecting them by the brain edema they induce even when the lesion itself is too small to be seen. The EEG may likely show the presence of seizure activity and even localize it to a particular region of the brain; it will not, however, answer the question of what pathologic process is responsible. Also, in this case, because a mass lesion is expected, performing a spinal tap is relatively contraindicated for the fear of inducing uncal herniation in a patient who may have increased ICP.

16. **(A)** The optimal management of any intracranial neoplasm includes use of corticosteroids. These significantly diminish the amount of tumor-induced brain edema and are remarkably effective in ameliorating symptoms caused by CNS neoplasms. The current recommendation for the treatment of multiple brain metastasis is treatment with a full course of fractionated radiation to the whole brain. This is geared to treat all visible lesions within the parenchyma as well as those that may still be too small to be detected. Intrathecal chemotherapy is effective in treating meningeal carcinomatosis, where the primary site of involvement is the meninges and the surface of the brain. The two available agents for this modality of treatment have very poor penetration into deeper regions of the brain when administered intrathecally.

17. **(B)** Surgical resection is recommended only for cases involving a single brain metastasis that is surgically accessible in patients with a reasonable life expectancy. It is also relatively indicated in patients with multiple brain lesions in whom one particular lesion is imminently life-threatening. Intravenous chemotherapy has, unfortunately, yielded poor results in the treatment of brain metastasis. This is particularly so in this patient, because her tumors are already likely to be resistant to the chemotherapeutic agents with which she has already been treated.

18. **(B)** Glioblastoma multiforme is a highly malignant neoplasm, arising from glial cells or their precursors within the CNS. It is the most common of all primary malignancies of the CNS and its peak incidence is within the fifth to seventh decade of life. A low-grade astrocytoma is a tumor derived from glial cells of astrocytes. Fig. 11–4, shows a large cystic giant astrocytoma on T2 weighted MRI where fluid is shown as a white area with midline shift (not glioblastoma multiforme presented in this question).

19. **(C)** Glioblastoma multiforme grows rapidly, and the tumor often contains a necrotic core that occurs as its growth surpasses its blood supply. Additional features on MRI include irregular shape, poor demarcation from surrounding

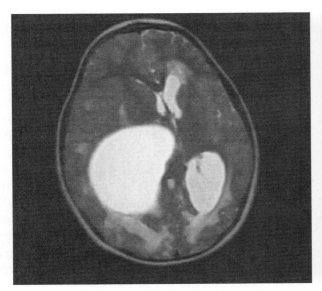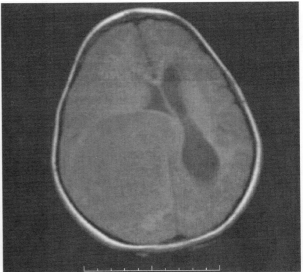

Figure 11–4.
Large cystic giant astrocytoma on T2 weighted MRI where fluid is shown as a white area. Midline shift.

brain tissue, and the presence of variable amount of surrounding white-matter edema.

20. **(D)** This cerebella-pontine angle tumor is most likely an acoustic neuroma. This is the most commonly encountered neoplasm in this region. It arises from the Schwann cells that form the myelin sheath of the vestibular division of the eighth cranial nerve (hence a more accurate name is vestibular schwannoma). This tumor typically arises within the internal acoustic canal and growths in the direction of least resistance—through the meatus into the cerebellopontine angle cistern.

21. **(C)** An astute neurologist once said that in neurologic diagnosis, as in real estate, location is everything. He alluded to the fact that in the diagnosis of neurologic ailments, one can often generate lists of possible diagnoses based solely on the location of the lesion in question. With unusual exceptions, each location within the CNS is likely to be associated with a certain type of neoplasm. The medulloblastoma (also called a primitive neuroectodermal tumor or PNET) is a highly aggressive and rapidly growing tumor that most often arises within the cerebellar vermis. It usually grows locally as a roughly spherical mass to bulge into and obliterate the adjacent fourth ventricle. Ependymoma or

choroid plexus papilloma should also be considered in the differential diagnosis.

22. **(B)** Choroid plexus papillomas are benign tumors of the CNS that arise from the cells that form the choroid plexus. These tumors can be found wherever choroid plexus is present, including the lateral and fourth ventricles. They cause symptoms of increased ICP, most commonly by causing massive degrees of hydrocephalus. This can be from two mechanisms—obstruction of normal CSF pathways or production by the tumor of excessive volumes of CSF. (Remember that CSF is produced mainly by the choroid plexus.) Ependymomas are also highly malignant tumors usually found in the fourth ventricle of children. Its precursor cell is the ependymal cell that lines the ventricular system. As medulloblastomas, these tumors are highly aggressive and fast growing. Contrary to the former, however, ependymomas tend to arise from the floor of the fourth ventricle (the dorsal surface of the brainstem).

23. **(D)** Obtain an MRI or myelogram of the entire spinal axis to rule out the possibility of "drop metastasis" from the medulloblastoma. The constellation of emerging new symptoms points toward spinal cord dysfunction; the

most likely cause is the presence of drop metastasis from the medulloblastoma. Primary CNS neoplasms rarely metastasize outside of their site of origin. Exceptions to this statement include both medulloblastoma and ependymoma. These tumors shed viable cells into the CSF, where they are transferred to such distant areas as the intracranial or, more commonly, the spinal subarachnoid space. There they can lodge and replicate to form tumor nodules that can compress adjacent neural structures. The test of choice for diagnosing the presence of these drop metastasis is a MRI of the spine with intravenous contrast or a myelogram.

24. **(D)** Treatment of drop metastasis consists primarily of complete craniospinal irradiation with local boosts to the areas where tumor nodules are detected. Chemotherapy, particularly a combination of procarbazine, lomustine (CCNU), and vincristine (PCV), is usually given to treat disease that is locally recurrent after maximal irradiation. Radiation-induced toxicity or radionecrosis is highly unlikely to be the cause of these newly developed symptoms. The first reason for this is that the child's new symptoms and findings appear to be exclusively spinal in origin. Second, radiation-induced necrosis, a feared complication of CNS irradiation, is never observed in such a short interval after completing treatment.

25. **(A)** Intubation will accomplish two purposes. First, it will protect the airway and prevent the possibility of aspiration. Second, it will allow controlled hyperventilation (PCO_2 of 25–30 mm Hg), which causes cerebral vasoconstriction, which, in turn, transiently lowers ICP and reduces intracranial intravascular blood volume. Mannitol will reduce intracerebral pressure and volume. The role of corticosteroids in the management of cerebral trauma is controversial at best. Their advocates propose that corticosteroids work by reducing the amount of traumatically induced brain edema. Even these investigators concur that their effect is not immediate and that they take at least 4–6 hours to work. The subdural space is between the inner layer of dura and the arachnoid.

26. **(E)** Mannitol is a complex sugar that remains in the intravascular space because of its high molecular weight. When it is given in large doses (1–2 g/kg of body weight), water is extracted from the cerebral interstitium by its osmotic effect, causing reduction in total brain volume. Both these measures are temporizing steps to allow enough time for definitive diagnosis and treatment to take place. The effect of hyperventilation on ICP rapidly wears off after a few hours. Over time, mannitol will diffuse into the cerebral interstitium, losing its effectiveness and even exacerbating cerebral edema. A note of caution, however, mannitol is an osmotic diuretic and as such must be given with extreme caution in the setting of hypotension due to excessive blood loss.

27. **(D)** This is the classic presentation of an acute epidural hematoma (Fig. 11–5) transient traumatic loss of consciousness, followed by a lucid interval and then by neurologic deterioration. Epidural hematomas are frequently associated with linear skull fractures, which cause injury to the middle meningeal artery located immediately deep to the overlying fracture. They are more common in younger individuals, because in younger people, the dura mater is less firmly adherent to the inner table of the skull. Todd's phenomenon is a transient focal weakness or paralysis that results after a seizure. The particular pattern of weakness is often a clue to the site of the seizure focus within the brain.

28. **(C)** Acute subdural hematomas (Fig. 11–1) occur most commonly when violent accelerations or deceleration injuries of the head cause tearing of the bridging veins within the subdural potential space. They generally imply a much more severe injury to the brain itself than in the case of their epidural counterpart. For this reason, they are associated with cerebral contusions in over 30% of cases.

29. **(A)** This entity is caused by sharp accelerations or decelerations of the head and its contents as seen in high-speed motor vehicle accidents. During impact, shock waves are generated that are able to travel through the semisolid substance of the brain. These shock waves penetrate and

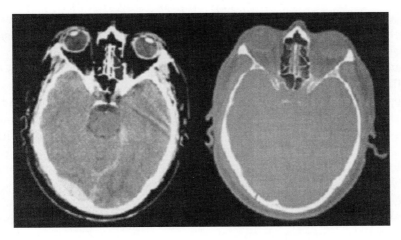

Figure 11–5.
Epidural hematoma. CT of the head windowed for brain (left) and bone (right) shows and epidural hematoma resulting from an underlying occipital skull fracture. This injury was caused by a blow to the back of the head. Notice the classic lens-shaped hematoma. The brain window also shows a thin left tentorial subdural hematoma appearing as a white line running from the midline posteriorly and curving toward the left of the pons. *(Reproduced, with permission, from Doherty GM: Current Surgical Diagnosis and Treatment, 12th ed. 876. McGraw-Hill, 2006.)*

cause shear and stretch injury to multiple deep axonal tracts. DAI represents a severe diffuse injury to the entire brain. For this reason, victims present with marked neurological dysfunction. CT scan typically shows no evidence or reason to suspect increased ICP; it merely shows punctate hemorrhages in many of the tracts that are affected.

30. **(C)** The presence of a Battle's sign and hemotympanum is highly suggestive of the possibility of a left temporal bone fracture. When this occurs, it is common for the dura mater at this site to be torn. This leads to leakage of CSF into the mastoid air cells and middle ear. CSF is subsequently able to reach the nasopharynx via the eustachian tube, a phenomenon called paradoxical rhinorrhea, which is a serious but usually self-limiting condition. Most cases of traumatic CSF leaks heal spontaneously within approximately 1 week. Patients require close in-hospital observation, however, because bacterial meningitis readily occurs in the presence of CSF leakage to the outside.

31. **(C)** Spina bifida occulta does not cause symptoms and is frequently found incidentally in the workup of other conditions. The presence of a tuft of hair and the radiographic abnormalities described above are consistent with the diagnosis of spina bifida occulta. This is a congenital abnormality that results from abnormalities in the development of mesodermal elements (sclerotome) which form the dorsal elements of the lumbosacral spine. A burst fracture of the spine is found after acute excessive axial loading of the spine. The features of such a fracture are reduced height of the affected vertebral body and displacement of bony fragments centrifugally in the axial plane (hence the term *burst*).

32. **(D)** Spondylolisthesis occurs when there is disruption, most often by a fracture, of the pars intra-articularis of the L5 vertebra. The pars is the bony element that is found between the ascending facets of L5 (that articulate with the L4 vertebra) and the descending facets of L5 (that articulate with S1). The functional result of this disruption is that the descending facets are "floating" and not able to function in stabilizing the L5–S1 joint. If this becomes progressive, then anterior subluxation of the L5 vertebral body with respect to that of S1 occurs.

33. **(D)** There is a high degree of correlation in the occurrence of defects in neural tube closure and Arnold-Chiari malformations, and all babies born with one should be examined for the other.

Development of communicating hydrocephalus is a feature of a type-II Arnold-Chiari abnormality. Stenosis of the aqueduct of Sylvius and the presence of an ependymoma in the fourth ventricles are other reasons for the development of hydrocephalus in children. There is, however, no incidental correlation between these and defects of neural tube closure.

34. **(C)** Abnormal elongation of the medulla and lower cranial nerves may be evident in Arnold-Chiari syndrome. Additional features include fusion of the corpora quadrigemina, leading to a "beaked" tectum; partial or complete absence of the corpus callosum; and microgyria. The corpora quadragemina are relay stations for hearing (inferior corpora quadragemina) and the light reflex (superior copora quadragemina), and they form the posterior surface of the midbrain.

35. **(A)** Noncommunicating hydrocephalus is defined as hydrocephalus caused by obstruction of CSF flow and obstruction within the ventricular system. In this case, the ventricular system is dilated upstream from the obstruction caused by stenosis of the aqueduct of Sylvius and collapsed distally. Communicating hydrocephalus occurs when the obstruction to CSF flow occurs within the subarachnoid space or at the level of its resorption into the bloodstream by the arachnoid granulations. In this case, all ventricles are dilated proportionately.

36. **(B)** Normal-pressure hydrocephalus is a condition seen in the elderly in which there is symmetrical enlargement of the entire ventricular system. When patients with this condition are studied by lumbar puncture, it is found that despite ventriculomegaly, the ICP is abnormally low. This syndrome presents with a characteristic triad of symptoms—dementia, ataxia, and urinary incontinence.

37. **(A)** Pseudotumor cerebri is a condition that most commonly occurs in young adults, particularly in females. In this condition, ICP as measured by a lumbar puncture is elevated, while the size of the cerebral ventricles on imaging studies is small or normal. It is a generally progressive condition that causes headache and

damage to the optic nerve, sometimes leading to loss of peripheral vision and blindness.

38. **(A)** This abnormality is relatively common and occurs in 1 of 1000 pregnancies. It occurs four times more commonly in whites than blacks and four times more commonly in female fetuses than in male fetuses. The abnormality can be identified on an x-ray, because the vault of the skull is absent. Anencephalus is caused by failure of the cephalic part of the neural tube to close off.

39. **(A)** This cystic structure is an arachnoid cyst. These are CSF-filled cysts that occur when leaves of arachnoidal tissue fuse, trapping CSF within them. These cysts slowly grow over time, sometimes attaining very large size. They cause symptoms by virtue of their large size, as they are able to compress adjacent structures. Patients with these cysts most commonly present with a history of chronic headache. Neurologic symptoms or deficits are unusual. Patients with arachnoid cysts frequently give a history of severe blows to the head and skull fractures, perhaps implying head trauma as a causative agent. The most common locations of arachnoid cysts are the middle cranial fossa, the cerebellopontine angle, and the suprasellar area. Dandy-Walker cysts are the result of an intrauterine developmental abnormality in which there is failure of proper formation of the foramina of Lushka and Magendie. As a consequence, the main egress of CSF out of the ventricular system is obstructed, leading to hydrocephalus and a massively enlarged, cyst-like fourth ventricle.

40. **(B)** Cystic astrocytomas are neoplasms of the CNS. They usually consist of a large, nonenhancing cyst on the wall of which is an enhancing tumor nodule. They are most commonly found within the substance of the cerebellar hemispheres of children and young adults. A Rathke's cleft cyst is a remnant of the embryologic Rathke's pouch. These are found within the sella turcica.

41. **(B)** CTS is a condition in which the median nerve is compressed at the level of the wrist by a thickened carpal flexor retinaculum. This

leads to numbness and painful paresthesia along the median nerve distribution within the hand. It also causes weakness and atrophy of the thenar muscles within the hand, innervated by the superficial recurrent branch of the median nerve. Once there is clinical suspicion, the best diagnostic test to confirm the presence of CTS is a nerve-conduction study. This study often shows a block or delay in conduction of the median nerve at the level of the carpal tunnel. Conduction within all branches of the ulnar nerve should be normal. This test is often also useful in distinguishing between CTS and the possibility of a C6 radiculopathy.

42. **(A)** The best prognostic indicator of survival and outcome in patients with missile wounds to the brain is the mental status and level of responsiveness after proper resuscitation. His initial poor neurologic grade can be attributed to cerebral injury itself or to cerebral hypoperfusion in a patient with clear hemodynamic shock. Initial presentation is, thus, of little value in judging the prognosis for these types of injuries. Other prognostic factors that have been identified as important in predicting the outcome of gunshot wounds to the head include:

     (a) Path of the bullet. A missile that crosses the midline or the midcoronal plane is associated with a much worse outcome than one that stays unilaterally.

     (b) The presence of an intracranial hematoma of greater than $2 \times 2 \times 2$ cm is ironically a positive prognosticator, because it represents a mass lesion that can be causing intracranial hypertension and can be more readily evacuated via a craniotomy.

43. **(B)** A markedly diminished level of consciousness coupled by a CT scan that shows a hematoma, edema, and subfalcian herniation indicate that the patient is suffering from intracranial hypertension. Hyperventilation and mannitol are quick and effective ways to reduce intracranial pressure temporarily. However, these measures are only temporary, and the patient needs urgent decompression by craniotomy. Placement of burr holes in the ER is of no

value in the management of these injuries. Placement of an ICP monitor may be helpful for the postoperative period, but is likely to be of limited help without prior craniotomy.

44. **(C)** The ideal intraoperative management of this patient would begin by performance of a wide craniotomy through which the intracerebral hematoma can be evacuated. Necrotic brain tissue if left alone is likely to worsen the occurrence of cerebral edema postoperatively, and for that reason, every measure should be taken to debride it as thoroughly as possible. Easily accessible bone and bullet fragments can also be removed. Bone and bullet fragments that are deeply located and difficult to locate should be left intact. Persistence in their removal often leads to a greater risk of brain injury by intraoperative manipulation and dissection. If problems with raised intracranial pressure are expected, placement of a suitable ICP monitoring device is highly recommended as part of the surgical procedure.

45. **(D)** This is the classic history for acute SAH—the acute onset of a massive headache. The acuity should suggest nothing other than a vascular phenomenon. Furthermore, the presence of a right occulomotor nerve palsy strongly suggests bleeding from an aneurysm of the right posterior communicating artery. Anatomically, most posterior communicating aneurysms point their domes laterally and inferiorly, in the direction toward the occulomotor nerve. In general, when the dome of the aneurysm ruptures, the jet of blood injures the adjacent nerve. In this situation, the lesion results in complete occulomotor nerve palsy with a fixed dilated pupil. It is a neurosurgic dogma that complete occulomotor palsy should be regarded as a ruptured posterior communicating artery aneurysm until proved otherwise. Acute bacterial meningitis also presents with headache and meningism. The onset of the symptoms is, however, much more gradual, and high fever is usually present.

46. **(B)** The best test in the diagnosis of an acute SAH is a nonenhanced CT of the brain. In this study, subarachnoid blood can easily be seen as a hyperdense substance filling the otherwise

hypodense cisterns of the subarachnoid space. Its sensitivity is greater 95%, but sensitivity falls to 50% by 1 week after the hemorrhage. Lumbar puncture can also be used to diagnose SAH, but it is an invasive procedure that should be reserved for cases in which the suspicion of such hemorrhage remains following a negative CT scan. MRI (with or without gadolinium), despite its exquisite sensitivity for the diagnosis of intracerebral lesions, is notoriously poor in its ability to detect acute blood within the subarachnoid space. EEG is of no value for the diagnosis of an acute SAH.

47. **(E)** Neostigmine and pyridostigmine are both anticholinesterase agents and can be used in the reversal of nondepolarizing muscle relaxants. Pyridostigmine causes less muscarinic effect than does neostigmine. The effect of pyridostigmine is more prolonged and produces fewer secretions and less severe bradycardia.

48. **(C)** Both narcotics and thiopental depress respiration, and the addition of N_2O further augments this depressant action. Thus, the response to hypercapnea is diminished.

49. **(C)** Diazepam is a benzodiazepine derivative that seems to have a calming effect on part of the limbic system, thalamus, and hypothalamus. It should be injected slowly (<1 mg/min) into a larger vein to avoid phlebitis and local irritation.

50. **(D)** Weight gain, DI, decreased memory, and visual field defect are consistent with a suprasellar hypothalamic lesion. Calcified cystic lesions in this location, particularly in adolescents, are characteristic of craniopharyngiomas. The rate of calcification in childhood is about 85% and in adult is about 40%. Craniopharyngiomas are pathologically benign but due to their location and their firm attachment to critical structures surrounding them can result in severe neurofunctional impairment. The cyst wall is lined with squamous epithelium and the fluid contains cholesterol crystals.

51. **(D)** DI is commonly precipitated by low level of ADH secretion. The clinical presentation does not manifest until over 85% of ADH secretory capacity is damaged. Rarely it is nephrogenic and is caused by lack of renal response to ADH hormone. Nephrogenic form is often produced by toxic effect of certain drugs or familial X-linked recessive genetic disorder. DI is defined by increased diluted urinary output, constant thirst for usually cold water, and high serum osmolality. If it is not properly treated it can lead to extreme dehydration and electrolyte imbalance. The best test is water deprivation for 4 hours while monitoring the urine output and urine and serum osmolality. If urine osmolality remains flat or changes less than 30 mOsm and the serum osmolality approaches 300 mOsm/L, the diagnosis of DI is confirmed. At this point the patient should be given 5 U of an exogenous pitressin subcutaneously. By comparing the urine osmolality after Pitressin to the initial values, the extent of the DI can be determined. The increase in urine osmolality by more than 67% is indicative of severe ADH deficiency. The increased levels of 6–67% is suggestive of partial deficiency.

52. **(B)** Trigeminal neuralgia or Tic Douloureux is clinically characterized by paroxysmal lancinating pain in the distribution of one or two division of trigeminal nerve. There is commonly no sensory or motor impairment on examination. The pain is triggered by certain mild stimuli such as touching, chewing, brushing teeth, and cold breeze. If any objective neurological findings are detected, other pathologies causing compression of the nerve at its exit zone from the brainstem must be suspected. Such pathologies as AVM, tumors, and aneurysm must be ruled out by MRI. This disease is assumed to be caused by a loop of a vessel, often superior cerebellar artery or posterior inferior cerebellar artery (PICA), compressing the trigeminal nerve as it emerges from brainstem.

53. **(B)** Most antiepileptic medications are effective to control the pain in this condition. The drug of choice is Carbamazepin which is effective in two-thirds of the patients. Phenytoin is an intravenous option in those who cannot take oral medication due to severe pain. Baclofen is an effective medication in conjunction with Carbamazepin. Gabapentin is another antiepileptic medication

which is useful in mild forms of the TN or in association with other medications. Other medications that are being used for this condition include Amitriptyline (Elavil) and Clonazepam (Klonopin).

54. **(D)** The most common cause of the spontaneous SAH is berry aneurysm and AVM. Aneurysms are often located on the circle of Willis in the subarachnoid space hence bleeding occurs in this space. Massive hemorrhages can break in the parenchyma and produce intraparenchymal clot. AVMs usually bleed in the parenchyma but frequently is superficial and present with associated SAH. Sickle cell angiopathy can also present as SAH from subpial vessels. In a patient with history of SCD, angiopathy as the cause of SAH should be considered. On other hand, bleeding is extremely rare in meningiomas and when it occurs it is often intratumoral or intraparenchymal and do not appear as a SAH.

55. **(C)** Four vessel angiography remains a gold standard vascular study for detecting aneurysms and AVMs. It provides the detail and definition that are required for surgical intervention. MRA and CTA are often very helpful to detect and provide some detail. The newer high speed CT scans with angiography software can produce the definition close to standard angiography. PET scan and spectroscopy are primarily used to determine the metabolic activities of the brain and are incapable of detecting vascular lesions.

56. **(E)** The rate of complications in cerebral angiography is relatively low and in experienced hands is less than 1%. Among the potential complications, cerebral ischemic or hemorrhagic stroke, vascular dissection, and aneurysmal rupture are frequently reported. In patients with SCD administration of the high-osmolar contrast often precipitate sickle cell crisis. Therefore, these patients should be pretreated with exchange transfusion and maintained in a well hydrated state. Steroids are also used prior to angiography to reduce the postangiography complications.

57. **(C)** History of recent onset of headache in adult should always raise the suspicion of neoplasm. Amyloid angiopathy and hypertension are frequent cause of the intracerebral hemorrhage in elderly, but the critical difference with neoplastic bleed is the presence of edema and mass effect which is disproportionate to the size of the hemorrhage. The presence of edema suggests a preexisting lesion with recent bleed. Although intraparenchymal hemorrhage can produce edema but it takes many hours to develop. Therefore, the presence of edema in early hours after the ictus is indicative of underlying pathology. AVMs and coagulopathies also can cause intraparenchymal bleed without surrounding edema which is the hallmark of an underlying lesion.

58. **(C)** MRI with contrast is the study of choice to determine the presence of underlying pathology. The pattern of enhancement can identify such lesions as primary brain tumor or hemorrhage in a metastatic lesion. Although lung and breast are the most common neoplasm that metastasis to brain, the incidence of bleeding is more common in melanomas and lymphomas. AVMs also have special MRI features that make the diagnosis possible. The vascular details nonetheless require angiographic studies. The vascular study is ineffective in determining the presence of neoplastic lesions unless an AVM or aneurysms are suspected. Transcranial Doppler is used to determine the circulation velocity in the intracranial vessels particularly in middle cerebral artery. This test is used to monitor the vasospasm occurring after aneurysmal SAH and has no role in identifying any other pathology.

CHAPTER 12

Trauma

C. Gene Cayten and Rao R. Ivatury

Questions

DIRECTIONS (Questions 1 through 87): Each of the numbered items is followed by five answers. Select the ONE lettered answer that is BEST in each case.

1. A 20-year-old unrestrained driver was involved in a motor-vehicle crash. A computed tomography (CT) of the abdomen revealed a large hematoma in the second portion of duodenum. The rest of the abdomen is normal. The initial management of this duodenal hematoma should be:

    (A) Operative evacuation
    (B) Nasogastric decompression, intravenous fluids, and gradual resumption of oral diet
    (C) Endoscopic retrograde cholangiopancreatogram (ERCP)
    (D) Laparotomy, pyloric exclusion, and gastrojejunostomy
    (E) Octreotide

2. In a patient who had a motor-cycle crash, a CT of the abdomen revealed a peripancreatic hematoma and indistinct pancreatic border. The most definitive test for a pancreatic injury requiring operative intervention is:

    (A) ERCP
    (B) Ultrasonography
    (C) CT scanning
    (D) Operative exploration
    (E) Amylase test of lavage fluid

3. A 30-year-old restrained driver was involved in a motor-vehicle crash. He is hemodynamically stable and has a large seat belt sign on the abdomen. His abdomen is tender to palpation. In this patient one should be most concerned about:

    (A) Liver and spleen injury
    (B) Transection of the head of the pancreas
    (C) Renal pedicle avulsion
    (D) Hollow-viscus injuries
    (E) Pelvic fracture

4. A 45-year-old man skidded from the road at high speed and hit a tree. Examples of deceleration injuries in this patient include:

    (A) Aortic valve rupture
    (B) Kidney injury
    (C) Posterior dislocation of shoulder
    (D) Mesenteric avulsion
    (E) Stomach rupture

5. A 25-year-old man fell down from his bicycle and hit a concrete wall on his left side. An ultrasound examination showed free fluid in the abdomen. A CT scan confirmed a grade III splenic injury. The most important contraindication for a nonoperative management of the splenic injury is:

    (A) Hemodynamic instability
    (B) Active bleeding on CT scan
    (C) Adult patient
    (D) Lack of availability of blood for transfusion
    (E) Extensive associated injuries

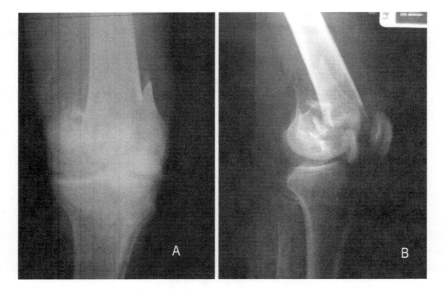

Figure 12–1.
Anteroposterior radiograph demonstrating a comminuted supracondylar femur fracture with intra-articular extension. *(Reproduced, with permission, from Doherty GM: Current Surgical Dignosis & Treatment. 1140. McGraw-Hill, 2006.)*

6. A 40-year-old man is involved in a car crash, presenting with blood pressure of 80 mm Hg. The patient is found to have subdural hematoma and a supracondylar fracture of the left femur FAST shows fluid within the abdomen. He is taken to the OR, where intra-abdominal bleeding is controlled, and the subdural hematoma is drained. The femur fracture (Fig. 12–1) should be treated by which of the following?

    (A) Long-leg cast
    (B) Steinmann pin insertion and traction
    (C) Operative reduction and internal reduction
    (D) Aspiration of knee joint
    (E) Operative reduction with internal fixation

7. An 18-year-old man is brought to the emergency department with a stab wound just to the right of the sternum in the sixth intercostal space. His blood pressure is 80 mm Hg. Faint heart sounds and pulsus paradoxus are noted. Auscultation of the right chest reveals decreased breath sounds. The *initial* management of this patient should be which of the following?

    (A) Aspiration of the right chest cavity
    (B) Aspiration of the pericardium
    (C) Echocardiogram

    (D) Pericardial window
    (E) Insertion of central venous access line

8. A 60-year-old woman runs her car off the road and it hits a telephone pole. She presents to the emergency department with severe anterior chest pain and a blood pressure of 110/80 mm Hg. A chest x-ray shows a questionably widened mediastinum. The next step in management should be which of the following?

    (A) Transthoracic echocardiogram
    (B) Pericardiocentesis
    (C) Aortogram
    (D) Central venous access line
    (E) CT of chest

9. An 18-year-old man presents to the emergency department with a gunshot wound to the left chest in the anterior axillary line in the seventh intercostal space. A rushing sound is audible during inspiration. Immediate management is which of the following?

    (A) Exploratory laparotomy
    (B) Exploratory thoracotomy
    (C) Pleurocentesis
    (D) Closure of the hole with sterile dressing
    (E) Insertion of chest tube

10. A 25-year-old man is shot in the left lateral chest. In the emergency department, his blood pressure is 120/90 mm Hg, pulse rate is 104 beats per minute (bpm), and respiration rate is 36 breaths per minute. Chest x-ray shows air and fluid in the left pleural cavity. Nasogastric aspiration reveals blood-stained fluid. What is the best step to rule out esophageal injury?

    (A) Insertion of chest tube
    (B) Insertion of nasogastric tube
    (C) Esophagogram with gastrografin
    (D) Esophagoscopy
    (E) Peritoneal lavage

11. A 32-year-old female falls from the tenth floor of her apartment building in an apparent suicide attempt. Upon presentation, the patient has obvious head and extremity injuries. Primary survey reveals that the patient is totally apneic. By which method is the immediate need for a definitive airway in this patient best provided?

    (A) Orotracheal intubation
    (B) Nasotracheal intubation
    (C) Percutaneous cricothyroidotomy
    (D) Intubation over a bronchoscope
    (E) Needle cricothyroidotomy

12. A 17-year-old girl presents to the emergency department with a stab wound to the abdomen and a blow to the head that left her groggy. Her blood pressure is 80/0 mm Hg, pulse is 120 bpm, and respiration rate is 28 breaths per minute. Her abdomen has a stab wound in the anterior axillary line at the right costal margin. Two large-bore intravenous lines, a nasogastric tube, and a Foley catheter are inserted. The blood pressure rises to 85 mm Hg after 2 L of Ringer's lactate. The appropriate management is which of the following?

    (A) Peritoneal lavage
    (B) Ultrasound of the abdomen
    (C) Laparoscopic assessment of the peritoneal cavity
    (D) Exploratory laparotomy
    (E) CT of the head

13. A 22-year-old woman presents to the emergency department with a chief complaint of severe left upper quadrant (LUQ) pain after being punched by her husband. Her blood pressure is 110/70 mm Hg, pulse is 100 bpm, and respiration rate is 24 breaths per minute. The best means to establish a diagnosis is which of the following?

    (A) FAST
    (B) Physical examination
    (C) CT of the abdomen
    (D) Peritoneal lavage
    (E) Upper gastrointestinal (GI) series

14. A 60-year-old man is attacked with a baseball bat and sustains multiple blows to the abdomen. He presents to the emergency department in shock and is brought to the operating room (OR), where a laparotomy reveals massive hemoperitoneum and a stellate fracture of the right and left lobes of the liver. Which of the following techniques should be used immediately?

    (A) Pringle's maneuver
    (B) Packing the liver
    (C) Suture ligation
    (D) Ligation of the right hepatic artery
    (E) Ligation of the proper hepatic artery

15. A 23-year-old man is shot with a handgun and found to have a through-and-through injury to the right transverse colon. There is little fecal contamination and no bowel devascularization. At operation, what does he require?

    (A) Right hemicolectomy with ileotransverse colon anastomosis
    (B) Right hemicolectomy with ileostomy and mucous fistula
    (C) Debridement and closure of wounds with exteriorization of colon
    (D) Debridement and closure of wounds
    (E) Segmental resection with primary anastomosis

16. A 20-year-old woman presents to the emergency department with a stab wound to the abdomen. There is minimal abdominal tenderness. Local wound exploration indicates that the knife penetrated the peritoneum. What is the ideal use of antibiotic administration?

    (A) Preoperatively
    (B) Intraoperatively, if a colon injury is found
    (C) Postoperatively, if the patient develops fever
    (D) Postoperatively, based on culture and sensitivity of fecal contamination found at the time of surgery
    (E) Intraoperatively, if any hollow viscus is found to be injured

17. A 70-year-old woman is hit by a car and injures her midabdomen. The best way to rule out a rupture of the second part of the duodenum is by which mode?

    (A) Repeated physical examinations
    (B) Ultrasound
    (C) Repeated amylase levels
    (D) CT with oral and intravenous contrast
    (E) Peritoneal lavage

Questions 18 and 19

18. A 35-year-old woman was punched in the right side of the abdomen and chest. There was some right upper abdomen tenderness but no guarding or rebound. Results of a gastrografin upper GI study showed a coiled-spring (stack of coins) appearance of the second and third part of the duodenum. What is the most likely diagnosis?

    (A) Rupture of the duodenum
    (B) Contusion to the head of the pancreas
    (C) Intraluminal blood clot
    (D) Retroperitoneal hematoma
    (E) Duodenal hematoma

19. Which would be the appropriate management of the patient described above?

    (A) Exploratory laparotomy and drainage
    (B) Duodenal diverticularization

    (C) Pyloric exclusion
    (D) Repeat upper GI series at 5- to 7-day intervals
    (E) CT-guided percutaneous drainage

20. A 15-year-old girl had an injury to the right retroperitoneum with duodenal contusion. What is the test required to exclude a rupture of the duodenum?

    (A) Serum amylase
    (B) Dimethyliminodiacetic acid (HIDA) scan
    (C) Gastrografin study
    (D) Upper GI with barium
    (E) ERCP

21. A 33-year-old man presents to the emergency department with a gunshot injury to the abdomen. At laparotomy, a deep laceration is found in the pancreas just to the left of the vertebral column with severance of the pancreatic duct. What is the next step in management?

    (A) Intraoperative cholangiogram
    (B) Debridement and drainage of defect
    (C) Distal pancreatectomy
    (D) Closure of abdomen with J-P drains
    (E) Vagotomy

22. A 40-year-old man is hit by a car and sustains an injury to the pelvis. Which of the following is most indicative of a urethral injury?

    (A) Hematuria
    (B) Scrotal ecchymosis
    (C) Oliguria
    (D) High-riding prostate on rectal examination
    (E) Intravenous pyelography (IVP) showing dye extravasation in the pelvis

23. For the patient described in question 18, urine did not extend to the leg because the membranous layer (Scarpa's fascia) is fused inferiorly with which of the following?

    (A) Femoral sheath
    (B) Fascia lata
    (C) Femoral fascia

(D) Deep inguinal ring

(E) Superficial inguinal ring

24. A 70-year-old man is brought to the emergency department following a car crash. X-rays revealed a fractured rib on the left and a fracture of the right femur. A CT scan of the abdomen showed a left-sided retroperitoneal hematoma adjacent to the left kidney and no evidence of urine extravasation. The hematoma should be managed by which of the following?

(A) Observation

(B) Exploratory laparotomy through a midline incision

(C) CT scan-guided aspiration

(D) Surgical exploration through a left-flank retroperitoneal approach

(E) Pneumatic antishock garment (PASG)

25. A 60-year-old man is hit by a pickup truck and brought to the emergency department with a blood pressure of 70/0 mm Hg. Peritoneal lavage showed no blood in the abdomen. The blood pressure is elevated to 85 systolic following the administration of 2 L of Ringer's lactate. An x-ray showed a pelvic fracture. What is the next step in management?

(A) Exploratory laparotomy with packing of the pelvis

(B) CT scan of the pelvis

(C) External fixation of the pelvis

(D) Open reduction and internal fixation (ORIF) of the pelvis

(E) Exploratory laparotomy with bilateral ligation of the internal iliac arteries

26. An 18-year-old man is brought to the emergency department after falling down a flight of stairs and losing consciousness for 3 minutes. A cervical collar is in place. The cervical spine is considered to be free of serious injury following which procedure?

(A) A physical examination revealing no pain or tenderness

(B) A lateral cervical spine x-ray

(C) Completely negative findings on neurological examination

(D) Anteroposterior (AP), lateral, and odontoid views of the neck

(E) Flexion and extension views of the neck

27. A 16-year-old boy presents to the emergency department with a stab wound to the anterior midneck. On physical examination, it is difficult to determine if the plane of the platysma has been violated. However, subcutaneous emphysema is found on palpation. What is the next management step?

(A) Esophagogram

(B) Arteriography

(C) Surgical exploration

(D) Esophagoscopy

(E) CT scan of the neck with oral and intravenous contrast

28. A 20-year-old woman presents to the emergency department after being hit in the face during a baseball game. On physical examination, the patient's blood pressure is 90 mm Hg, and there is significant bleeding from the nose that cannot be controlled either by fracture reduction or by anterior and posterior nasopharyngeal packing. What is the next step in management?

(A) External carotid artery ligation

(B) Bilateral internal maxillary artery ligation

(C) Angiographic evaluation and embolization

(D) Foley catheter balloon tamponade of bleeding

(E) Insertion of nasogastric tube

29. A 65-year-old man is brought to the hospital after being hit by a car. His blood pressure is 150/90 mm Hg, and pulse is 120 bpm. There is deformity just below the left knee and no distal pulses palpable in that leg. Plain films show proximal tibia and fibula fractures. What is the next step in management?

    (A) Operative intervention to restore flow with an arterial shunt
    (B) Angiography
    (C) Doppler ultrasound
    (D) Operative reduction and internal fixation
    (E) Heparinization

30. A 70-year-old man is brought into the emergency department following his injury as a passenger in a car crash. He complains of right side chest pain. Physical examination reveals a respiratory rate of 42 breaths per minute and multiple broken ribs of a segment of the chest wall that moves paradoxically with respiration. What should the next step be?

    (A) Tube thoracostomy
    (B) Tracheostomy
    (C) Thoracentesis
    (D) Endotracheal intubation
    (E) Intercostal nerve blocks

31. A 30-year-old man is brought to the emergency department in respiratory distress following a shotgun wound to the face. There is a possible cervical spine injury. Which is the best way to gain rapid control of the airway?

    (A) Nasotracheal intubation
    (B) Percutaneous jet ventilation
    (C) Cricothyroidotomy
    (D) Endotracheal intubation
    (E) Aspiration of blood from pharynx and jaw thrust

32. A 14-year-old boy is hit in the right eye with a stick. There is extensive ecchymosis. On physical examination, upward gaze is found to be lost. The most likely diagnosis is injury to which of the following (Fig. 12–2)?

    (A) Superior rectus muscle
    (B) Inferior rectus muscle
    (C) Superior oblique muscle
    (D) Levator palpebrae superioris muscle
    (E) Medial rectus muscle

33. Following a car crash in which her face hit the steering wheel, a 37-year-old woman presents to the emergency department with facial deformity. Facial x-rays showed a transverse fracture through the articulation of the maxillary and nasal bones with the frontal bone. The fracture also passed below the zygomatic bone. What is the diagnosis?

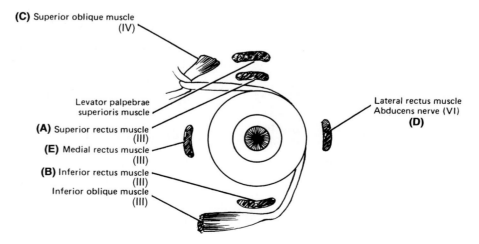

Figure 12–2.
The muscles of extraocular movement. *(Reproduced, with permission, from Lindner HH: Clinical Anatomy. Appleton & Lange, 1989.)*

(A) Sphenoid wing fracture

(B) LeFort II fracture

(C) Petrous temporal fracture

(D) Palatal split

(E) Mandibular disruption

34. A 43-year-old man is hit in the face with a baseball bat and presents to the emergency department with massive facial swelling, ecchymosis, and an elongated face. There is mobility of the middle third of the face on digital manipulation of the maxilla. What is the likely diagnosis?

(A) Lambdoid injury

(B) Odontoid fracture

(C) LeFort III fracture

(D) Palatal split

(E) Mandibular disruption

35. A 26-year-old man is stabbed in the right intercostal space in the midclavicular line and presents to the emergency department. On examination, subcutaneous emphysema of the right chest wall, absent breath sounds, and a trachea shifted to the left are noted. What is the most likely serious diagnosis?

(A) Pneumothorax

(B) Tension pneumothorax

(C) Massive hemothorax

(D) Hemopneumothorax

(E) Chest wall laceration

Questions 36 and 37

36. A 31-year-old man is shot in the back of the left chest, and the bullet exits the left anterior chest. The patient's blood pressure is 130/90 mm Hg, respiration rate is 28 breaths per minute, and pulse is 110 bpm. A chest x-ray reveals hemothorax. A chest tube is inserted and yields 800 mL of blood; the first and second hour drainage is 200 mL/h and 240 mL/h, respectively. What is the next step in management?

(A) Place a second chest tube.

(B) Collect the blood for autotransfusion.

(C) Transfuse and observe drainage for another hour.

(D) Insert a Swan-Ganz catheter.

(E) Perform a left thoracotomy.

37. In the patient described above the most likely cause of the bleeding in the patient is injury to which of the following?

(A) Pulmonary artery

(B) Lung parenchyma

(C) Internal thoracic (mammary) and/or intercostals arteries

(D) Pulmonary vein

(E) Left atrium

38. A 60-year-old man crashes his car into a bridge abutment and is found slumped over his steering wheel. In the emergency department, the signs and symptoms of pericardial tamponade are evident. These findings are most likely attributable to which of the following?

(A) Coronary artery laceration

(B) Left atrial rupture

(C) Right atrial rupture

(D) Coronary vein laceration

(E) Intrapericardial vena cava injury

39. Following an injury to the shoulder joint, a New York Yankees catcher developed a "catcher's mitt hand" or shoulder and hand syndrome. There was swelling of the right upper extremity, skin atrophy, and vasomotor instability. He also complained of a burning sensation in the involved extremity. What would be the next step in management?

(A) Immobilization of right arm in cast

(B) To avoid physical therapy for 3 months

(C) Forceful shoulder joint manipulation

(D) Prednisone for 2 weeks in resistant cases

(E) Surgical procedure on wrist joint

40. A 47-year-old woman involved in a skiing accident suffered a severe blow to the middle upper abdomen. Physical examination revealed diffuse tenderness, but there was no evidence of rebound tenderness or guarding. What test would be performed to rule out traumatic pancreatitis?

   (A) Peritoneal lavage
   (B) Serum amylase
   (C) CT scan with oral and intravenous contrast
   (D) Upper GI study
   (E) ERCP

41. A 19-year-old man presents to the emergency department with a gunshot wound through the umbilicus. The systolic blood pressure is 70 mm Hg on palpation, and his abdomen is tightly distended. Large-bore intravenous lines are placed, and Ringer's lactate is infused. What should be the next step?

   (A) Peritoneal lavage
   (B) CT scan of the abdomen
   (C) Exploratory laparotomy
   (D) Transfusion of the patient until the systolic blood pressure reaches 90 mm Hg
   (E) PASG

42. A 34-year-old man is brought into the emergency department with a large open knife wound to the left thigh. The patient's systolic blood pressure is 90 mm Hg. Blood is spurting from the wound. What is the initial management step?

   (A) Clamp the bleeding artery with a vascular clamp.
   (B) Apply a tourniquet 7.5 cm above the wound.
   (C) Apply direct pressure with sterile gauze.
   (D) Apply PASG, and inflate both legs.
   (E) Insert central venous access line.

43. A 40-year-old construction worker is pulled from the rubble after a building collapses and pins his right lower leg. X-rays in the emergency department reveal a comminuted fracture of the right tibia and fibula. The dorsal pedis and posterior tibial pulses are palpable. The patient complains of severe pain that is accentuated with dorsiflexion of the foot. The calf feels tense. What is the appropriate step?

   (A) ORIF of fracture
   (B) ORIF of fracture plus three-compartment fasciotomy
   (C) Closed reduction and observation
   (D) ORIF only if pulses become weak
   (E) Arteriogram

44. An 18-year-old woman who is 8-month pregnant is brought into the emergency department. She was hit by a car and now complains of abdominal pain. Her blood pressure is 80/60 mm Hg, pulse is 120 bpm, and respiration rate is 30 breaths per minute. Large-bore intravenous lines are placed through the antecubital fossa. The fetal heart rate is 160 bpm. What is the next step?

   (A) Infuse 2000 mL of Ringer's lactate over 10–15 minutes.
   (B) Apply a PASG, inflating only the legs.
   (C) Displace the uterus to the left.
   (D) Order an ultrasound of abdomen and pelvis to rule out free blood.
   (E) Perform peritoneal lavage 2 cm above the umbilicus.

45. A 60-year-old man is a front-seat passenger in a car crash. He is found to have three fractured ribs on the right, rupture of the liver, pelvic fracture, right femoral fracture, and a left tibial fracture. The patient is given broad-spectrum antibiotics, and his injuries are managed by surgery, requiring 12 U of blood. The patient improves initially, but on the third postoperative day, he develops hypoxia (PaO_2, 55 mm Hg), with confusion, tachypnea, and petechia. What is the most likely diagnosis?

   (A) Recurrent intra-abdominal hemorrhage from dilutional thrombocytopenia
   (B) Transfusion reaction
   (C) Antibiotic allergy
   (D) Fat embolus
   (E) Disseminated intravascular clotting (DIC)

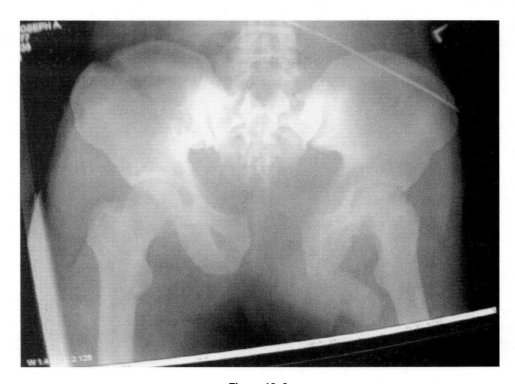

Figure 12–3.
AP radiograph of a patient with a fractured pelvis. There is widening of the symphysis pubis and a displaced fracture of the right ilum. *(Reproduced, with permission, from Brunicardi FC et al.: Schwartz's Principles of Surgery, 8th ed. 1683. McGraw-Hill, 2005.)*

46. A 43-year-old woman is thrown from a car following a car crash. She presents to the emergency department with a fracture of the pelvis (Fig. 12–3). Her blood pressure is 80/60 mm Hg, pulse is 110 bpm, and respiratory rate is 26 breaths per minute. Bright red blood is found on rectal examination and bony fragments can be palpated through the rectal wall. The patient remains hypotensive despite 3 L of Ringer's lactate and 2 U of type-specific blood. What is the most important step in management?

    (A) Exploratory laparotomy and colostomy
    (B) External fixation of the pelvic fracture
    (C) PASG
    (D) Fresh-frozen plasma
    (E) Wiring of symphysis pubis

47. With regard to neck injuries, which of the following is true?

    (A) The internal jugular vein may be ligated unilaterally without unfavorable sequelae.
    (B) Unilateral ligation of the common carotid artery results in a neurologic deficiency in 90% of cases.
    (C) Esophageal injuries should be drained externally only when extensive devitalization is present.
    (D) Tracheostomy is indicated in dealing with most laryngeal or tracheal injuries.
    (E) Injuries to the trachea must be drained externally.

48. The injury most often missed by selective nonoperative management of abdominal stab wounds is to which of the following?

    (A) Colon
    (B) Spleen
    (C) Ureter
    (D) Diaphragm
    (E) Small bowel

49. A 40-year-old woman is brought to the emergency department following a car crash in which she was the driver. In the emergency department, her blood pressure is 80/60 mm Hg, pulse is 128 bpm, and respiratory rate is 32 breaths per minute. She complains of right lower chest wall and severe right upper quadrant (RUQ) tenderness. Her breath sounds are questionably diminished. The immediate priority is to perform which of the following?

    (A) Peritoneal lavage
    (B) Chest x-ray
    (C) CT scan of chest and abdomen
    (D) Thoracentesis with an 18-gauge needle
    (E) Endotracheal intubation

50. A 30-year-old woman is brought to the emergency department after she stepped on a rusty nail and sustained a puncture wound to the foot. The patient has been on a therapeutic dose of steroids for the past 5 years for ulcerative colitis. Her last tetanus toxoid booster was 8 years ago. What should the patient receive?

    (A) Tetanus toxoid booster
    (B) Human immunoglobulin
    (C) Antibiotics with anaerobic coverage
    (D) Tetanus toxoid plus human immunoglobulin
    (E) Tetanus toxoid plus human immunoglobulin and antibiotics with aerobic and anaerobic coverage

51. A 24-year-old woman with blunt trauma to the head sustained in a car accident presents with a history of loss of consciousness for approximately 10 minutes at the scene of the accident. She is currently fully awake, oriented, and responsive. With regard to the appropriate care of this woman, which of the following statements is true?

    (A) In this setting, a fully awake patient who has a normal examination does not require hospital admission for observation.
    (B) If skull x-rays show no fracture, the likelihood of a significant intracranial injury is low, and hospital admission is unwarranted.

    (C) If fundoscopic examination of this patient shows no papilledema, elevated intracranial pressure can be ruled out.
    (D) The initial effects of elevated intracranial pressure are bradycardia and hypertension.
    (E) If this patient were to exhibit a sudden fall in blood pressure and alteration in mental status, spinal cord, or brainstem injury would be most likely.

52. A 12-year-old girl is brought into the emergency department after an unprovoked attack and bite by a raccoon. The bite is on the left lower leg. Which treatment should be provided?

    (A) Administration of human rabies immunoglobulin (HRIG) into the left gluteal area
    (B) Administration of a five-dose course of human diploid cell rabies vaccine (HDCV)
    (C) Administration of a 5-day course of HDCV and a 3-day course of HRIG
    (D) Administration of a 5-day course of HDCV and a single dose of HRIG with up to half of the dose administered directly around the wound
    (E) Administration of a 5-day course of HDCV and a single dose of HRIG administered into the gluteal area

53. An 18-year-old man is bitten on the leg by what appears to be a rattlesnake. A tourniquet has been placed above the wound, and the patient arrives at the emergency department 70 minutes after the injury. There are two fang marks with 15 cm of edema and erythema surrounding the wound. What should immediate treatment include?

    (A) Suction applied through longitudinal incisions directly through the fang marks
    (B) Suction applied through longitudinal incisions proximal to the bite
    (C) Excision of the fang mark, including skin and subcutaneous tissues
    (D) Administration of four ampules of antivenin
    (E) Removal of tourniquet

54. A 20-year-old woman presents to the emergency department with a stab wound to the neck above the angle of the mandible. The patient's blood pressure is 110/80 mm Hg, pulse rate is 100 bpm, and respiration rate is 24 breaths per minute. Between initial presentation and insertion of intravenous lines, the hematoma in the upper neck enlarges significantly. What should be the next step in the patient's management?

(A) Barium swallow
(B) Flexible endoscopy
(C) Operative exploration
(D) Doppler ultrasound
(E) Angiography

55. A 65-year-old man is brought into the emergency department with a gunshot wound to the neck. His blood pressure is 80/50 mm Hg. The patient undergoes rapid resuscitation and is brought immediately to the OR, where a carotid artery injury is found in zone II (between the angle of mandible and cricoid) (Fig. 12–4). The patient has no internal carotid flow; just before surgery, his neurological status deteriorates, and he becomes unresponsive. The operative management should be which of the following?

(A) Immediate intravascular bypass shunt
(B) Ligation of the internal carotid artery
(C) Primary anastomosis
(D) Interposition saphenous vein graft
(E) Patch vein graft

56. A 19-year-old man is brought to the emergency department with a stab wound at the base of the neck (zone I) (Fig. 12–4). The most important concern for patients with such injuries is which of the following?

(A) Upper extremity ischemia
(B) Cerebral infarction
(C) Exsanguinating hemorrhage
(D) Mediastinitis
(E) Tracheal stenosis

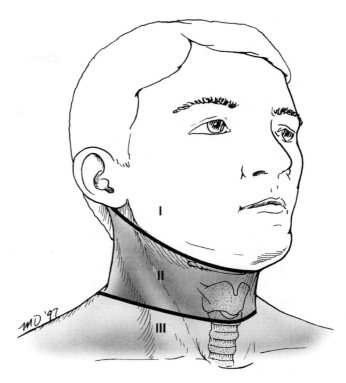

Figure 12–4.
For the purpose of evaluating penetrating injuries, the neck is divided into three zones. Zone I is below the clavicles an is also known and the thoracic outlet. Zone II is located between the clavicles and hyoid bone, and Zone III is above the hyoid. *(Reproduced, with permission, from Brunicardi FC et al.: Schwartz's Principles of Surgery, 8th ed. 140. McGraw-Hill, 2005.)*

57. A 42-year-old man is hit on the left side of his body by a car and is brought to the emergency department with fractures of the left tenth, eleventh, and twelfth ribs and left tibia and fibula fractures. The patient's blood pressure is 120/90 mm Hg, pulse rate is 100 bpm, and respiration rate is 24 breaths per minute. He has hematuria and left flank pain. Intravenous lines are inserted. IVP shows no excretion from the left kidney but normal excretion from the right. What would be the next step in management?

(A) Exploratory laparotomy
(B) CT scan with intravenous contrast
(C) Arteriography
(D) Cystogram
(E) Peritoneal lavage

58. A 26-year-old man is brought to the emergency department with a stab wound to the right side of the back just medial to the posterioraxillary line. His blood pressure is 120/80 mm Hg, pulse rate is 98 bpm, and respiration rate is 22 breaths per minute. Physical examination reveals no abdominal tenderness, guarding, or neurologic changes. Local exploration of the stab wound is performed using local anesthesia. The track to the wound ends in the paraspinal muscles. What would be the next step in management?

(A) Admit the patient for 24 hours of observation.

(B) Perform peritoneal lavage.

(C) Perform CT scan with rectal and intravenous contrast.

(D) Discharge to outpatient clinic for follow-up monitoring.

(E) Perform ultrasound.

59. A 25-year-old woman is brought to the emergency department with multiple gunshot wounds to her abdomen. Her blood pressure is 70 mm Hg. Her abdomen is massively distended. Large intravenous lines are placed, and a nasogastric tube and Foley catheter are inserted. The patient is brought immediately to the OR. After 2 L of normal saline, her blood pressure is 75/0 mm Hg, pulse rate is 140 bpm, and respiration rate is 30 breaths per minute. The next step in management should be which of the following?

(A) Open the abdomen and use a large Richardson retractor to compress the abdominal aorta against the vertebrae just below the diaphragm.

(B) Perform left thoracotomy, and cross-clamp the descending aorta just above the diaphragm.

(C) Apply the PASG to elevate blood pressure before incision.

(D) Infuse 4 U of whole blood before incision.

(E) Perform exploratory laparotomy and pack obvious bleeding sites.

60. A 30-year-old woman involved in a car crash is brought into the emergency department. Her blood pressure is 90/60 mm Hg, pulse rate is 120 bpm, and respiration rate is 18 breaths per minute. On peritoneal lavage, she is noted to have free blood in the peritoneal cavity. At the time of exploratory laparotomy, a liver laceration is noted, and there is a 2.5-cm-diameter contusion to an area of small bowel. How should the small-bowel contusion be treated?

(A) Transillumination evaluation of hematoma with meticulous hemostasis

(B) Resection of the bowel with single-layer anastomosis

(C) Inversion of the area of contusion with a row of fine nonabsorbable mattress sutures

(D) Resection of the bowel and ileostomy

(E) Observation (no surgical therapy)

61. A 19-year-old man is brought into the emergency department with a gunshot wound that occurred 4 hours before admission. At exploratory laparotomy, an injury is noted in the transverse colon with extensive tissue destruction. There is a large amount of fecal contamination. Management of this injury should include which of the following?

(A) Debridement and closure of wound with a proximal colostomy

(B) Resection with proximal colostomy and distal mucous fistula

(C) Resection of the injured colon with primary anastomosis and proximal colostomy

(D) Resection of the wound with primary anastomosis and proximal cecostomy

(E) Exteriorization of repaired colon

62. A 60-year-old man is brought into the emergency department after being hit by a car. His blood pressure is 70 mm Hg palpable, and abdomen is massively distended and tender. A large, stellate fracture of the right lower liver is noted, and despite repeated attempts at suturing, bleeding persists. The anesthesiologist notes that the pH of arterial blood is 7.2 and that the patient has become hypothermic. A total of 8 U of blood have been transfused. What is the next step in management?

(A) Insert an atriocaval shunt.

(B) Perform a right hepatic lobectomy.

(C) Pack the RUQ for 15–20 minutes while the anesthesiologist transfuses more blood.

(D) Perform a right hepatic artery ligation.

(E) Firmly pack the RUQ, close the abdomen, and plan to return to the OR within 36–72 hours.

63. A 40-year-old man sustained injuries to the liver, gallbladder, small intestine, and colon from gunshot wounds. At the time of surgery, a cholecystostomy was placed in the injured gallbladder to expedite operative management. Four weeks later, the patient is doing well. Which is the next step in management?

(A) Remove the cholecystostomy tube.

(B) Perform a cholangiogram through the cholecystostomy tube.

(C) Perform a cholecystectomy.

(D) Perform a choledochoduodenostomy.

(E) Perform a permanent cholecystostomy.

64. A 22-year-old man is found to have a complete transection of the common bile duct following a gunshot wound to the abdomen. There is also a through-and-through wound to the edge of the right lobe of the liver that is not bleeding at the time of surgery. How should the bile duct injury be managed?

(A) Choledochojejunostomy and cholecystectomy

(B) Whipple operation

(C) Primary repair with a cholecystostomy tube decompressing the gallbladder

(D) Cholecystectomy alone

(E) Choledochoileostomy

65. An 18-year-old man presents to the emergency department with a stab wound to the abdomen.

His blood pressure is 80/50 mm Hg. He is brought immediately to the OR, where an enlarged hemoperitoneum is found at laparotomy. Primary repair of the hepatic artery is performed, but because of ongoing blood loss resulting in an unstable hemodynamic situation, the portal vein injury is simply ligated. Bleeding is well controlled. The patient is brought to the recovery room, where his blood pressure drops to 80/60 mm Hg and central venous pressure is 2 cm H_2O. What should be the next step in management?

(A) Transfusion of whole blood to elevate blood pressure

(B) Reexploration to determine site of bleeding

(C) Reexploration to repair portal vein

(D) Vasopressor to increase blood pressure

(E) Ringer's lactate to increase blood pressure

66. A 25-year-old man presents to the emergency department with a gunshot wound to the abdomen. On exploratory laparotomy, he is found to have multiple small-bowel enterotomies, transverse colon enterotomy, and a partial injury just to the left of the midline of the pancreas. The pancreatic duct appears intact. What is the appropriate management of the pancreatic injury?

(A) Closed-suction drainage and lavage

(B) Drain with sump drains

(C) Distal pancreatectomy

(D) Operative pancreatogram followed by distal pancreatectomy if ductal injury is noted

(E) Transection of injured area of pancreas with Roux-en-Y (jejunal) anastomosis to the transected tail of the pancreas

67. A 29-year-old woman is brought to the emergency department with a gunshot wound to the abdomen. Her blood pressure is 80/60 mm Hg, pulse rate is 118 bpm, and respiration rate is 24 breaths per minute. She is brought immediately to the OR, where a large amount of blood and clots are found within the abdomen. After initial packing of the abdomen and stabilization of the patient, a retroperitoneal hematoma is found just above the renal veins. Proximal and distal control of the inferior vena cava is obtained and the blood pressure comes up to 100/60 mm Hg. Which is the most appropriate management?

    (A) Vascular repair of the injury
    (B) Packing of the area with a definitive plan to return to the OR in 48 hours
    (C) Ligation of the inferior vena cava
    (D) Use of intracava shunt to allow venous return while repairing the injury
    (E) Use of Gore-Tex interposition graft to restore continuity

68. A 26-year-old woman in her sixth month of pregnancy is brought to the emergency department. She had been punched in the abdomen. She is found to have generalized abdominal pain, tenderness, abdominal distention, ileus, and absent fetal heart sounds. The patient's blood pressure is 80/60 mm Hg; despite administration of 3 L of Ringer's lactate, her blood pressure only comes up to 90/60 mm Hg. What is the next step in management?

    (A) Application of PASG
    (B) Transfusion of 2 U of blood and reevaluate
    (C) Exploratory laparotomy and vaginal hysterectomy
    (D) Exploratory laparotomy with evacuation of the uterus and closure of the uterus disruption
    (E) CT scan of the abdomen

69. A 52-year-old secretary generally wears high heels and tight-fitting shoes. She saw her practitioner because of foot pain. His diagnosis of plantar fasciitis is characterized by which of the following?

    (A) It is an uncommon cause of persistent heel pain.
    (B) It causes pain on the lateral aspect of the calcaneum.
    (C) It results in part from poor selection of footwear.
    (D) It does not reveal abnormality on x-ray.
    (E) It occurs usually at rest.

70. A 43-year-old male clerk cuts his right hand on a broken glass door. In evaluating the hand, what should be kept in mind?

    (A) The proximal wrist crease corresponds with the wrist joint.
    (B) The distal wrist crease corresponds with the deep palmar arch.
    (C) Hypothenar muscles are the short muscles of the thumb.
    (D) The ulnar nerve supplies the medial three and one-half fingers on the palmar surface.
    (E) The radial artery is the sole source of arterial supply to the hand.

71. A newborn boy was examined to exclude congenital dislocation of the hip (CDH). Which of the following tests is relative to the management of CDH?

    (A) The diagnosis should be established between 2 and 4 years of age.
    (B) Abduction of the flexed hip causes a click (Ortolani's sign) (Fig. 12–5).
    (C) Abduction of the hip is not limited.
    (D) Apparent lengthening of the thigh with the hip and knee flexed may be seen.
    (E) Open reduction usually is required.

72. A football player extends his right arm to make a tackle but experiences intense pain on tackle contact with subsequent inability to move the right arm. Examination reveals swelling and tenderness about the shoulder with loss of the normal deltoid contour. Which is the most likely diagnosis?

    (A) Brachial plexus injury
    (B) Anterior dislocation of the shoulder

end of the humerus. Which of the following is the most serious complication of this fracture?

(A) Nonunion of fracture fragments

(B) Nonunion of fracture fragments with deformity

(C) Disruption of the growth plate at the distal end of the humerus

(D) Forearm compartment syndrome (Volkmann's ischemia)

(E) Ankylosis of the elbow joint

74. A 25-year-old man experiences pain in the right knee while skiing, causing his knee to twist and him to fall to the ground. His knee is swollen. He cannot bear full weight or fully extend or bend his leg. There is tenderness over the medial joint line (Fig. 12–6). Emergency-room x-ray findings were normal, and the range of motion (ROM), although restricted, is stable to varus and valgus stress. Straight-leg raise is unrestricted. Which is the most likely type of injury?

(A) Anterior cruciate ligament

(B) Tuberosity

(C) Transverse genicular ligament

(D) Medial meniscus

(E) Posterior cruciate ligament

75. A 50-year-old man hears a "snap" and then feels pain in his right leg while lunging for a forearm drive playing tennis. He walks off the court with difficulty, but his leg is swollen and painful. Findings on x-rays of the leg and ankle in the emergency room are negative. Foot sensation is normal, but findings on the Thompson test (failure of plantar flexion to occur after squeezing the gastrocnemius) are positive. What is the diagnosis?

(A) Gastrocnemius muscle tear

(B) Acute thrombophlebitis

(C) Rupture of the Achilles tendon

(D) Acute compartment syndrome

(E) Fibula fracture

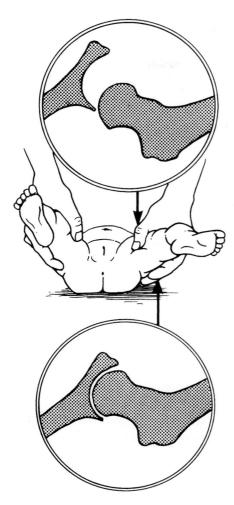

Figure 12–5.
In Ortolani's sign, abduction and lifting with the fingers produces a corresponding jerk when the dislocated femoral head slides back into the acetabulum. *(Reproduced, with permission, from Doherty GM: Current Surgical Dignosis & Treatment. 1170. McGraw-Hill, 2006.)*

(C) Fracture of the proximal posterior portion of the humerus

(D) Deltoid muscle rupture

(E) Posterior dislocation of the shoulder

73. A 7-year-old boy falls off his bicycle, landing on the left elbow. He presents to the emergency room with massive, tense swelling of the elbow with painful and restricted elbow motion. X-rays show a displaced fracture of the distal

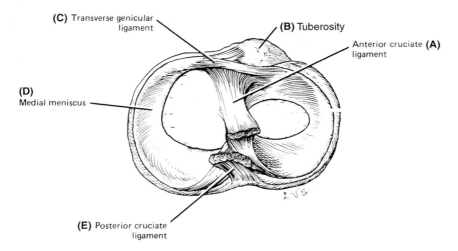

(C) Transverse genicular ligament

(B) Tuberosity

Anterior cruciate **(A)** ligament

(D) Medial meniscus

(E) Posterior cruciate ligament

Figure 12–6.
Superior aspect of the right tibia showing ligaments. (*Reproduced, with permission, from Lindner HH: Clinical Anatomy. Appleton & Lange, 1989.*)

76. A 40-year-old housewife trips over the garden hose, landing on the patio with an outstretched hand. Swelling and pain in the wrist rapidly occur, but findings on emergency room x-rays are negative for fracture or dislocation. In addition to the swelling, there is restriction of wrist dorsiflexion and palmar flexion as well as some tenderness of the anatomic snuffbox at the base of the thumb. What is the best treatment?

    (A) Splint the wrist for 4 days until the swelling and wrist pain subside.
    (B) Apply a cast to the wrist and repeat the wrist x-ray in 10–14 days.
    (C) Apply a cast to the wrist for 8 weeks.
    (D) Apply an Ace wrap to the wrist and remove daily for range of motion and exercise in warm water.
    (E) Perform open exploration of the wrist.

77. A 55-year-old right-handed woman has left elbow pain laterally after cleaning up a flooded basement by wringing out water-soaked rags. X-ray findings are negative. There is tenderness and slight swelling over the lateral epicondyle of the humerus. Anatomically, this condition can be explained by which of the following?

    (A) Sprain of the lateral collateral elbow ligament
    (B) Rupture of the triceps muscle

    (C) Tendinitis of the wrist extensors
    (D) Synovitis of the left elbow joint
    (E) Rupture of pronator teres muscle

78. A 16-year-old cross-country runner experiences right midleg pain during workouts. Sometimes the pain prevents him from completing the prescribed mileage. There is midtibial tenderness but no deformity. ROM of the ankle and knee are full and painless. There is no calf tenderness or fullness, and the Achilles tendon is intact. X-ray findings for the tibia and fibula, including both the ankle and knee joints, are normal. What should the patient be advised to do?

    (A) Rest, take anti-inflammatory agents, and use crutches for 2 weeks.
    (B) Wear a short leg cast for 3 weeks.
    (C) Rest, take anti-inflammatory agents, use crutches, and undergo a bone scan.
    (D) Continue running but increase stretching exercises before and after workout and apply analgesics to the painful area for 20 minutes after workout.
    (E) Use steroids.

79. A 47-year-old man awakens with low back pain after a weekend of gardening. He recalls no specific incident of trauma and has never had back pain before. There is no radiation of the

pain and no disturbance of normal bowel or bladder function. The ROM of the low back is painful and restricted in all planes, and there is paraspinal tenderness from L2 to L5 on the right. Scoliosis and kyphosis are absent. Findings on straight-leg-raising test are negative, reflexes are active and equal, and the patient can walk on his heels and toes. Findings on x-rays of the lumbar spine are normal. Which is the best treatment?

(A) Bed rest for 48 hours, anti-inflammatory agents, heat to the low back, and nonnarcotic analgesics

(B) Bed rest for 7–10 days, heat to the lower back, anti-inflammatory agents, muscle relaxants, and analgesics

(C) Hospitalization for pelvic traction, physical therapy, anti-inflammatory agents, intramuscularly analgesics, and muscle relaxants

(D) Immediate magnetic resonance image (MRI) for the lumbar spine

(E) Lumbar puncture

80. An 86-year-old woman experiences left hip pain after a fall at home. She cannot ambulate, her hip area is swollen and painful, and her left lower extremity is shortened and externally rotated. Before the fall, she was ambulatory and had no complaint of hip, pelvic, or knee pain. In addition to the fracture of the proximal portion of the left femur, the x-ray would show which of the following?

(A) Arthritis of the left hip
(B) Calcific bursitis of the left hip
(C) Osteoporosis
(D) Fracture of the pelvis
(E) Dislocation of the head of the femur

81. A 70-year-old man has had a long-term "bow-legged" condition but recently his right knee has become warm, swollen, and tender. He reports no recent trauma and gets no relief with rest or Tylenol (paracetamol). He is otherwise in good health and takes no medication. X-rays

show arthritis of the knee. Which would be the best treatment?

(A) Bed rest, anti-inflammatory agents, analgesics, and a knee brace

(B) Use of a cane for ambulating, restriction of knee-bending activities, and implementation of muscle-strengthening exercises

(C) Intra-articular steroid injection, bed rest, and analgesics

(D) Long-leg cast and crutches for 3 weeks, analgesics, and anti-inflammatory agents

(E) Urgent surgical correction

82. A 64-year-old woman is admitted to the emergency department with multiple injuries. She requires a central venous pressure line. To minimize the possibility of infection, the principal management of the catheter should be which of the following?

(A) Repeated attempts via the same cannula in the neck

(B) After failure at one site, use of same cannula at another site

(C) Use of multiport catheters

(D) Avoidance of wound contamination by application of tincture of iodine for more than 4 seconds

(E) Selection of subclavian vein over femoral vein

83. A 40-year-old woman was involved in a car crash. She was unconscious for 5 minutes. X-ray revealed a depressed fracture in the frontal region. Which of the following statements is true of skull fracture?

(A) It always requires surgical exploration.
(B) It is compound if multiple.
(C) It requires burr holes if compound.
(D) In the anterior cranial fossa, it may produce rhinorrhea.
(E) It requires steroid administration.

84. A 32-year-old man underwent laparotomy for trauma because of multiorgan injuries. He was discharged after 2 weeks in the hospital only to be readmitted after 3 days because of abdominal pain and sepsis. The CT scan showed an accumulation of fluid in the subhepatic space. This space is likely to be directly involved following an injury to which of the following?

    (A) Inferior pole of the right kidney
    (B) Stomach
    (C) Superior mesenteric artery
    (D) Inferior mesenteric vein
    (E) Right psaoas muscle

85. Following a bullet wound penetrating the descending colon, necrotizing fasciitis of the anterior abdominal wall occurred postoperatively. Which of the following is true for this condition?

    (A) It does not involve the superficial fascia.
    (B) It causes extensive localized abscess.
    (C) It is silent without pain in the majority of patients.
    (D) It is treated by wide excision and broad-spectrum antibiotics.
    (E) It is treated by immediate incision and drainage.

86. A 30-year old man sustained a pelvic fracture with a large pelvic hematoma. Rectal examination reveals a large laceration in the rectal wall and a nonpalpable prostate. His vital signs have stabilized with multiple transfusions. This patient requires which of the following?

    (A) Resuscitation, blood transfusions, external fixature, and exploratory laparotomy
    (B) Resuscitation, angiography, embolization of the pelvic bleeders, exploratory laparotomy
    (C) Resuscitation, broad-spectrum antibiotics, retrograde cystourethrogram, CT of abdomen and pelvis, suprapubic cystostomy, and diverting colostomy

    (D) Exploratory laparotomy, urinary diversion, sigmoid colostomy, presacral drainage, and debridement of the rectal wall
    (E) ORIF of pelvic fracture by a posterior approach, colostomy, and suprapubic cystostomy.

87. Which is true of intraperitoneal colon injuries?

    (A) They should never be repaired primarily.
    (B) They may be treated by exteriorization of the repair.
    (C) They should be treated with resection and colocolostomy.
    (D) They require drainage after repair.
    (E) Most can be treated by debridement and repair.

DIRECTIONS (Questions 88 through 101): Each set of matching questions in this section consists of a list of lettered options followed by several numbered items. For each numbered item, select the appropriate lettered option. Each lettered option may be selected once, more than once, or not at all. Select the most appropriate option for each case.

Questions 88 through 90

    (A) Peritoneal lavage
    (B) Wound exploration
    (C) Sonogram
    (D) Paracentesis
    (E) CT with intravenous and oral contrast
    (F) IVP
    (G) Exploratory laparotomy
    (I) Angiogram

88. A 16-year-old boy presents to the emergency department with a gunshot wound to the abdominal cavity.

89. A 60-year-old woman presents with a stab wound to the back just above the iliac crest. She is in stable condition.

90. A 26-year-old man presents with a tangential small-caliber gunshot wound of the anterior abdominal wall.

Questions 91 through 93

  (A) Splenorrhaphy with one suture
  (B) Partial splenectomy
  (C) Splenectomy
  (D) Splenorrhaphy with Dexon mesh
  (E) Packing
  (F) Subphrenic abscess
  (G) Pancreatitis
  (H) Left lower lobe pneumonia
  (I) Postsplenectomy sepsis
  (J) Gastric wall ulcer
  (K) Left colon perforation
  (L) Pneumococcal infection

91. A 48-year-old woman was brought to the emergency department after sustaining a stab wound to the left side of the abdomen. Exploration of the abdomen shows 1000 mL of blood, clot, and feces. There is a bleeding laceration across the middle third of the spleen but not involving the pedicle, a 3-cm laceration of the left transverse colon, and through-and-through lacerations of the stomach and the left lobe of the liver. What should be the management of the splenic injury?

92. One week following splenectomy, a 12-year-old girl presents with nausea, vomiting, headache, and confusion. What is the most likely diagnosis?

93. Nine days following splenectomy, a 13-year-old patient presents with fever and leukocystosis. The chest x-ray shows free air under the diaphragm. What is the most likely diagnosis?

Question 94

  (A) Flail chest
  (B) Empyema
  (C) Diaphragm rupture
  (D) Cervical rib
  (E) Hemothorax
  (F) Chylothorax
  (G) Pectus excavation
  (H) Paradoxical respiration

94. A 60-year-old man is in a car crash in which he is the driver. He did not have a seat belt or an airbag. He is found to have multiple rib fractures over his right chest. His pulse is weaker during inspiration. What are the most likely diagnoses?

Questions 95

  (A) Sacroiliac joint
  (B) Neck of femur
  (C) Lateral meniscus
  (D) Intertrochanteric
  (E) Pubic tuberosity
  (F) Spine of ischium
  (G) Ischial cruciate ligament
  (H) Anterior cruciate ligament
  (I) Posterior cruciate ligament
  (J) Biceps femora
  (K) Pectineal line

95. An 81-year-old female falls and presents to the emergency department. What injury to this tissue or structure causes lower leg extremities to be externally rotated?

DIRECTIONS (Questions 96 through 98): The response options for items 96–98 are the same. You will be required to select one answer from each item in the set. For each patient with dyspnea, select the most likely diagnosis.

Questions 96 through 98

  (A) Tension pneumothorax
  (B) Cardiac tamponade
  (C) Spontaneous pneumothorax
  (D) Open pneumothorax
  (E) Massive hemothorax
  (F) Flail chest
  (G) Rupture diaphram

96. A 23-year-old man, tall and thin, was jogging one evening when he suddenly felt a sharp pain in the left chest, worse on taking a deep breath and shortness of breath.

97. A 45-year-old man was a passenger in a car when he was T-boned by a truck at a high speed. He is short in breath, complains of severe pain in the chest, and is hypoxic on the pulse oximeter. The breath sounds are diminished on the left and the percussion note is completely dull. He rapidly becomes tachycardic and hypotensive.

98. A 25-year-old woman was stabbed by her boyfriend in the left chest. On examination, she has a 1-cm stab wound just inferior to her left breast in the mid-clavicular line. There is jugular venous distension and breath sounds are completely absent on the left side. She is becoming extremely dyspneic and hypoxic.

DIRECTIONS (Questions 99 through 101): The response options for items 99–101 are the same. You will be required to select one answer from each item in the set. For each patient who was involved in a motor-vehicle crash, match the most likely injury.

Questions 99 through 101

   (a) Diffuse axonal injury
   (b) Acute extradural hematoma
   (c) Acute subdural hematoma
   (d) Tentorial herniation
   (e) Flail chest
   (f) Posterior dislocation of the hip
   (g) Fracture of the pelvis
   (h) Diaphragmatic rupture

99. A 45-year-old man with a skull fracture of the temporal bone

100. A 23-year-old man with a head-on collision, bent steering wheel and knee imprint on dashboard.

101. A 30-year-old with a side impact injury, has multiple rib fractures on the left side with pain and hypoxia.

Answers and Explanations

1. **(B)** Intramural duodenal hematoma may occur secondary to blunt trauma of the abdomen. Usually this hematoma is submucosal and the injury is not transmural. It may cause a temporary obstruction of the duodenum and usually responds to nasogastric suction and intravenous fluids. Only if the patient has persistent obstruction (as demonstrated by an upper GI study) beyond 2 weeks, a surgical approach may be required.

2. **(A)** The most definitive test for a lesion requiring operative correction is demonstration of a disrupted major pancreatic duct. While CT scanning may give a suggestion of a ductal injury, and operative exploration of the area of injury may be inconclusive, ERCP is very reliable in showing a disrupted duct. Amylase testing of lavage effluent is nonspecific.

3. **(D)** While all the injuries listed are potential problems in this patient, the most severe is blunt hollow viscus injury. A delay in diagnosis beyond 12 hours is associated with increased morbidity and mortality. There may be very few physical signs of a viscus perforation and CT findings may be subtle and not definitive. A seat belt sign across the abdomen should raise suspicion of this injury and prompt an aggressive pursuit of diagnosis by serial examination and a consideration of a peritoneal lavage or repeat CT scan.

4. **(E)** Deceleration injuries occur when the body is subjected to a sudden stop when traveling at a high speed (e.g., high-speed automobile hitting a tree, fall from a height). As the impacting part of the body comes to a sudden halt, the organs behind continue to travel forward, thus causing shearing injuries at the junction of mobile and fixed parts; such as mesenteric avulsion. The other choices are possible but much less common.

5. **(A)** While all other choices may be relative, hemodynamic instability is the prime contraindication for nonoperative treatment.

6. **(B)** The priorities in patient care are to control hemorrhage in the abdomen and decompress the subdural hematoma. The optional initial surgical therapy of the supracondylar femur fracture is the insertion of a Steinmann pin for traction. If traction fails to produce adequate alignment, open reduction can be performed at a later date.

7. **(A)** In a patient presenting with a chest wound in shock, the priorities are airway, breathing, and circulation. Thus, aspiration of the right chest to rule out a tension pneumothorax should be performed first. Aspiration of the pericardium does not definitively rule out cardiac injury; a pericardial window provides both diagnosis and decompression. An echocardiogram is not indicated in an unstable patient.

8. **(C)** The most definitive test for aortic injury is the aortogram, even though only 20–30% of patients with widened mediastinum demonstrate it. A transthoracic echocardiogram does not image the aorta wall; however, a transesophageal echocardiogram may have more value in experienced hands.

9. **(D)** The immediate treatment is the closure of the hole by any means available. Sucking chest wounds allow shift of the mediastinum to the opposite side. Thoracotomy is not usually required. Laparotomy is indicated for a gunshot wound below the fourth intercostal space, but it should follow respiratory stabilization. A chest tube will be required, following closure of the sucking wound, to prevent a tension pneumothorax.

10. **(D)** Either an esophagoscopy or a barium swallow—or both—can be used to rule out esophageal injury. The esophagogram should not be performed with Gastrografin because of its deleterious effects if aspirated into the lungs. Nasogastric tube aspiration showing blood is suggestive of an esophageal injury in this patient but is not specific. Peritoneal lavage is sensitive for an intra-abdominal injury, causing bleeding.

11. **(A)** In a patient with significant blunt mechanism of injury and head injury, the cervical spine should be protected against further injury. In an apneic patient with the potential for cervical spine injury, orotracheal intubation may be attempted with in-line stabilization of the neck. If this is unsuccessful, percutaneous cricothyroidotomy is the best definitive step.

12. **(D)** A patient without other sources of blood loss who presents to the emergency department with a stab wound to the abdomen and in shock should have an expeditious exploratory laparotomy. Hemorrhage control should take precedence over definitive management of a concomitant head injury. The other tests will waste precious time and are contraindicated in a patient in shock.

13. **(C)** The best means to establish the diagnosis is CT scan of the abdomen. It will demonstrate solid-organ injury and the appropriate amount of fluid (blood) in the peritoneal cavity. It also serves as a baseline for a patient being treated conservatively for spleen and liver injuries.

14. **(B)** The initial operative step is packing of the liver to obtain control of the bleeding. A Pringle maneuver can then be performed. In

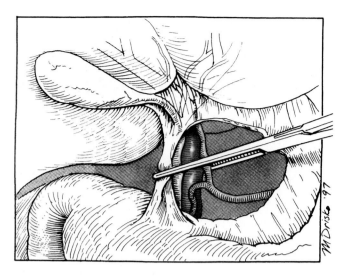

Figure 12–7.
The Pringle maneuver. *(Reproduced, with permission, from Brunicardi FC et al.: Schwartz's Principles of Surgery, 8th ed. 160. McGraw-Hill, 2005.)*

this procedure, the proper hepatic artery is compressed between one finger inserted into the foramen omentalis (Winslow, epiploic) and another anterior to the free edge of the lesser (gastrohepatic omentum) (Fig. 12-7). Selective right hepatic artery is rarely useful, and ligation of the proper hepatic artery is contraindicated.

15. **(D)** Most gunshot injuries to the right side of the colon should be closed primarily. Resection is required only where there is extensive devitalization of tissue or injury to the mesocolon causing devascularization of the bowel.

16. **(A)** Antibiotics should be given preoperatively to all patients with wounds penetrating the peritoneal cavity. Intraoperative and postoperative antibiotics fail to reduce postoperative abscesses and wound infections adequately.

17. **(D)** CT scan with oral and intravenous contrast is the most sensitive and specific study to diagnose injuries to the retroperitoneal duodenum. Findings on physical examination and peritoneal lavage are generally negative because of the retroperitoneal location of the posterior wall of the second portion of the duodenum. Rising amylase levels may increase suspicion of the injury but are not specific.

18. **(E)** The coiled-spring or stacked-coin appearance of the duodenum is diagnostic of a duodenal hematoma.

19. **(D)** Oral feeds and fluids are withheld, and hyperalimentation is administered. The upper GI study is repeated at 5- to 7-day intervals. Surgery can usually be avoided.

20. **(C)** Rupture of the duodenum would show in an extravasate Gastrografin study. Contusion of the head of the pancreas might show a widening of the duodenal C-loop. If barium enters the peritoneal cavity, it causes severe peritonitis.

21. **(C)** Distal pancreatectomy is the procedure of choice for distal pancreatic injuries. It is essential to avoid creation of an intestinal anastomosis (such as in pancreaticojejunostomy), which can leak. An intraoperative pancreatogram is indicated to rule out more proximal duct injuries. Debridement and drainage of the defect alone may result in a pancreatic fistula.

22. **(D)** A high-riding prostate on rectal examination indicates that the urethra has been torn and the prostate rides up with the bladder. The definitive study for suspected urethral injury is a urethrogram. Inability to void and a crushed pelvis also should raise the possibility of a urethral injury.

23. **(B)** Urine may extend in the subcutaneous layer to the anterior abdominal wall and scrotal skin. Fusion of Scarpa's fascia (part of superficial fascia) with fascia lata (deep fascia) explains why urine does not extend down the thigh (Fig. 12–8).

24. **(A)** A small nonexpanding hematoma with no associated urine extravasation can be managed by observation with repeat CT scan or ultrasound. If the patient becomes hypotensive, exploration through a midline incision would be indicated.

25. **(C)** Early external fixation of the pelvis has been shown to reduce bleeding and mortality in patients in shock consequent to pelvic fractures. An unstable patient should not be sent for a CT scan. Selective angiography with embolization of the bleeding vessel may also be helpful in these patients. Laparotomy usually results in uncontrollable pelvic bleeding.

26. **(D)** Clearing the cervical spine usually consists of obtaining normal findings on AP, lateral,

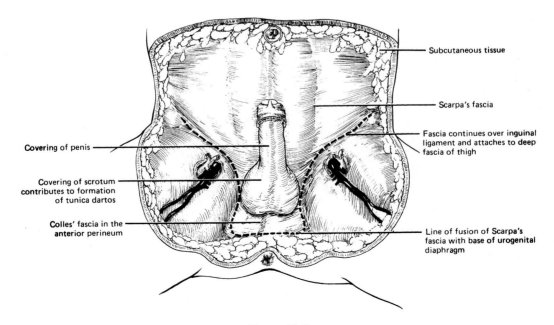

Figure 12–8.
Scarpa's fascia showing continuation into the anterior male perineum. *(Reproduced, with permission, from Way LW: Current Surgical Diagnosis & Treatment, 10th ed. Appleton & Lange, 1994.)*

and odontoid views of the cervical spine. Flexion and extension views are rarely indicated and must be performed under careful supervision. Negative findings on physical examination alone are not reliable in a patient with an impaired sensorium.

27. **(C)** Midneck (zone II) stab wounds should be surgically explored if subcutaneous emphysema or expanding hematoma are found. Zone II midneck lesions are those between the lower border of the mandible and hyoid cartilage. Further studies are indicated if the findings just listed are not present or the platysma has not been clearly violated.

28. **(C)** Because it is not possible to identify the specific vessels injured by physical examination, angiography with embolization is indicated. Insertion of a nasogastric tube in patients with midfacial trauma should be avoided because of the presence of a false passage to the brain.

29. **(B)** In a stable patient presenting with peripheral vessel occlusion following blunt trauma, angiography is indicated to plan the appropriate operative approach. An angiogram can also document preexisting arterisclerosis, collateral circulation, and distal runoff. Doppler ultrasound is useful to localize the injury site but gives less information regarding collateral circulation. Immediate operation to control bleeding and restore flow is indicated if the patient's condition is unstable.

30. **(C)** Thoracentesis should be performed first to rule out a tension pneumothorax or hemothorax. However, if the patient does not respond rapidly, early endotracheal intubation is necessary for patients with a flail segment of the chest wall. Intercostal nerve blocks and other means to control pain are important but should be performed after respiratory problems have been brought under control.

31. **(C)** In a patient with a massive midface injury, cricothyroidotomy or tracheostomy should be performed, depending on the urgency of the need for airway control (Fig. 12–9). Cricothyroidotomy can usually be performed more quickly than tracheostomy. Nasotracheal and endotracheal intubation may push blood and debris into the trachea.

32. **(A)** Loss of upward gaze is attributable to impairment of the superior rectus muscle and occasionally the inferior oblique muscle. Loss of upward gaze of the eye should not be confused with failure to elevate the upper eyelid (levator palpebrae superioris muscle), which contains both striated and nonstriated components.

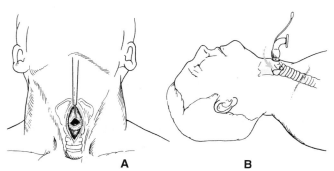

Figure 12–9.
Cricothyroidotomy is recommended for an emergency surgical airway. Vertical incisions are perferred to avoid injury to the anterior jugular veins, which are located just lateral to the midline. Hemorrahage from these vessels will obscure vision and prolong the procedure. When making an incision in the cricothyroid membrane, the blade of the knife should be angled inferiorly to avoid injury to the vocal cords. A. Heavy silk suture for traction on the thyroid cartilage. B. Insertion of the cricothyroid tube. *(Reproduced, with permission, from Brunicardi FC et al.: Schwartz's Principles of Surgery, 8th ed. 130. McGraw-Hill, 2005.)*

33. **(B)** The bones injured describe a Le Fort II fracture,(Fig. 12–10) occasionally associated with a palatal split, where the right and left maxillary are completely separated at the midline or the hard palate. Gently rocking the maxillary arch causes the maxilla and nasofrontal areas to move in concert. If there is a Le Fort III fracture, the entire face is detached from the cranial base.

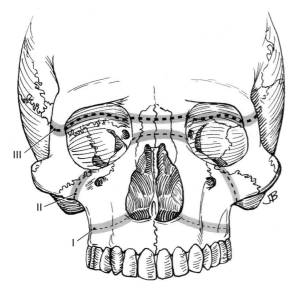

Figure 12–10.
Classic Le Fort fracture patterns. *(Reproduced, with permission, from Brunicardi FC et al.: Schwartz's Principles of Surgery, 8th ed. 514. McGraw-Hill, 2005.)*

34. **(C)** The physical findings are characteristics of a Le Fort III fracture (Fig. 12–10). In this injury, the fracture passes through maxilla and nasal bones and above the zygomatic bone.

35. **(B)** Shift of the trachea strongly suggests a tension pneumothorax. Subcutaneous emphysema is also more common with a tension pneumothorax than with the other conditions listed. Simple pneumothorax and chest wall laceration are much less serious injuries than tension pneumothorax.

36. **(E)** A patient bleeding at a rate of more than 200 mL/h should have an emergency thoracotomy. Autotranfusion of blood collected through chest tube should be considered for lesser

degree of bleeding but is less reliable to succeed if bleeding does not decrease.

37. **(C)** Bleeding that is sufficient to require thoracotomy usually comes from vessels in the systemic circulation, particularly the internal thoracic (mammary) and intercostal arteries.

38. **(A)** Tamponade from blunt trauma to the heart is usually attributable to myocardial rupture or coronary artery laceration. The left coronary artery gives off the left anterior interventricular artery that passes between the left and right ventricle on the anterior surface of the heart. The right main coronary artery passes in the sulcus between the right atrium and the right ventricle on the anterior surface of the heart.

39. **(D)** Prednisone for 2 weeks in resistant cases is given and then tapered. The "shoulder–hand" syndrome is a reflex autonomic dystrophy occurring after an injury (usually shoulder) that causes immobilization of the ipsilateral extremity. Treatment is directed toward gradual physical therapy and nonsteroidal analgesic drugs. Stellate ganglion block may be helpful in resistant cases.

40. **(C)** CT scan with oral and intravenous contrast gives the best sensitivity and specificity in diagnosing blunt trauma to the pancreas. ERCP could be useful in studying the integrity of the pancreatic duct, but a CT scan is more accurate in revealing traumatic pancreatitis without major ductal injury. An upper GI series may show widening of the duodenal C-loop. An isolated serum amylase elevation is not diagnostic of pancreatic injury. Repeated testing of amylase levels, if amylase levels increase with time, may be more diagnostic of traumatic pancreatitis than a single value.

41. **(C)** The patient should be brought to the OR prepared and draped, with the nasogastric tube and Foley catheter inserted, and then anesthetized immediately prior to laparotomy. Some surgeons initially control the aorta through a thoracotomy incision through the seventh intercostal space. Transfusion before control of bleeding causes more bleeding.

42. **(C)** Apply direct pressure with sterile gauze. Direct pressure is the best choice. Attempting to clamp vessels can cause further vascular or nerve injury. Tourniquet is used only if direct pressure fails. As soon as direct pressure is attempted, a second person should insert a large-bore peripheral intravenous line.

43. **(B)** A tense calf with comminuted fractures (fractures exposed to exterior) and pain on dorsiflexion necessitates a fasciotomy because of the very high probability of a compartment syndrome. Arterial injury is possible (but rare) in lower leg injuries if the pulses are palpable.

44. **(C)** Displace the uterus to the left. The first step in restoring cardiac return in a patient in the third trimester who has become hypovolemic is to displace the gravid uterus off the vena cava by pushing it to the left. The other choices (except for the use of the PASG) should be considered following displacement of the uterus.

45. **(D)** Fat embolus is usually associated with long bone or pelvic fractures and is associated with petechiae. Transfusion and antibiotic reactions causing hypotension would occur relatively quickly following administration.

46. **(B)** The most likely cause of the patient's persistent hypotension is the pelvic fracture; therefore, external fixation should be performed promptly. While the patient is undergoing external fixation in the OR, an exploratory laparotomy and colostomy should be performed for the rectal injury.

47. **(A)** In the patient who has no neurologic deficit preoperatively, every effort should be made to repair a carotid artery injury. Four-vessel angiography should be performed in stable patients with injuries in zones I and III. Careful judgment should be exercised in selecting patients with zone II injuries who are to have angiography (i.e., suspected injuries to bilateral carotid arteries or vertebral arteries) and in selecting those for observation. Carotid artery ligation might also be employed in patients who are unstable without a high incidence of neurologic deficit.

48. **(D)** Selective management of abdominal stab wounds, especially to the lower chest and upper abdomen, relies on physical examination and diagnostic peritoneal lavage (DPL) to identify the need for operative exploration. Small, isolated diaphragmatic lacerations may be asymptomatic and may not result in red blood cell counts required to cause a positive DPL These small diaphragmatic wounds are best detected by laparoscopy. Missed diaphragmatic injuries may cause late diaphragmatic hernias with potential morbidity and mortality.

49. **(D)** In a patient with respiratory distress and shock, adequate breathing is of higher priority than circulation. Insertion of an 18-gauge needle to rule out and/or treat a pneumothorax takes precedence over diagnostic tests.

50. **(E)** Tetanus toxoid plus human immunoglobulin and antibiotics with aerobic and anaerobic coverage. Patients who are taking steroids or who are immune suppressed should receive human immunoglobulin even though previously immunized. Tetanus booster and antibiotic therapy are also necessary.

51. **(D)** In general, most patients with significant head injury should be admitted for observation. Skull x-rays cannot be relied upon for the diagnosis of intracranial injury, because lesions may still be present, even with normal skull x-ray. Elevated intracranial pressure may be present, even with the absence of papilledema. Bradycardia and hypertension (not hypotension) are the features of elevated intracranial pressure.

52. **(D)** Raccoons should be regarded as rabid animals unless the geographic area is known to be free of rabies. A 5-day course of vaccine and a single dose of HRIG should be administered. They should not be administered jointly into the gluteal area, because administration in this area results in lowering neutralizing antibody titers. Where feasible, up to half of the dose of HRIG should be infiltrated into the area around the wound.

53. **(D)** This patient's response is considered moderate to great in regard to envenomation and requires 3–5 vials of antivenin IV in 500 mL of normal saline. The tourniquet should not be removed until the antivenin therapy is instituted. Incision and suction will be of benefit only if accomplished within 30 minutes of sustaining the bite, and excision of the bite area is valuable only if performed within 1 hour.

54. **(E)** In considering management of neck wounds, three zones are described. Zone III refers to the area above and posterior to the angle of the mandible (see Fig. 12–4). Angiographic definition of the site and extent of arterial injury is important because of the difficulty in exposure of internal carotid injuries near the base of the skull. Such injuries may require the use of extracranial–intracranial arterial bypass.

55. **(B)** Even those who advocate reconstruction of carotid arteries in patients with neurological deficit do not recommend attempted reconstruction in patients who are comatose. If the patient were not comatose, proximal and distal control with stenting and interposition graft would be the procedure of choice.

56. **(C)** Exsanguinating hemorrhage is the predominant risk, because bleeding may not be easily recognized, given that bleeding into the pleural cavity and mediastinum can occur. The abundant collateral blood supply generally protects against upper extremities or cerebrovascular compromise.

57. **(C)** Arteriography is used to assess possible renal artery injury in these circumstances. It is used if the kidney is not visualized with an IVP or CT a scan. Operative intervention without arteriography is not necessary in a stable patient. Peritoneal lavage is useful in determining the presence of intraperitoneal bleeding; if arteriography shows a need for surgery, peritoneal lavage will not be necessary.

58. **(D)** A patient with definitive negative findings on wound exploration can be discharged from the hospital for outpatient follow-up care. It is sometimes difficult to determine the depth of a stab wound to the back because of the thickness of the paraspinal muscles. Some authors have found that nearly 20% of patients with such injuries have negative findings on exploration. Such patients can be discharged. Deeper stab wounds to the back may injure peritoneal structures without penetration of the peritoneal cavity. Thus, peritoneal lavage is less useful than a CT scan with intravenous, oral, and (particularly) rectal contrast to rule out retroperitoneal colon injuries.

59. **(A)** Open the abdomen and use a large Richardson retractor to compress the abdominal aorta against the vertebrae just below the diaphragm. The advantages of occluding the subdiaphragmatic aorta (as opposed to the supradiaphragmatic aorta) are that it: (a) avoids opening another major cavity; and (b) results in less diminution of blood flow to the spinal cord and renal circulation. Further attempts to resuscitate the patient with whole blood will not be successful until bleeding sites are controlled; such measures may even increase bleeding by elevating blood pressure, which reopens vessels that have already stopped bleeding. Attempting to control individual bleeding sites with packing is difficult in a patient with multiple gunshot wounds who is exsanguinating.

60. **(D)** Contusion of the small bowel may be larger than apparent and may lead to necrosis and perforation. Contusions of 1 cm or less in diameter may be turned in with mattress sutures. However, larger contusions should be resected. The advantage of a single-layer anastomosis is the speed of performance and the reduced likelihood of compromising the muscularis mucosa.

61. **(B)** The necrotic bowel is resected, the proximal end is constructed as an end colostomy, and the distal end is constructed as a mucous fistula. This is the best procedure, because it will avoid an anastomosis in a contaminated abdomen. Any procedure that involves either wound closure or anastomosis in an abdomen with extensive fecal contamination presents a significant risk of leakage and therefore should not be performed. Exteriorization should not be performed unless ischemic bowel is resected.

62. **(E)** Once a patient shows acidemia and hypothermia from significant blood loss, further operative manipulations will not likely result in control of persistent bleeding. It is best to pack the RUQ firmly and return to the OR in 36 hours. It is possible that the patient has a retrocaval hepatic vein injury, but attempting to insert an intracaval shunt in the presence of acidemia and hypothermia is not likely to be successful. Hepatic artery ligation has been used infrequently in recent years, because in most cases, hepatic bleeding is venous and, therefore, not altered by the ligation.

63. **(B)** A cholecystocholangiogram must be performed to ensure that the gallbladder is not leaking, and that there is free flow of dye in the duodenum if no abnormality is detected on the cholangiogram, the cholecystomy tube is removed. The patient should undergo follow-up gallbladder studies several months later, but routine removal of the gallbladder is not necessary.

64. **(A)** Although it may be technically possible to perform a primary anastomosis for a complete transection, these invariably lead to bile duct structure. It is important to remember that debridement of the duct following a gunshot wound increases the tension on the anastomosis. The best method for the early treatment of injuries to the common bile duct is a duct-to-small bowel anastomosis.

65. **(A)** Obstruction to the portal outflow causes acute splenic hypervolemia simultaneously with systemic hypovolemia. If not treated by overtransfusion of blood volume (in some cases, almost equal to the patient's normal blood volume), death may occur from hypovolemia. Vasopressors should never be used to correct blood pressure in the face of hypovolemia.

66. **(A)** Routinely performing distal pancreatectomy for all penetrating injuries to the body or tail of the pancreas significantly prolongs the operative time and contributes to additional hemorrhage and possible hypothermia. Approximately 25% of patients undergoing distal pancreatectomy develop an intra-abdominal abscess. Distal pancreatectomy is the procedure of choice if there is an obvious disruption of the pancreatic duct in the body or tail. Closed-suction drainage is preferred to suction drainage because of the lower incidence of abscess formation with closed-suction drainage. If there is an injury to the duodenum, a pancreaticogram can be performed through the injury site; however, a normal duodenum should not be opened to secure an intraoperative pancreaticogram.

67. **(A)** Although injuries in the inferior vena cava can be ligated if the repair is unduly time consuming for the patient with continued hypotension, every attempt must be made to repair a suprarenal vena cava injury. Packing of the injury should be performed only if acidemia and/or hypothermia develop, because packing of the vena cava is not likely to be effective for a very long period. If an interposition graft is necessary, vein graft should be obtained from the infrarenal cava or iliac veins. A synthetic graft is likely to thrombose. An intracaval shunt generally requires a thoracotomy to gain proximal control and is reserved for retrohepatic injuries to the vena cava.

68. **(D)** Exploratory laparotomy with evacuation of the uterus and closure of the uterus disruption is the procedure of choice despite continued hypotension. Blood administration should be instituted but is not as critical as gaining surgical hemostasis. A PASG may have a limited temporizing effect but should not be used as an alternative to exploratory laparotomy. Any patient with abdominal trauma who is hypotensive should not be sent for a CT scan.

69. **(C)** Plantar fasciitis may occur either with or without a calcaneal spur. Plantar fasciitis is more likely when footwear is inappropriate or there is excessive exercise (e.g., in athletes). There is pain either after exercise (in a patient who has had a period of rest) or at the end of prolonged activity. Tenderness is over the medial aspect of the plantar fascia close to the calcaneum. X-ray may reveal a tear in the periosteum or a calcaneal spur.

70. **(A)** The proximal wrist crease corresponds with the wrist joint, and the distal crease of the wrist corresponds with the proximal portion of the flexor retinaculum. The hypothenar muscles are on the ulnar side, and the thenar muscles are on the thumb side of the hand. The ulnar artery contributes predominantly to the superficial and the radial artery to the deep palmar arches in the hand.

71. **(B)** It is important to recognize congenital dislocation of the newborn soon after birth. Delay in initiating appropriate treatment may lead to permanent hip joint disease. There may be apparent shortening of the thigh, although with the hip and knee flexed.

72. **(B)** The mechanism of injury (abduction and external rotation) combined with the characteristic observable deformity of deltoid contour loss makes anterior dislocation the best choice. The common site of shoulder joint dislocation is inferior, because the rotator cuff muscles are absent there.

73. **(D)** Ischemia contracture may result in deformity and disability of the hand, which impairs function of the entire upper extremity, not only of the elbow area.

74. **(D)** Restriction of motion ("locking"), effusion ("swelling"), and medial joint-line tenderness are the hallmarks of meniscal tears. Stability-to-stress testing eliminates collateral ligament rupture, and the ability to elevate the straight leg eliminates patella dislocation and quadriceps tendon ruptures. In addition, patella dislocation would also be characterized by gross patella deformity laterally.

75. **(C)** Of all the conditions listed, only an Achilles tendon rupture will result in positive findings on the "squeeze" test (Thompson's sign), whereby a squeezing of the gastrocnemius muscle fails to cause plantar flexion of the foot.

76. **(B)** Tenderness in the anatomic snuffbox (the interval between the extensor pollicis longus and the extensor pollicis brevis and abductor pollicis longus tendons) may signify a fracture of the carpal scaphoid (navicular) bone. Initial x-ray findings are often negative, but the fracture line often shows up in a repeat x-ray taken after 10–14 days.

77. **(C)** The act of wringing rags results in repeated and forceful wrist dorsiflexion, causing increased pressure on the wrist extensor muscles, which have their tendinous origins from the lateral humeral epicondyle. This results in an inflammatory condition at the bone tendon junction, lateral epicondylitis, or "tennis elbow." Although this condition is common in tennis players, it occurs more frequently in the general population.

78. **(C)** Although rest, anti-inflammatory agents, and crutches adequately treat the symptoms, the diagnosis of a stress fracture can be made only with a bone scan if the initial x-ray findings are negative for fracture.

79. **(A)** In the absence of bladder or bowel disturbance, or sciatic symptoms, a neurological defect caused by a herniated disk is unlikely. A short period of rest, along with heat, anti-inflammatory agents, and analgesics, is the best treatment for a soft-tissue inflammatory lesion of the lumbar region.

80. **(C)** Postmenopausal osteoporosis is the common denominator in all fractures involving elderly women. In this particular fracture, it is the twisting effect on an osteoporotic femur that causes the fracture rather than the impact of the fall itself.

81. **(B)** Acute synovial reactions of weight-bearing joints with underlying arthritis are a common occurrence. It is usually related to minor traumatic events. Complete immobilization may increase joint stiffness secondary to arthritis, but partial reduction of stressful motions (avoiding kneeling and squatting) and continued muscle activity would be beneficial. These will allow the synovial reaction to subside while decreasing the weakening and stiffness caused by the underlying arthritis.

82. **(E)** Where possible, a single-lumen cannula should be inserted into the vein to avoid repeated attempts. The tincture of iodine should remain in contact with the skin for 30 seconds before venipuncture. Unsterile adhesive must not be placed over the entry site.

83. **(D)** Skull fractures should be explored only if they are compound, if a depressed fracture is present, or if an intracranial lesion requires exploration. Compound fracture implies that the fracture site communicates with the exterior. Rhinorrhoea is caused by leakage of CSF through a fractured cribriform plate.

84. **(B)** Subhepatic space infection usually occurs after surgery or peritonitis in the supracolic compartment. It is an unlikely complication of biliary pancreatitis. Infections in the subhepatic space may extend to the infracolic compartment via the paracolic gutter (of Morrison). This implies a perforation of the stomach.

85. **(D)** In addition to necrosis of the superficial and deep fascia, thrombosis of the microcirculation of the subcutaneous tissue occurs. Mortality rates have been reduced from 80% in the past to less than 12% in recent series. Polymicrobial infection is more commonly encountered, and gram-positive and gram-negative organisms are found in 70% of cases. Treatment is based on adequate debridement and use of appropriate broad-spectrum antibiotics.

86. **(D)** The patient needs a urinary diversion for the uretheral injury and a colostomy for the rectal injury.

87. **(E)** The modern treatment of civilian injuries of the colon emphasizes primary repair in the vast majority. The results are excellent in terms of suture line complications. Colocolostomy is reserved for a select few patients with the most optimal circumstances. Exteriorization after repair is no longer advised.

88. **(G)** All gunshot wounds clearly entering the abdominal cavity should be treated by emergency exploratory laparotomy. Over 80% of the time, injuries requiring repair will be found.

89. **(E)** A CT scan with intravenous and oral contrast can best rule out possible retroperitoneal injury caused by a stab wound.

90. **(B)** Wound exploration that convincingly documents failure of penetration through the posterior rectus fascia will most likely exclude abdominal injury from a tangential gunshot wound. A patient with negative findings on wound exploration can be discharged and followed as an outpatient. Peritoneal lavage would also rule out an intra-abdominal injury; however, it would require a subsequent period of hospital observation. A laparotomy would provide the most definitive evidence that an intra-abdominal injury did not occur, but a negative finding on laparotomy has a definitive associated complication rate.

91. **(C)** In a patient with significant bleeding, peritoneal contamination, and multiple injuries, splenectomy is indicated. Prompt packing of the liver injury and splenectomy are the first considerations at laparotomy.

92. **(I)** Postsplenectomy sepsis presents with sudden onset of nausea, vomiting, headache, confusion, and sometimes coma. Abdominal findings may be essentially normal following splenectomy. Inhibition of opsonization of leukocytes is evident with increased susceptibility to pneumococcal infection.

93. **(K)** Colon perforation is likely to show free air under the left hemidiaphragm. A subphrenic abscess presents with fever, leukocytosis, and a left pleural effusion. Gastric wall necrosis may likewise result in perforation with free air. There is air below the diaphragm following laparotomy, but it usually manifests symptoms clearly within the first week after operation.

94. **(A)** Flail chest should be suspected in multiple rib fractures where the individual rib is divided in two places. Paradoxical movement results in lung compression as the flail segment moves inward during inspiration.

95. **(C)** Both subcapital and intertrochanteric fractures present with external rotation of the lower extremity. The lateral rotators are attached to the bone distal to the fracture line to cause this typical clinical sign. Trochanteric fractures have a better prognosis, because the blood supply to the proximal segment remains intact.

96. **(C)** The history is typical of spontaneous pneumothorax. Physical examination will reveal diminished breath sounds on the side of collapse and x-ray will confirm the diagnosis. A tension pneumothorax will cause hypotesios.

97. **(E)** Lateral impact may cause fracture ribs causing pain, difficulty in breathing, and may be associated with significant hemorrhage from intercostal vessels. The physical signs described are those of a massive hemothorax.

98. **(A)** Precordial stab wound, distended jugular veins, and hypotension should suggest a cardiac tamponade. It must be kept in mind that the same signs are those of a tension pneumothorax. Dyspnea and deviation of trachea to the opposite side, absent breath sounds, and hyperresonant percussion note should suggest the correct diagnosis.

99. **(B)** A temporal skull fracture crossing the middle meningeal artery grove with lucid interval are pathognomonic of an extradural hemorrhage.

100. **(F)** Head-on collision and bent steering wheel should raise suspicion for head injuries, facial fractures, and deceleration injuries. The impact of knee against the dash-board forces the head of the femur posteriorly in the acetabular socket and may cause acetabular fracture.

101. **(E)** Multiple rib fracture with often multiple fractures in the same segment of a rib may cause flail chest and contribute to pain and hypoxia. It is the underlying pulmonary contusion that will determine the extent of respiratory failure.

CHAPTER 13

Pediatric Surgery

Tyr Ohling Wilbanks and Meno Leuders

Questions

DIRECTIONS (Questions 1 through 34): Each of the numbered items in this section is followed by five answers. Select the ONE lettered answer that is BEST in each case.

1. A full term neonate is found to have a swollen right scrotom. Gentle persistent pressure easily reduces an air filled structure back into the abdomen. The condition recurs promptly as the infant begins to cry. This

   (A) Mandates immediate surgical repair
   (B) Is the same defect as a communicating hydrocoele
   (C) Should have a tension-free mesh repair
   (D) Should prompt exploration of the left groin
   (E) Is generally irreducible in children

2. A 1-month-old infant presents to your office with an umbilical hernia. It is reducible but prolapses again almost immediately. It is TRUE that this defect

   (A) Is present in all children at birth
   (B) Will not close spontaneously
   (C) Should be repaired if still present at 3 months of age
   (D) Should be repaired at this time if it is >1 cm in diameter
   (E) Is likely to become incarcerated

3. You are called to the emergency room to see a 5-year-old child who has been vomiting for two days. She is thin, pale, lethargic, and febrile to 102.4°F. She has a respiratory rate of 39 beats per minute (bpm) and a diffusely tender, rigid abdomen without localizing signs. You should

   (A) Order an abdominal/pelvic CT scan with oral contrast to clarify the diagnosis.
   (B) Realize that her omentum is likely to "wall off" and contain the infection.
   (C) Order a barium enema to rule out intussusception.
   (D) Start fluid resuscitation and observe on broad-spectrum IV antibiotics.
   (E) Take her immediately to the operating room for abdominal exploration.

4. A 7-week-old girl is referred by her pediatrician for projectile vomiting over the past week. Her weight has remained stable, her fontanelles are not sunken and she sucks avidly. Her abdomen is soft with visible peristalsis in the epigastrium without evidence of a mass. A diagnosis of pyloric stenosis, in this case (Fig. 13–1)

   (A) Should lead to immediate surgical pyloromyotomy
   (B) Should not require any laboratory testing
   (C) Should prompt an order for an abdominal ultrasound
   (D) Should not be entertained until she has been tried on a new formula
   (E) Would be unlikely in the absence of an "olive"

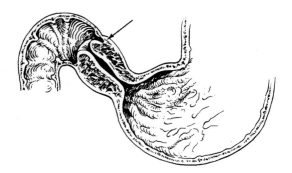

Figure 13–1.
Hypertrophic pyloric stenosis. Note that the distal end of the hypertrophic muscle protrudes into the duodenum (arrow), accounting for the ease of perforation into the duodenum during pyloromyotomy. *(Reproduced, with permission, from Doherty GM: Current Surgical Diagnosis and Treatment, 12th ed. 1315. McGraw-Hill, 2006.)*

5. A previously healthy 2 ½-year-old is admitted by the pediatrician for bilious vomiting and severe abdominal pain. Despite reports of the child being inconsolable you find him sleeping very soundly in his mother's arms. His abdomen is soft with a suggestion of right upper quadrant fullness. He has heme-negative, soft stool in the rectum. He is afebrile and his white blood cell (WBC) is 7800. Abdominal x-ray shows dilated loops of small bowel. You consider a diagnosis of intussusception

   (A) To be unlikely in the absence of "current jelly" stools
   (B) And arrange prompt surgical exploration and reduction
   (C) And order an ultrasound
   (D) And order an air contrast enema
   (E) And order a CT scan with rectal contrast

6. An 8–year-old presented with a 1-day-history of vomiting without diarrhea progressing to severe right lower quadrant. You make the diagnosis of early appendicitis and take her to the operating room. Upon delivering the cecum, you find a normal appearing appendix immediately adjacent to multiple large lymph nodes in the mesentery of the appendix and terminal ileum. The tissues appear "boggy" and indurated. The most likely diagnosis is

   (A) Acute lymphoma
   (B) An intussesception, which was reduced as you delivered the cecum

   (C) Mesenteric adenitis
   (D) Subclinical appendicitis with reactive adenopathy
   (E) Campylobacter enterocolitis

7. A 2-year-old toddler weighing 11 kg is admitted for observation of abdominal pain. There has been vomiting or diarrhea and the child had been eating normally 7 hours previously. Electrolytes are as follows: Na, 135 mEq/L; K, 3.9 mEq/L; HCO_3, 19 mEq/L; CL 110 mEq/L. The most appropriate IV fluid orders would be

   (A) D5 ¼ NS @ 22 mL/hour
   (B) D5 ½ NS @ 22 mL/hour
   (C) D5 NS @ 22 mL/hour
   (D) D5 ¼ NS @ 44 mL/hour
   (E) D5 ½ NS @ 44 mL/hour

8. A frustrated young mother calls emergency medical services (EMS) to report hearing a series of thumps down the staircase before finding her 15-month-old son lying at the foot of the stairs crying. He is brought to the emergency department boarded and collared. He is still crying, moving all extremities, has a heart rate of 135 bpm and a blood pressure of 80/95 mm Hg. Which test should be done first?

   (A) Cervical spine films to rule out cervical spine injury
   (B) Skull films to rule out skull fracture
   (C) Head CT to rule out intracranial hemorrhage
   (D) Abdominal CT to rule out ruptured spleen
   (E) Skeletal survey to rule out child abuse

9. A 15 kg, 7-year-old girl is in the emergency room with dramatic blood loss from a scalp laceration after blunt trauma. Suturing the laceration has achieved hemostasis but she is lethargic and clammy with digital and perioral cyanosis. Her heart rate is 110 bpm and blood pressure is 80/40 mm Hg. The most appropriate initial fluid order is

   (A) 450 mL of type specific blood over ½ hour
   (B) 150 mL of D5 ¼ NS over ½ hour

(C) 150 mL of type specific blood over ½ hour

(D) 300 mL of D5 ¼ NS over ½ hour.

(E) 300 mL of type specific blood over ½ hour

10. You are called to see a 4-hour-old neonate in the well-baby nursery who has developed bilious vomiting after taking his first feeding. He was born at 39-week gestation, has not yet passed meconium and has an unremarkable examination. An upper gastrointestinal (GI) series would be the study of choice to rule out which of the following clinical conditions?

(A) Ileal atresia

(B) Meconium ileus

(C) Duodenal web

(D) Malrotation

(E) Tracheoesophageal fistula

11. A 2-month-old former preemie presents to your office with an easily reducible right inguinal hernia. He was born at 30-week gestation, was on continuous positive airway pressure (CPAP) for 4 days, was treated for hyperbilirubinemia, and was discharged home after 24 days. Since going home he has been thriving, eating avidly, and now weighs 3.6 kg. His parents are well informed and although they want the hernia repaired as quickly as possible; they are concerned about the risks of general anesthesia. You tell them that

(A) They should wait another 5 ½ months until he is 60 weeks of gestational age.

(B) They should wait until he weighs 5 kg.

(C) They should wait another 3 months until he is 50 weeks of gestational age.

(D) They can schedule him as soon as possible because he weighs >2.5 kg.

(E) They can schedule him in 2 weeks because at that point he will have reached gestational term age of 40 weeks.

12. A 12-year-old boy crashes his bicycle and drives one of the handle bars into his left upper quadrant. He complains of abdominal and left shoulder pain. He weighs 41 kg. On exam his heart rate is 111 bpm, his blood pressure is 95/50 mm Hg ,and he is tender in the left upper quadrant. After a 450 mL bolus of Ringer's lactate he is calmer, his heart rate is 85 bpm and his blood pressure is 105/55 mm Hg. You order an abdominal computerized axial tomography (CAT) scan. Nonoperative management in the intensive care unit (ICU) would be justified if

(A) You find a grade I splenic laceration on the CAT scan with some active extravasation of IV contrast

(B) If he becomes restless, recurrently tachycardic, and hypotensive while on the way to CAT scan

(C) He requires 2 U of packed red blood cells (PRBCs) to maintain his vital signs in the 3 hours after the CAT scan demonstrates a grade I splenic laceration

(D) FAST exam before the CAT scan demonstrates free fluid around the spleen

(E) It fails to increase his blood pressure

13. A 9 ½-year-old girl presents to your office with an approximately 1 ¼-cm nodule in her neck, just to the left of the midline and below her cricoid cartilage. It is nontender and moves when she swallows. It has been enlarging over the last several months and was not seen by the pediatrician at her 9-year-old check up. There is no family history of endocrine disorders. The most likely diagnosis is

(A) Reactive viral lymphadenopathy

(B) Papillary thyroid cancer

(C) A brachial cleft cyst

(D) A follicular adenoma of the thyroid

(E) A thyroglossal duct cyst

14. A 3-year-old, recently adopted Romanian boy is referred after his initial pediatrician's assessment for an undescended testicle. On exam his left testicle is normal and in place. He has no evidence of hernias. However, his right hemiscrotum is empty and there is a testicule sized mass plapable at the pubic tubercle. The most appropriate next step is

    (A) Observation until age 5
    (B) Right orchiopexy
    (C) Right orchiopexy and right inguinal hernia repair
    (D) Right orchiopexy and right testicle biopsy
    (E) An abdominal ultrasound

15. A 6-year-old girl presents with a left breast mass. Her mother first noticed it a day before and is very concerned because both the child's maternal grandmother and maternal aunt have had breast cancer. It is firm, smoothly circumscribed, and slightly eccentric under the left areola. The right breast is unremarkable. You suggest

    (A) Immediate excisional biopsy
    (B) A mammogram
    (C) Repeat examination in 1 month
    (D) Genetic testing for breast cancer (BRCA) 1 and 2 mutations
    (E) Sterotactic needle biopsy

16. A 9-month-old is brought in by EMS after falling from his changing table. He is poorly responsive and being mask ventilated. You opt to intubate him prior to sending him to CAT scan. Compared to an adult an important consideration in his intubation is

    (A) Selecting an cuffed tube, the size of his little finger
    (B) The relatively large size of the infant cricoid compared to the thyroid cartilages
    (C) Decreased forward flexion of the neck and trachea while supine
    (D) More rapid desaturation after cessation of bag/mask ventilation
    (E) It takes a shorter time to intubate an infant

17. You are called to see a 7-day-old girl in the neonatal ICU who is having bilious aspirates from her feeding tube. She was born at 32-week gestation with Apgars of 8/10 and has been doing well after requiring CPA for only 18 hours. She has been afebrile, her WBC has been stable ~18,000, but she has been having increased numbers of apneic and bradycardic episodes. Abdominal x-ray suggests traces of pneumotosis. The most appropriate next step is:

    (A) Initiate CPAP for her respiratory difficulties leading to air aspiration
    (B) Hold feedings and start antibiotics
    (C) Send stool for *P. intestinalis* and start antibiotics
    (D) Check her liver function tests
    (E) Exploratomy laparotomy

18. You are called to the emergency room to see a 7-week-old boy with blood in his bowel movements (BMs). On examination the child is active, responsive, and appears well perfused. His heart rate is 124 bpm and his blood pressure is 80/45 mm Hg. The most likely diagnosis is

    (A) Meckel's diverticulum
    (B) Juvenile polyposis
    (C) Allergy to his formula
    (D) Peptic ulcer disease
    (E) Anal fissure

19. A 4-year-old girl is referred to your office by the pediatrician for the finding of an abdominal mass on her 4-year-old well child visit. She had been consistently in the seventy-fifth pecentile for height and weight and although she is still in the seventy-fifth pecentile for height she is only in the fortieth percentile for weight. She has been eating normally and having normal daily BMs. On examination you palpate an 8-cm right midabdominal mass. It is firm, nontender, and poorly mobile. The most likely diagnosis is

    (A) Constipation with a distended cecum
    (B) Wilms' tumor
    (C) Neuroblastoma
    (D) Lymphoma
    (E) Hempatoblastoma

20. A 12-year-old girl presents to the emergency department following a skiing crash in which the left side of her midtorso hit a tree. She presents with left side lower chest and upper abdominal pain. She also complains of left shoulder pain. The most likely diagnosis is which of the following?

(A) Rib fractures
(B) Liver injury
(C) Ruptured diaphragm
(D) Splenic injury
(E) Ruptured stomach

Questions 21 and 22

A mentally retarded 7-year-old child with cerebral palsy is admitted for repair of a left indirect inguinal hernia. Clinical palpation reveals a large left retroperitoneal abdominal mass.

21. What is the most common presentation for a patient with a Wilm's tumor?

(A) Unilateral flank mass
(B) Back pain
(C) Hematuria
(D) Urinary tract infection (UTI)
(E) Weight loss

22. Before radiologic investigation, which is the best method to distinguish a Wilm's tumor from a neuroblastoma?

(A) Shifting dullness
(B) Physical examination of the abdomen
(C) Catecholamine levels
(D) Auscultation for bowel sounds
(E) Cortisol administration

23. A mother brings her 3-year-old daughter to the pediatric emergency room with a complaint of a tender and firm lump in her right labia. According to the mother the lump has been there for 3 months but now it cannot be "pushed back in". The girl is apprehensive and tender in the right lower quadrant for several hours. A likely diagnosis is:

(A) Appendicitis
(B) Direct inguinal hernia
(C) Inguinal lymphadenopathy
(D) Indirect incarcerated hernia containing an ovary
(E) Indirect incarcerated hernia containing bowel

24. An otherwise healthy 3-week-old baby boy comes to the emergency room with this mother. The baby has been vomiting for 1-day, initially formula then more and more bilious material. He appears dehydrated, last diaper was changed 16 hours ago. There is now some blood stool from his anus. His fontanelle is depressed. His SMA7 shows a moderate metabolic acidosis and his WBC is 17,000. After initial fluid resuscitation what diagnostic test is useful to make the diagnosis here?

(A) CT scan of chest and abdomen
(B) Barium enema
(C) Upper GI series
(D) Serial abdominal exams
(E) Right upper quadrant ultrasonography (USG)

25. Clinical symptoms and presentations of malrotation least likely include

(A) Volvulus
(B) Chronic abdominal pain
(C) Failure to thrive
(D) Intestinal atresia
(E) Diarrhea

26. A newborn full-term baby boy with diagnosis of imperforate anus (Fig. 13–2) is also at risk to have a

(A) Dextrocardia
(B) Rib cage anomaly
(C) Tracheoesophageal fistula
(D) Ulnar skeletal deformity
(E) Proximal limb malformation

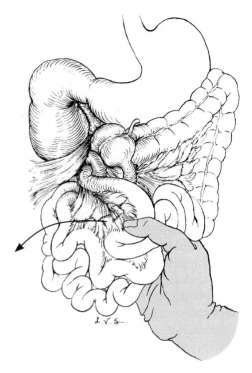

Figure 13–2.
Malrotation of the midgut with volvulus. Note cecum at the origin of the superior mesenteric vessels. Fibrous bands cross and obstruct the duodenum as they adhere to the cecum. Volvulus is untwisted in a counterclockwise direction. *(Reproduced, with permission, from Doherty GM: Current Surgical Diagnosis and Treatment, 12th ed. 1297. McGraw-Hill, 2006.)*

27. The most common pathogen in neonatal sepsis is

    (A) *Haemophilus influenzae*
    (B) Pneumococcus
    (C) *Klebsiella pneumoniae*
    (D) *Escherichia coli*
    (E) *Staphylococcus epidermidis*

28. A 3.3 kg, 36-week baby girl was born prematurely after labor caused by ruptured membranes. The prenatal ultrasound revealed a polyhydramnion at 26 weeks. Fetal echocardiogram was normal and amniocentesis was without genetic aberrance. On examination there was a normal anus, an nasogastric tube (NGT) drained bile stained fluid. The baby passed some mucus from below but no typical dark meconium. A chest and abdominal x-ray showed a "double bubble sign". What is the most likely diagnosis?

    (A) Acute pancreatitis
    (B) Neonatal Hirschsprung's disease
    (C) Duodenal atresia
    (D) Malrotation of midgut
    (E) Duodenal duplication

29. A 6-year-old girl is referred to you by her pediatrician complaining of a pain in her throat and presenting with an anterior cervical midline mass for several weeks. After a course of antibiotics the inflammation and erythema resolved but the mass still persisted. The mother is concerned. She remembers a time when the child was 3-years-old complaining of similar symptoms, but then it spontaneously resolved. Physical chest exam is normal but the mass appears to rise upward when the girl sticks out her tongue. What is the most common diagnosis?

    (A) Lingual thyroid
    (B) Branchial cleft remnant
    (C) Thyroglossal duct cyst
    (D) Uncomplicated cervical neck abscess
    (E) Thyroiditis

30. A 7-year-old boy was involved in a motorcycle crash while seated in the back of a minivan without restraints. His vital signs in the emergency room are stable but he is complaining of left upper quadrant abdominal pain. The FAST scan shows scanty fluid around in the left colic gutter. An abdominal and pelvic CT scan with iv and po contrast is performed and the radiologist suggests a "blush" (arterial extravasation) in the splenic parenchyma. The spleen itself sustained a deep parenchymal tear and is classified as a grade III injury. The child remains hemodynamically stable. What is recommended next?

    (A) Continuous hemodynamic monitoring, celiac angiogram, and angio embolisation of splenic artery.
    (B) Immediate exploration in the operation room

(C) If hemodynamic instability develops, aggressive fluid resuscitation including a repeated bolus of 20 mL/kg lactated Ringer's solution followed by a liver spleen scan

(D) Monitoring only

(E) Pneumovax and elective splenectomy in 6 weeks

31. In the emergency room department a 2-year-old girl is brought after she is passing three episodes of maroon colored stools. A similar episode occurred the night before. She is afebrile and has no abdominal pain. Dark clotted blood mixed with fresh blood is seen in her diaper. Her heart rate is 116 bpm and a blood pressure measured at 76/42 mm Hg. Appropriate fluid resuscitation with infusion of 20cc/kg of normal saline ensues. Vital signs normalize. Coagulation studies, crossmatch, complete blood count (CBC) are ordered and an insertion of a nasogastric tube is performed. There is no blood in the NGT and golden bile is aspirated. What is the differential diagnosis in this GI bleed?

(A) Anal fissure

(B) Meckel's diverticulum

(C) Colon polps

(D) Intussusception

(E) Bleeding gastric ulcer

32. Which is not a long-term complication of a 1-year-old baby boy having undergone corrective hepatoportoenterostomy (Kasai procedure) for biliary atresia?

(A) Recurrent episodes of cholangitis

(B) Hepatic cirrhosis and portal hypertension despite adequate bile drainage

(C) Upper GI bleeding episodes from esophageal varices

(D) Need for hepatic transplantation after initial Kasai procedure has failed

(E) Anastomotic leakage of portoenterostomy

33. Shortly after an uncomplicated birth a full-term baby boy develops respiratory distress and excessively spits after an unsuccessful feeding trial, requiring endotracheal intubation. A chest x-ray is performed and shows signs of aspiration in the right basilar and apical lung fields. There is air in the stomach, which appears hyperinflated. A trial of NGT placement is unsuccessful. What diagnosis is suspected?

(A) Duodenal atresia

(B) Hypertrophic pyloric stenosis

(C) Tracheoesophageal fistula without esophageal atresia

(D) Distal tracheoesophageal fistula with proximal esophageal atresia

(E) Achalasia

34. A 11-year-old boy with past medical history of sickle cell disease (homozygote form) comes to the pediatric emergency room with left upper abdominal pain, fever, and episodes of vomiting. He is complaining of previous episodes in the past that occurred after heavy meals. A chest x-ray shows the normal heart silhouette in the right chest. A routine abdominal ultrasound shows absence of a gallbladder in the right upper quadrant. The liver parenchyma is seen on the opposite side. Also, the radiologist calls you confused, indicating a thick-walled, fluid-filled cystic structure with echodense particles on the left side, which appears tender on palpation. A liver function test is normal except for an alkaline phospatase of 187. WBC is 17.6. What is the most likely diagnosis?

(A) The patient has constipation and should get an enema to clear out his fecal impaction from the left colon.

(B) Preventing a sickle cell crisis, the patient should be placed on additional nasal oxygen, copious hydration, pain medication, and maintaining a hematocrit of >28%.

(C) In addition to preventing a sickle cell crisis, the patient seems to have acute cholecystitis and needs IV antibiotics followed by cholecystectomy.

(D) The patient has situs inversus totalis and cholecystectomy is contraindicated.

(E) Cholelithiasis requiring delay in cholecystectomy until symptoms are totally resolved.

Answers and Explanations

1. **(B)** Congenital inguinal hernias are more common in premature infants, in males, and on the right side. The defect involves the failure of the processus vaginalis to fuse leaving an open communication from the abdomen to the tunica albuginea. The semantic difference between a scrotal hernia and a communicating hydrocele is that the hernia contains abdominal contents while the hydrocoele contains only fluid. The abdominal musculature is normal and no repair is required beyond high ligation of the sac. Previously, the historically high risk of anesthesia prompted contralateral exploration to avoid a second anesthetic. With modern anesthesia the risk of ischemic injury to the spermatic cord out weighs the risk of anesthesia. That risk, however, increases below 50 weeks of gestational age (i.e., from conception). Although some authorities would repair this child promptly, many would wait until he has passed the 50-week mark. At that time, some would perform flexible fiber-optic peritoneoscopy through the open right sac during the repair to evaluate the contralateral side, while others would elect to simply observe that side for the clinical appearance of a hernia.

2. **(A)** The umbilical hernia is the only hernia universally present at birth due to the need for umbilical cord patency up to that instant. After birth, the vast majority of umbilical hernias close by age 3–5 years. The risk of incarceration is low and repair is usually reserved for children older than 3–5 years of age or those with a fascial defect >1–2 cm in diameter.

3. **(E)** Conditions other than appendicitis, such as mesenteric adenitis, could possibly present like this; but this child's pale countenance and tachypnea suggest impending septic shock. While a 10–20-mL/kg fluid bolus and antibiotics should be rapidly administered; this child clearly has a acute surgical abdomen and requires urgent exploration. The thicker adult omentum will frequently contain a perforated appendix, creating an abscess. A young child's omentum is typically thin and flimsy and perforation usually leads rapidly to diffuse peritonitis. Barium enema to rule out intussuscepting, which would be unlikely in a child this old, is contraindicated in the presence of peritoneal signs. If further imaging were desired, USG is fast, generally well tolerated, and can be quite revealing in thin, young children. CAT scanning would involve radiation exposure, can be difficult to read in which this child would likely vomit up.

4. **(C)** Although pyloric stenosis is typically seen in 4-week-old male infants, it can certainly be seen in females and in those older and younger. The hypertrophied pylorus, which presents as an olive-sized mass in the epigastrium, is frequently "hiding" below the liver or the distended stomach and can only be appreciated in ~50% of patients. Electrolyte distrubances and volume depletion are more common in infants who have been vomiting for several weeks and can lead to cardiovascular collapse on the induction of anesthesia. Although this expected weight and the diagnosis should prompt a check of her electrolytes and surgery should be delayed until any deficits are gradually corrected. Formula intolerance and pylorospasm are also causes of chronic vomiting and the diagnosis of hypertrophic pyloric stenosis should be confirmed by an ultrasonogram

showing a pyloric wall thickness of >3 mm and channel length of >16 mm.

5. **(D)** This is a typical presentation for intussusception. Between episodes of colicy pain, the exhausted child may rest comfortably. Although USG can be used to screen for intussusception a negative study with such a compelling clinical scenario would not be definitive. An air contrast (or barium) enema with no more than 120 mm Hg pressure would provide a definitive diagnosis and possibly be therapeutic. This should certainly be tried before subjecting the child to laparotomy. A CAT scan would involve as much radiation without being as definitive and without any hope of therapeutic benefit. Peritoneal signs, fever, leukocytosis, and bloody stools are all late signs suggesting intestinal necrosis and would be contraindications to rectal studies. In those cases prompt exploration is indicated.

6. **(C)** Had you observed the USG yourself, you might have noted that the noncompressable structure(s) appeared more spherical than tubular. Lymphoma is unlikely in this age group, especially with this acute presentation. You would expect a bacterial enterocolitis to produce more fever, leukocytosis, and diarrhea. While both subclinical appendicitis and a reduced intussusception are theoretically possible, streptococcal infection is another possibility but also tends to produce more fever and leukocytosis and less adenopathy. It would be a strong second choice and the child should also have had a rapid strep test.

7. **(D)** Children's kidneys do not acquire significant ability to concentrate sodium until well after the age of 2 years. D5 $\frac{1}{4}$ NS is the most appropriate maintenance fluid for young children with normal electrolytes. The baseline fluid requirement for children is 100 mL/kgd for the first 10 kg, 50 mL/kgd for the second 10 kg, and 25 mL/kgd for each kg thereafter. (nb: Premature infants will require significantly more.) This child's requirement can be calculated as follows: 10 kg × 100 mL/kgd + 1 kg × 10 mL/kgd = 1050 mL/d = 44 mL/h.

8. **(C)** Due to the ligamentous flexability and platicity of the cartilaginous infant skeleton, both bony spinal injuries and skull fracutre are uncommon. However, because of the easy deformability of the skull, brain injury can easily occur, especially since infants are "top heavy". Their heads are relatively large compared to their bodies and they tend to fall head-first. His vital signs are not surprising for a crying infant and while splenic injury should be considered, it is less likely than the possible brain injury. Likewise, one should always consider child abuse, but the mother's agitation and story are not unreasonable and unless further history in uncovered skeletal survey is probably not warranted at this time.

9. **(E)** This child is in the early stages of profound shock as manifested by the signs of vasoconstriction. Her blood pressure is not that abnormal for her age but hypotension may be a late or even preterminal symptom of hypovolemic shock in young children. Given the apparent severity of the blood loss, type-specific blood is probably more appropriate volume replacement than crystalloid. A standard bolus for volume replacement should be 10–20 mL/kg. Once again, given the apparent severity of volume depletion, the 20-mL/kg bolus (300 mL) would be more appropriate.

10. **(E)** Upper GI series in the obvious study for tracheoesophageal fistulae and duodenal webs. It would also diagnosis an ileal atresia. Although a distal ileal lesion might be difficult to delineate it would still be the best test. Because of its utility in diagnosing these other conditions it is also the test of choice for malrotation, which can be diagnosed by demonstrating the sweep of the duodenum and ligament of Treitz to be to the right rather than the left of the spine. It would also more readily rule in or out a midgut volvulus, which is the complication of malrotation, about which we are most concerned in this patient. Only the meconium ileus (which consists of inspissated nuggets of hard meconium obstructing the distal colon) would be better diagnosed (and possibly treated) with a water-soluble rectal contrast study.

11. **(A)** Because of the immaturity of their reticular activating systems, infants of less than 50-week gestatonal age are at increased risk for apneic episodes in the first 24 hours after general anesthesia. Although herniorrhaphy would usually be performed as day surgery, infants of less than 50-week gestational age or weighing <2.5 kg should be admitted for 24 hours of postoperative monitoring or have their elective operations delayed until they have achieved those landmarks. However, former preemies are at increased risk and apneic complications have been seen up to 55 weeks of gestional age. The conservative recommendation for these infants is to wait until they are of 60-week gestational age.

12. **(D)** Nonoperative management of splenic trauma is usually successful in grade I lacerations and would be the standard of care in a hemodyamically stable patient. This boy responded well to a modest fluid bolus but if he becomes unstable on the way to CAT scan it would be hazardous to allow him to go into full-blown shock while in the scanner. Likewise, he should be explored (or embolized, depending on the resources available) for other signs of active bleeding including requiring >20 mL/kg PRBC to maintain his vital signs or seeing active extravasation on contrast on the CAT scan. Seeing fluid around the spleen on the FAST exam simply supports the clinical diagnosis of ruptured spleen but not an indication for intervention in the absence of hemodynamic instability.

13. **(B)** While reactive lymphadenopathy is by far the most common cause of neck masses in children; a lymph node should not move with deglutition and is more likely to be tender. A branchial cleft syst should be more lateral and the thyroglossal duct cyst should be higher and in the midline (although they can sometimes present off the midline). One might also have expected some prior evidence of both of these congenital cysts, although that is not always the case. The location and characteristics strongly suggest a thyroid nodule. While follicular adenomas are much more common in adults than cancers they are rarer in children and a rapidly growing solitary nodule is likely to be a papillary carcinoma, the most common thyroid cancer in children.

14. **(C)** Although waiting until age 1 is acceptable, there should be little further delay. Waiting until puberty would subject the child to a high probability of abnormal development. Abdominal USG can be useful to search for an intra-abdominal testicle but this child's testicle was palpable. Since all cryptorchid testicles are accompanied by an inguinal hernia; heniorraphy should always accompany an orchiopexy for cryptorchism. Testicular biopsy is unnecessary and may be injurious. The risk of malignancy, although increased 20-fold, does not manifest itself until at least the early twenties.

15. **(C)** Breast cancer is vanishingly rare in children with on ~60 cases reported in the English literature even in patients with the BRCA mutations. Therefore, needle biopsy and mammogram are unlikely to be helpful. The most likely tumor in this case is a benign fibroadenoma. Removal of breast masses in prepubescent girls carries a strong possibility of damage to the involved breast bud with subsequent hypoplasia of the adult breast. In this case, it would be better to defer excision until after puberty unless the mass continues to enlarge or becomes symptomatic.

16. **(E)** When spine, an infant's relatively large occiput, large tongue,and small mandible resulted in an obstructed airway due to forward flexion of the neck. Padding should be placed beneath the infants shoulder and back to allow the head to fall back into the physiologic "sniffing" position. The infant cricoid cartilage is also smaller than the thyroid, making the subglottic space funnel shaped rather than tubular. Pediatric endotracheal (ET) tubes are therefore uncuffed and size is detemined by measuring the child with the Braslow tape or comparing the tube to the patient's little finger. Due to their higher cardiac indices and more rapid medabolisms, children require a more rapid respiratory rate and will desaturate more quickly once respirations are held.

17. **(B)** Necrotizing enterocolitis (NEC) is primarily a disease of preemies occurring in anywhere from 3% to 10% of the population. It is believed to be initiated by an unfavorable combination of mucosal injury, bacterial overgrowth, and ready nutrients (in the form of infant formula). Early manifestations are bilious nasogastric/ orogastric (NG/OG) aspirates and early signs of infection. Later gas may be seen in the walls of the intestines (pneumotosis intestinalis or pneumotosiscoli) on abdominal x-ray. The final, preterminal stages would be free air and peritonitis. Initial treatment is to be withhold enteral nutrients and start broad-spectrum antibiotics aimed at the typical GI pathogens. Surgical exploration is reserved for more severe symptoms such as clinical deterioration, free air, or abdominal wall erythema.

18. **(C)** An allergic colitis due to milk or soy protein allergy is the most common cause of GI bleeding in the neonate. Anal fissures (easily diagnosed by examination) are the next most common in neonates and probably the most common in infants. Juvenile polyps (which are solitary in 80% of the cases) are a more common cause in older children.

19. **(C)** While constipation with a distended cecum is probably the most common cause of an abdominal mass, this child has a history of normal BMs and a relatively fixed mass. Lymphoma is the most common solid tumor of childhood after brain tumors; but it is more common in older ages and does not typically present in the abdomen. Neuroblastoma is the most common abdominal tumor and would lead to the differential. Wilm's tumor (or nephroblastoma) would be the next most common abdominal tumor occurring about 75% as frequently as neuroblastoma. Hepatoblastomas are far less comon than either of these two tumors.

20. **(D)** The spleen is the most common solid organ injured by blunt trauma. Though gastric rupture could cause the clinical presentation described, it is very rare. Rib fracture in the midtorso alone generally does not cause the referred shoulder pain, because blood does not collect under the left diaphragm, as seen in splenic injuries.

21. **(A)** The most common presentation for a patient with a Wilm's tumor is a unilateral flank mass.

22. **(B)** Wilm's tumor is usually diagnosed in well-appearing children between the ages of 6–10. The initial complaint is unilateral flank mass usually palpated during bathing or dressing of child. Neuroblastoma, a tumor of adrenal gland origin, tends to secret dopamine. These children appear emaciated and are typically 2–3 years younger in age group. CT scan is essential in both cases prior to any surgery. Although large Wilm's tumors push the intra-abdominal content to the contralateral side, the tumor itself rarely crosses the midline. On the contrary, neruoblastoma typically crosses the midline. Lymphomas in general involve the nodal tissue surrounding the great vessels and push the abdominal viscera anteriorly and laterally.

23. **(D)** Most inguinal incarcerated hernias contain bowel but a nonreducible mass involving the labia speaks for an incarcerated ovary.

24. **(C)** This is a true pediatric surgery emergency; malrotation, bilious vomiting with severe metabolic acidosis, lethargy, and dehydration is a hallmark of this serious condition. Initially vomiting of the baby could first result in a masked metabolic alkalosis caused by loss of chloride and potassium. Later, however, metabolic acidosis caused by hypoperfusion, shock, and lactic acidosis prevails. The treatment is fluid and electrolyte resuscitation and prompt operative exploration, detorsion with bowel resection if necrotic bowel is present. Time is of the essence! Thirty percent of patients with malrotation present within the first week of life, 55% in the first month, and nearly all of them in the first year.

25. **(D)** All of the above can be seen in malrotation. In the case of this 3-week-old baby boy the presence of intestinal atresia is less likely since symptoms of obstruction would have occurred much earlier.

26. **(C)** It is also commonly known as VATER association. (vertebral, anorectal malformations, tracheoesophageal fistula, renal and distal limb malformations) The most common abnormalities are cardiac in origin and involve ventriculoseptal defect (VSD) and atrial septal defect (ASD).

27. **(E)** Staph. Epi is the most common pathogen on neonatal ICUs and wards and also associated as a pathogen for necrotizing enterocolitis. Indwelling catheters or a break in the fragile neonatal skin is often responsible. Often there is a rash, with peeling of hand and feet due to a staphylococcal toxin. Candida is a pathogen in babies who undergo prolonged courses of antibiotics. Enteral bacteria are second in line after staphylococci.

28. **(C)** The most common form of duodenal atresia is where the obstruction occurs below the ampulla of Vater. Hence bilious NGT output is reported in the scenario. Also the most common variant is characterized by a membranous intraluminal atresia (type I). Nearly 35% of babies with congenital duodenal obstruction have syndrome and of those a majority have associated cardiac defects. If the duodenal obstruction is incomplete, we call this a duodenal stenosis. Clinically this manifests much later in life and is characterized by failure to thrive, chronic vomiting, electroyte anomalities and is called a duodenal windscok variant. Here a membranous web in the most often second and third part of the duodenum is causing clinical symptoms of high, incomplete bowel obstruction. The treatment is resection of the web and a side-to-side duodenoduodenostomy.

29. **(C)** Embryologically the thyroglossal duct cyst (Fig. 13–3) runs from the pyramidal lobe of the thyroid to the foramen cecum at the base of the tongue. It needs complete excision including part of the hyoid bone to avoid recurrence. An ectopic lingual thyroid is located at the base of the tongue and virtually never seen in the above described anterior midline location. Cervical lymphadenitis needs to be ruled out and a several microbial stains performed if an abscess develops. Masses caused by atypical mycorbacterial do not respond to antibiotic

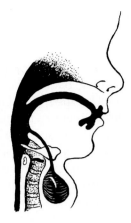

Figure 13–3. Thyroglossal cyst and duct course through the hyoid bone to the foramen cecum of the tongue. *(Reproduced, with permission, from Doherty GM: Current Surgical Diagnosis and Treatment, 12th ed. 1281. McGraw-Hill, 2006.)*

therapy and need to be excised. Brachial cleft remnants are almost always seen in the alter neck and divided in several types depending on their branch origin. They, however, can also get infected in manifest sometimes in form of a lateral neck abscess.

30. **(A)** While all blunt abdominal trauma patients developing hemodynamic instability should go to the operating room without delay; in this case it would be more beneficial to perform angioembolisation in a hemodynamically stable child. Plain films are of little value unless there is free air, prompting urgent colostomy. If there is no homodynamic instability in this child, every attempt should be made to preserve the spleen and avoid appendectomy. Pneumovax should be given in the perioperative period of a life saving splenectomy or when significant splenic tissue loss occurred. There is no role for an elective splenectomy in this trauma setting.

31. **(E)** Most common cause of lower GI bleed in this 2-year-old girl is a juvenile polyp. Anal fissures are also very common offenders of lower GI bleed, but perianal pain is a hallmark and not present in this case scenario. Meckel's diverticulum is the second most common cause in this age group involving a large amount of blood. Intussusception has to be excluded but in the absence of abdominal pain highly unlikely. Every attempt should be made to exclude an upper GI bleeding source, that is peptic ulcer disease or sequela of portal hypertension manifesting in esophageal varices (as seen in biliary atresia or chronic active viral hepatitis). Meckel's diverticula are true diverticula and derive their blood supply directly from the aorta as a remnant of a right vitelline artery. GI bleeding occurs as a result of heterotopic gastric mucosa.

32. **(E)** The etiology of biliary atresia remains unknown, but recent studies have linked into a prenatal rheo virus infection. An initial ultrasound is helpful to delineate extrahepatic bile anatomy in cases of unexplained nonphysiological hyperbilirubinemia. An magnetic resonance cholangiopancreatography (MRCP) is also helpful. If a hepatic HIDA scan shows uptake into the hepatocytes but fails to show a normal extrahepatic excretion pattern, a percutaneous liver biopsy is indicated. Typically there is a lymphocytic infiltration of the periportal field and absence of paucity of bile ducts. The most common type of biliary atresia (85%) is characterized by the atresia of the entire extrahepatic

duct system. The gallbladder is shrunken to a small strand of fibrous tissue including common bile duct and common hepatic duct. After the patient's first 3 months of life the success rate of operative hepatoportoenterotomy (Kasai procedure) falls significatly. Thirty-three percent deteriorate despite surgery. The Kasai operation remains the initial surgical treatment of biliary atresia. Long-term complications of hepatic cirrhosis, portal hypertension, bleeding esophageal varices, and recurrent bouts of cholangitis often force the patient to be scheduled for a hepatic liver transplant later in life.

33. **(D)** This case presentation is typical for a type C tracheoesophageal fistula with a proximal atresia of (Fig. 13–4) the esophageus. All the clinical symptoms can be explained. It is essential to hemodynamicaly stabilized the baby initially followed by an urgent corrective surgery. Often the tracheal fistula causes a big problem for anesthesia in terms of overinflation of the stomach and decrease in pulmonary compliance. Concomitantly a gastrotomy is performed alongside a right lateral thoracotomy. After extrapleural dissection and exposure of the right posterior mediastinum a ligation of right azygos vein and tracheoesophageal fistula is undertaken. The proximal esophageal pouch is gently

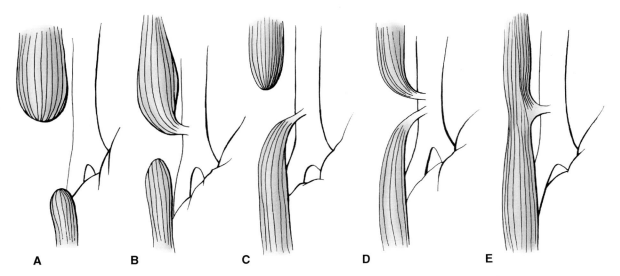

Figure 13–4.
A: Pure (long-gap) esophageal atresia. **B:** Esophageal atresia with proximal tracheoesophageal fistula. **C:** Esophageal atresia with distal tracheoesophageal fistula. **D:** Esophageal atresia with proximal and distal fistulae. **E:** Tracheoesophageal fistula without esophageal atresia. *(Reproduced, with permission, from Sabiston DC: Textbook of Surgery. Saunders, 1991.)*

mobilized and a primary esophageal anastomosis is often successful. In case of long-gap esophageal atresia, a transverse colon interposition is also used to bridge the gap. Type C is most common followed by a singular proximal esophageal without fistula. The H-type occurs in 1% of all cases and is difficult to diagnose, since these babies often develop chronic pulmonary infections without typical GI symptoms.

34. **(C)** This patient has situs inversus totalis and acute cholecystitis. After ensuring proper treatment of his sickle cell disease, he should receive IV antibiotics and be prepared for laparoscopic cholecystectomy. The surgical instrumentarium is to be placed in a mirror image but essentially the same rules and standards apply. The gallstones here probably contain bilirubin stones from frequent hemolytic episodes. It is also important to maintain a HCT of >28% and if necessary transfusions with Hb-A blood are carried out preoperatively.

CHAPTER 14

Practice Test

James E. Barone and C. Gene Cayten

Questions

DIRECTIONS (Questions 1 through 48): Each of the numbered item in this section is followed by five answers. Select the ONE lettered answer that is BEST in each case.

1. A 25-year-old woman complains of intermittent vague right upper quadrant (RUQ) pain. She has been on oral contraceptive tablets for 6 years. A CT scan of her abdomen shows multiple low-density solid masses occupying the entire right lobe of her liver as well as most of the left lobe. What is the best treatment for this patient?

   (A) Hepatic embolization
   (B) Discontinuation of oral contraceptives and a repeated CT scan of her abdomen in 3–6 months
   (C) CT-guided percutaneous needle biopsy of several liver masses
   (D) Laparoscopic biopsy of the liver masses and cholecystectomy
   (E) Gold therapy parenterally

2. A 76-year-old woman undergoes successful endoscopic stenting of the common bile duct (CBD) for obstructive jaundice secondary to an inoperable cholangiocarcinoma. Two weeks later, she consults her physician because of a fever of 102°F, general malaise, nausea, and RUQ discomfort. On physical examination, icteric sclera and RUQ tenderness are noted. Laboratory test results show leukocytosis, anemia, and an elevated serum bilirubin level. Chest x-ray shows no acute infiltrate, but the right diaphragm is elevated. What is the most likely diagnosis?

   (A) Cholangitis
   (B) Liver abscess
   (C) Acute calculous cholecystitis
   (D) Liver metastasis
   (E) Pneumonia

3. A 78-year-old woman develops a liver abscess following stent drainage of jaundice. What is the preferred therapy?

   (A) Oral administration of antibiotics
   (B) Aspiration of abscess
   (C) CT-guided percutaneous drainage alone
   (D) Administration of antibiotics and CT-guided percutaneous drainage
   (E) Surgical drainage

4. A 35-year-old man presents with a bleeding duodenal ulcer documented by endoscopy. The patient is somewhat unstable, and bleeding does not stop despite transfusing 8 U of blood. What is the most appropriate surgical therapy?

   (A) Further blood transfusion alone
   (B) Oversewing the ulcer alone
   (C) Oversewing the ulcer and performing a gastrojejunostomy
   (D) Oversewing the ulcer and performing a vagotomy and pyloroplasty
   (E) Oversewing the ulcer and performing a proximal gastrectomy

5. After undergoing a gynecologic operation, a 36-year-old patient developed β-streptococcal septicemia. Which is true of β-streptococcal infection?

   (A) It does not spread rapidly along lymphatic channels.
   (B) It is mainly resistant to penicillin.
   (C) It may spread rapidly through tissue planes.
   (D) It is unlikely to cause overwhelming infection from an intravenous site.
   (E) It commonly causes urinary tract infection (UTI).

6. A 44-year-old man develops intra-abdominal sepsis after undergoing difficult bowel resection and anastomosis. He is initially given ceftizoxime sodium (Cefizox), which is in effective because of overgrowth of which of the following?

   (A) *Pseudomonas*
   (B) *Staphylococcus aureus*
   (C) *Neisseria gonorrhoeae*
   (D) *Bacteroides fragilis*
   (E) *Haemophilus influenzae*

7. A 64-year-old man is noted on CT scan to have a liver abscess. He is diagnosed as more likely to have a pyogenic than amebic liver abscess. Why?

   (A) He emigrated from Mexico.
   (B) Jaundice is absent.
   (C) He has associated diarrhea.
   (D) He has a history of biliary tract disease.
   (E) There is a rapid response to metronidazole.

8. What is true of *Candida sepsis*?

   (A) It carries a relatively low mortality risk.
   (B) It is treated with actinomycin.
   (C) It can be partly prevented by ketoconazole.
   (D) It is caused by spore-forming organisms.
   (E) It is seen usually in conditions not requiring antibiotics.

9. A 43-year-old man had a previous injury to his wrist. The ulnar nerve was severed, as indicated by which of the following?

   (A) Claw hand involving the ring and little fingers
   (B) Claw hand involving the index and middle fingers
   (C) Atrophy of the thenar muscles
   (D) Absent sensation in the index finger
   (E) Inability to flex the distal phalanx of the index finger

10. After falling on the pavement, a 72-year-old woman is found to have a fracture of the radius and ulna (Colles' fracture). What is true of this fracture?

   (A) The fall occurs on the dorsum of the wrist.
   (B) Open reduction is most commonly indicated.
   (C) Younger men are generally affected.
   (D) The distal radial metaphysis is displaced dorsally.
   (E) The ulnar shaft is fractured proximally.

11. An 83-year-old retired navy general is scheduled to undergo aortoiliac bypass surgery for intermittent claudication. The factor(s) that would most likely cause concern because of the potential for development of cardiac complications is (are):

   (A) Signs of left ventricular failure
   (B) The patient's advanced age (>80 years) and jugular venous distention
   (C) History of angina and myocardial infarction (MI) 6 months previously
   (D) Left ejection fraction of over 50%
   (E) Aortic stenosis

Questions 12 and 13

A 24-year-old bank clerk is admitted to the hospital with left-sided blindness. She had emigrated from Africa and had been treated for sickle-cell disease. Examination reveals bleeding into the posterior (vitreous) chamber of the eye. Funduscopy cannot be done because of the presence of blood inside the eye.

12. What should be the next step in management?

    (A) Needle aspiration of the anterior chamber of the eye
    (B) Exploration of the posterior chamber
    (C) Administration of cortisone
    (D) Administration of steroids
    (E) Observation

13. The patient should be advised that repeated crisis may occur with which of the following?

    (A) Alkalosis
    (B) Moderate warmth
    (C) Pregnancy
    (D) Anemia
    (E) Oxygen administration

14. A 62-year-old woman underwent a modified mastectomy operation 5 years ago. One month before hospital admission, she undergoes repeated paracentesis of her left pleural cavity for a malignant effusion. The effusion recurred, as seen on x-ray, and she complains of dyspnea. What would appropriate therapy include?

    (A) Diuretic therapy
    (B) A salt-free diet
    (C) A low-albumin diet
    (D) Thoracoscopy, removal of fluid, and injection of talc into the left pleural cavity
    (E) Thoracotomy and pneumonectomy

15. A 43-year-old man sustains a fracture of the tibia. There are no neurologic or muscular lesions noted on careful examination. An above-knee cast is applied. After 6 weeks, the plaster is removed. It is noted that he has a foot drop and is unable to extend his ankle because of pressure injury to which of the following?

    (A) Posterior tibial nerve
    (B) Saphenous nerve

    (C) Femoral nerve
    (D) Deep fibula (peroneal) nerve
    (E) Nerve to the soleus muscle

16. A 62-year-old woman with multiple myeloma is given pamidronate calcium biphosphonate. This treatment has been shown to do what?

    (A) Increase survival
    (B) Improve quality of life and protect against skeletal fractures
    (C) Stimulate osteoclast
    (D) Increase hypercalcemia
    (E) Replace chemotherapy

17. A recently arrived 62-year-old emigrant from Greece complains of upper abdominal pain and fever. Ultrasound reveals a large liver cyst that, on serological testing, is shown to be hydatid disease. What should he undergo?

    (A) Cortisone therapy
    (B) Percutaneous drainage
    (C) Laparotomy and open drainage
    (D) Laparotomy and needle aspiration
    (E) Laparotomy and excision of cyst and perioperative albedazole

18. A 34-year-old woman with Crohn's disease has undergone her fifth operation with small-bowel resection. She has hemoglobin of 7 g/dL. An upper gastrointestinal (GI) series shows an apple-core lesion due to adenocarcinoma of the small bowel (Fig. 14–1). What is the most likely cause of her anemia?

    (A) Erythropoietin deficiency
    (B) Thyroid overactivity
    (C) Megaloblastic anemia
    (D) Aplastic anemia
    (E) Inability to absorb fat soluble vitamins

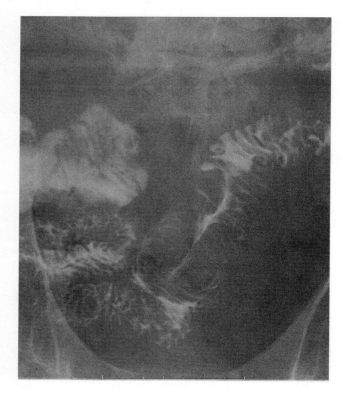

Figure 14–1.
Upper GI series shows apple-core lesion of mid-small bowel.

19. A 42-year-old man who has consumed several bottles of whiskey weekly for the past 20 years presents with hematemesis due to gastric varices. After appropriate resuscitation surgery is undertaken, what should he undergo?

    (A) Total gastrectomy
    (B) Splenectomy
    (C) Portal vein ligation
    (D) Hepatic vein ligation
    (E) Placement of an emergency portacaval shunt

20. A 12-year-old boy is admitted to the hospital with severe abdominal pain. He is noted to have slight jaundice. His hematocrit is 30, and reticulocytes are evident in a peripheral smear. His father underwent a splenectomy at age 25. Which test would clarify the cause of anemia?

    (A) Barium enema
    (B) Hemoglobin electrophoresis
    (C) Serum iron

    (D) Coombs' test
    (E) Red blood cell (RBC) osmotic fragility test

21. A 58-year-old woman has a gastric ulcer, achlorhydria, and vibration sense loss in the lower extremities. She has a megaloblastic anemia. What test would help support a diagnosis of pernicious anemia?

    (A) Response to injection of radioactive B_{12}
    (B) Endoscopic retrograde cholangiopancreatography (ERCP)
    (C) Prothrombin time (PT)
    (D) Radiolabeled B_{12} given orally
    (E) Response to trial of folic acid

22. A black ambulance driver presents with upper extremity pain, abdominal pain, jaundice, and splenomegaly. He appears cyanotic and gives a history of chronic obstructive pulmonary disease (COPD). X-rays show osteomyelitis, which, on needle aspiration, grows *Salmonella*. He has mild jaundice and a nonhealing ulcer on the left leg. His mother had anemia and died after suffering a stroke. His hematocrit is 28, and his blood shows sickle cells. What should the treatment do and not do?

    (A) Not include antibiotic treatment of osteomyelitis
    (B) Always include blood transfusion when his hematocrit is <30
    (C) Include administration of folic acid
    (D) Avoid the use of nasal oxygen
    (E) Include intravenous iron

23. Laparoscopy in abdominal trauma may be indicated in which of the following?

    (A) To exclude diaphragmatic injury
    (B) In patients with multiple previous abdominal operations
    (C) If there is limited cardiovascular reserve
    (D) If severe diffuse peritonitis exists
    (E) In hemodynamically unstable patients

24. A 42-year-old woman presents with a 3-cm breast mass of 3-month duration. Mammography shows microcalcification and features

suggestive of malignancy. The diagnosis is confirmed by which of the following?

(A) Needle biopsy
(B) Open biopsy from the edge
(C) Mammography
(D) Lymph node biopsy
(E) Thermography

25. A 45-year-old male is admitted to the emergency department subsequent to a high-speed motor vehicle accident. He was reportedly driving while intoxicated with alcohol and hit the embankment of an overpass. Examination reveals an unconscious male with a swollen neck and inspiratory stridor. Oxygen saturation is rapidly decreasing. What is the first concern?

(A) Immobilize the neck to avoid further neurologic injury.
(B) Obtain a whole body CT scan to assess full extent of injury.
(C) Call an otolaryngologist to evaluate the airway further.
(D) Perform a cricothyrotomy.
(E) Locate family members to obtain consent for any possible surgical intervention.

26. A 28-year-old woman has new onset hypertension and a bruit on abdominal examination. An arteriogram shows fibromuscular dysplasia (FMD) of the right renal artery. What is the best treatment option?

(A) Aortorenal saphenous vein bypass
(B) Patch angioplasty of the renal artery
(C) Percutaneous transluminal angioplasty
(D) Transaortic renal endarterectomy
(E) Hepatorenal bypass

27. A 42-year-old woman undergoes hysterectomy under spinal anesthesia. She develops severe respiratory distress after completion of the procedure.

What is the most common cause of respiratory arrest during administration of spinal anesthesia?

(A) Paralysis of the intercostal muscle
(B) Paralysis of the diaphragm (phrenic nerves)
(C) Centrally induced mechanism secondary to decreased cardiac output
(D) Diffusion of anesthetic to the level of the pons
(E) Diffusion of anesthetic to the level of the medulla

Questions 28 through 29

A 35-year-old man is brought to the emergency department after having been assaulted. A witness claims that he was hit on the head with a baseball bat and after the blow he was unconscious for approximately 10 minutes. The patient has a large bruise behind the left ear (Battle's sign) the site of impact being just a few centimeters above that. He is a little somnolesent but responds to questions and follows commands appropriately and accurately. He has no neurologic deficit other than mild weakness throughout the entire left half of the face. Inspection reveals dripping of a blood-tinged fluid coming from the patient's nose, which occurs particularly after attempts to rise from the recumbent position. A CT scan of the brain with bone windows shows no injury to the brain itself. There is a linear, nondepressed fracture transversely on the left petrous bone. There is opacification of the ipsilateral mastoid air cells, and there is a small amount of air intracranially at the tip of the left temporal fossa. The diagnosis of a traumatic cerebrospinal fluid (CSF) leak is obvious.

28. The most likely site of injury leading to cerebrospinal fluid rhinorrhea is an occult fracture in the frontal basal skull of which of the following?

(A) Semicircular canal
(B) Cavernous sinus
(C) Eustachian auditory tube
(D) Odontoid process
(E) Superior orbital fissure

29. Weakness of the left side of the face is due to an injury of the left facial nerve as it courses through the petrous temporal bone. The patient will manifest which of the following?

   (A) Absent gag reflex
   (B) Dilated pupil (mydriasis)
   (C) A bad taste sensation over the posterior third of the tongue
   (D) Deafness
   (E) Dryness of the cornea

30. Which of following treatments should be recommended?

   (A) Trendelenberg's position (lowering the head of the bed)
   (B) Urgent craniotomy to repair leakage of the CSF
   (C) Lumbar spinal drainage if the leakage persists
   (D) Encourage mobilization
   (E) Insertion of a nasopharyngeal ribbon

31. A young couple has been unsuccessful in conceiving a child over a 4-month period. The 28-year-old wife had been extensively investigated by a female reproductive specialist, and no abnormalities were detected. The husband, who initially refused to undergo semen analysis now agreed to this investigation, which revealed a low volume and azotemia. Follicle-stimulating hormone (FSH) level is normal. What is the most likely diagnosis?

   (A) Bilateral testicular atrophy
   (B) Congenital absence of the vas deferens
   (C) Hydrocele
   (D) Varicocele
   (E) Emotional disturbance

32. In evaluating a breast lesion in a female athlete, the surgeon notes that the tumor is in the anterior axillary line. To which site does the lateral edge of normal breast tissue extend?

   (A) The lateral edge of the pectoralis major muscle
   (B) The medial edge of the pectoralis minor muscle

   (C) Cover the medial third of the serratus anterior muscle
   (D) The semispinalis capitis
   (E) The posterior axillary fold

33. A 45 year old woman presents with a bloody nipple discharge. The most likely cause of this problem is:

   (A) Fibrocystic breast disease
   (B) Intraductal papilloma
   (C) Pituitary tumor
   (D) Invasive ductal carcinoma
   (E) Lobular carcinoma

34. A 74-year-old man presents with severe constant pain in the lower extremities associated with numbness and paresthesia of the plantar and lateral aspect of both feet. It is aggravated by walking or prolonged standing and occasionally made better by lying down. A magnetic resonance image (MRI) shows lumbar stenosis. He will have which of the following?

   (A) Spasticity
   (B) Hyperreflexia
   (C) Vertebral artery occlusion
   (D) Multiple roots involved bilaterally
   (E) Cancer is inevitably found

35. A 9-year-old boy has a 70% body surface area (BSA) burn that requires daily debridement in the Hubbard tank. To ease the pain of this debridement, what is the best selection?

   (A) Diazepam (Valium) and morphine
   (B) Innovar
   (C) Thiopental (Pentothal)
   (D) Nitrous oxide
   (E) Ketamine (Ketalar)

36. An 83-year-old retired scientist has inoperable prostatic cancer. His prostate specific antigen (PSA) levels begin to increase, and x-rays of his pelvis reveal metastatic bone disease. What is the characteristic feature of prostatic metastasis?

   (A) "Bossing" of the frontal and parietal lobes
   (B) Osteoblastic lesions

(C) Osteopetrosis and vascular necrosis of the head of the femur

(D) Fracture

(E) Onion peel lesion

37. A 62-year-old man develops abdominal pain after eating. An arteriogram reveals absence of blood flow in the celiac artery. Collateral branches supply the stomach through which of the following?

(A) Intercostal arteries

(B) Right renal artery

(C) Superior mesenteric artery

(D) Inferior epigastric artery

(E) Left colic artery

38. A 33-year-old man is involved in a motor vehicle accident. At operation, hepatic laceration and severe bleeding are noted. Which of the following would be relatively well tolerated by the patient?

(A) Persistent hepatic bleeding

(B) Portacaval shunt

(C) Portal vein ligation

(D) Hepatic arterial ligation

(E) Esophageal variceal bleeding

39. In evaluation of a patient who had previous surgery, acid secretion studies are performed. In the normal individual, what does gastrin do?

(A) It decreases basal (baseline) acid.

(B) It causes basal acid to remain constant.

(C) It causes basal acid to rise substantially within 1 hour.

(D) It causes a rise in basal acid after a latent period of 6 hours.

(E) It causes a fall and then a rise in basal acid.

40. In fluid replacement following a 20% BSA burn, the fluid requirement for the initial 24-hour period is dependent on which of the following?

(A) Patient's weight

(B) Serum Na

(C) CO level

(D) Acid base status

(E) Lactate level

41. A 20-year-old man with a duodenal ulcer complains of pain when eating food as well as during the early hours of the morning. During the cephalic phase of digestion, the stomach is stimulated by which of the following?

(A) Olfactory nerve

(B) Right glossopharyngeal nerve

(C) Sympathetic chain

(D) Left splanchnic nerve

(E) Vagus nerve

42. A 42-year-old construction worker noted a swelling in the right submandibuler region. Biopsy reveals malignancy, and surgical excision is advised. The patient is informed that one of the risks of this operation is which of the following?

(A) Horner syndrome

(B) Excessive sweating in the temporal region

(C) Deformity of the angle of the mouth

(D) Submandibular duct calculus

(E) Trismus

43. A 33-year-old man treated for lymphoma has increased levels of uric acid. This finding is usually caused by:

(A) Increased secretion of uric acid by the kidneys

(B) Increased production of uric acid

(C) Hypercalcemia

(D) Severe disease in the proximal interphalangeal (PIP) joints

(E) Side effects of chemotherapy

44. In osteoarthritis, there is which of the following?

(A) Degeneration of cartilage

(B) Slipped epiphysis

(C) Symmetrical polyarthritis and marked inflammatory synovitis

(D) Always a history of trauma

(E) Usually a prescription for colchicine

45. A 12-year-old boy is admitted to the hospital with a tentative diagnosis of osteomyelitis of the distal radius. What is found in this condition?

    (A) Tenderness is characteristically minimal.
    (B) There is an abscess in the soft tissue over the radius.
    (C) Hematogenous penicillin resistant *S. aureus* infection is likely to be present.
    (D) Fracture of the bone is always present.
    (E) There is tenosynovitis of the flexor tendons.

46. A student develops Bell's palsy of the facial nerve. During examination, she may also be found to have which of the following?

    (A) Loss of sensation in the skin over the cheek
    (B) Loss of sensation in the skin over the upper lip
    (C) Loss of cornea sensation
    (D) Dryness and damage to the cornea
    (E) Absent pupil reflex

47. A fracture of the femur occurs through the diaphysis of the femur. This injury involves which of the following?

    (A) Head of the femur
    (B) Acetabulum
    (C) Midshaft
    (D) Medial condyle
    (E) Anterior cruciate ligament

48. A 14-year-old boy is seen by his physician because of pain in the right hip. He is noted to have a limp on walking. His symptoms gradually developed over the past 3 months. The most likely cause of his symptoms is which of the following?

    (A) Volkmann's ischemia
    (B) Congenital dislocation of the hip
    (C) Slipped capital femoral epiphysis
    (D) Fracture of the proximal end of the fibula
    (E) Referred from a prostate lesion

DIRECTIONS (Questions 49 through 51): Each set of matching questions in this section consists of a list of lettered options followed by several numbered items. For each numbered item, select the appropriate lettered option.

Question 49

    (A) Pituitary ablation by surgery
    (B) Pituitary suppression with luteninizing hormone (LH) agonists
    (C) Prostatectomy
    (D) Cyclophosphamide (Endoxana)
    (E) Methotrexate
    (F) Thyroidectomy
    (G) Toxoids
    (H) Aromatase inhibitors (Anastrazol)
    (I) Parathyroidectomy

49. A 45-year-old man with abdominal pain, kidney stones, and peptic ulcer disease may very likely require which?

Question 50

    (A) Mucinous cystadenocarcinoma
    (B) Serous cystadenocarcinoma
    (C) Corpus luteum cyst
    (D) Dermoid cyst
    (E) Benign serous cyst
    (F) Pseudocyst
    (G) Endometriosis cyst
    (H) Hydatid cyst

50. The most common cyst in the ovary in a premenopausal patient is which?

Question 51

    (A) Is a condition in which it is safe to leave microscopic disease at the cut edges
    (B) Shows favorable response to radiotherapy
    (C) Has a 5-year survival rate of about 12%
    (D) Rates are increased in patients with duodenal ulcer

(E) Is a condition in which extensive removal of drainage lymph nodes should not be done

(F) Is associated with hyperchlorhydria

(H) Is associated with diverticulitis

51. What is true of pepsinogen?

DIRECTIONS (Questions 52 through 92): Each of the numbered item in this section is followed by five answers. Select the ONE lettered answer that is BEST in each case.

52. A 43-year-old woman presents with (RUQ) abdominal pain, and vomiting. She has had three children. The white blood cell (WBC) count is $14.3 \times 10^9/L$ and liver function tests are normal. To establish the diagnosis in this patient, the test of choice is:

(A) Computerized axial tomography (CAT) scan

(B) Ultrasound

(C) Hydroxy iminodiacetic acid (HIDA) scan

(D) MRI

(E) Endoscopic retrograde cholangiopancreatography (ERCP)

53. A 51-year-old woman underwent a Billroth II subtotal gastrectomy for carcinoma of the stomach 6 days ago. She had been recovering well except for persistent ileus. On morning rounds, you notice a large amount of serosanguinous drainage on her gown. The most likely diagnosis is:

(A) Wound dehiscence

(B) Wound infection

(C) Leak at the gastrojejunostomy anastomosis

(D) Leak from the duodenal stump

(E) Ascites

54. A 67-year-old, 60-kg homeless man has been in the intensive care unit (ICU) for a week after an emergency laparotomy and sigmoid resection for perforated diverticulitis. His serum albumin is 1.1 g/dL. He was just weaned from mechanical ventilation. His colostomy is not functioning. You start total parenteral nutrition (TPN) to deliver 1800 kcal/24 h. Two days later, the patient is in respiratory distress and requires reintubation and mechanical ventilation. You should check the level of serum

(A) Phosphate

(B) Magnesium

(C) Calcium

(D) Selenium

(E) Glucose

55. A 65-year-old man is 30 hours post-op sigmoid colon resection for diverticulitis. He says he feels well and he has a heart rate of 85 bpm, a blood pressure (BP) of 115/80 mm Hg, and a fever of 101.6°F. The most likely cause of the fever is:

(A) Clostridial myonecrosis

(B) Wound infection

(C) UTI

(D) Pneumonia

(E) Noninfectious

56. A 28-year-old, 70-kg man who was shot in the abdomen underwent a resection of his pancreas and duodenum for a shattered head of the pancreas. He required 14 U of packed RBCs and 25 L of crystalloid for resuscitation. Two days later he has hypoxemia and bilateral fluffy infiltrates on chest x-ray. The diagnosis of ARDS is made. Mechanical ventilation is begun via an endotracheal tube. Which of the following orders for ventilator settings is most appropriate?

(A) Tidal volume 650 mL, PEEP 8

(B) Tidal volume 450 mL, PEEP 5

(C) Tidal volume 800 mL, PEEP 0

(D) Tidal volume 650 mL, PEEP 0

(E) Tidal volume 450 mL, PEEP 0

57. A 38-year-old woman underwent an open cholecystectomy a week ago. She is found to have a subhepatic abscess and bacteremia. The preliminary blood culture report states that the organism cultured is an aerobic gram-negative rod. Of the antibiotics listed below, which would be the best choice?

    (A) Aztreonam
    (B) Clindamycin
    (C) Metronidazole
    (D) Vancomycin
    (E) Methicillin

58. A patient in the surgical ICU is in septic shock after surgery for perforated diverticulitis. His temperature is 102.3°F and his heart rate is 120 bpm. He is requiring dopamine for BP support. Which of the following drugs would be appropriate for use in this situation?

    (A) Recombinant activated protein C
    (B) Antitumor necrosis factor(TNF)antibody
    (C) Interleukin-1 (IL-1) receptor antagonist
    (D) Antiendotoxin antibody
    (E) Sodium nitroprusside

59. A patient is recovering from acute respiratory distress syndrome (ARDS). The patient no longer requires sedation and is being considered for weaning from the ventilator and possible removal of the endotracheal tube. Which of the following parameters is an indicator of potentially successful weaning?

    (A) PaO_2/FiO_2 ratio of 230
    (B) Rapid shallow breathing index of 125
    (C) Minute ventilation of 8.6 L/min
    (D) Mean airway pressure of 27 cm H_2O
    (E) Negative inspiratory force of 14

60. A 19-year-old male is admitted with a 2-cm stab wound of the sigmoid colon on the antimesenteric border. A small amount of solid feces is noted. No other injuries are present. Vital signs are stable throughout the case. The correct procedure is:

    (A) Repair the wound in two layers
    (B) Exteriorize the wound as a colostomy

    (C) Repair the wound in two layers with transverse colostomy
    (D) Resect the segment of sigmoid and perform a primary anastomosis
    (E) Resect the wound and perform a Hartmann procedure

61. An elderly woman underwent a radical mastectomy with radiation to the axilla 20 years ago. For 25 years, she has had an open wound that has never healed. It is not a recurrence of breast cancer. It is most likely:

    (A) Basal cell carcinoma
    (B) Squamous cell carcinoma
    (C) Hypertrophic granulation tissue
    (D) Malignant melanoma
    (E) Pyoderma gangrenosum

62. A 63-year-old man is admitted for an elective colon resection for recurrent attacks of sigmoid diverticulitis. You want to administer prophylactic antibiotics. In choosing a regimen you should be aware that the most common organism found in the colon of normal individuals is:

    (A) *Escherichia coli*
    (B) *Clostridium difficile*
    (C) *Pseudomonas* species
    (D) *Bacteroides* species
    (E) *Enterobacter cloacae*

63. A mountain climber arrives in your emergency department with frostbite of the left hand. The best method of rewarming the extremity is:

    (A) Forced warm air convection
    (B) To administer IV fluids warmed to 37°C
    (C) Radiant heat
    (D) Vigorous massage
    (E) Immersion in water warmed to 40°C

64. Two weeks after birth, a baby has persistent tachypnea, tachycardia, diaphoresis, and cyanosis. Workup reveals a patent ductus arteriosus. This can be closed with the use of:

    (A) Indomethacin
    (B) Acetaminophen

(C) Aspirin

(D) Cyclosporine

(E) Prostaglandin E1

65. A 65-year-old man presents with squamous cell carcinoma of the anus. He is in good health other wise. Metastatic workup is negative. The treatment of choice for this cancer is:

(A) Radiation

(B) Chemotherapy

(C) A & B

(D) Abdomino-perineal resection

(E) Wide local excision

66. The most likely cause of the finding pictured in Fig. 14–2 in a patient who has undergone no procedures is:

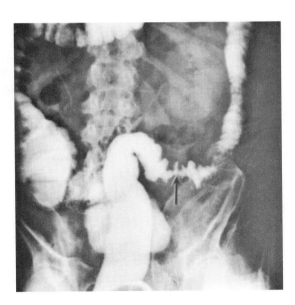

Figure 14–2.
Barium enema x-ray. Note the long segment of narrowing, the spasm, and the deformity (arrow) produced by an intramural abcess. *(Reproduced, with permission, from Doherty GM: Current Surgical Diagnosis and Treatment, 12th ed. 715. McGraw-Hill, 2006.)*

(A) Renal stone

(B) Bladder tumor

(C) Motion artifact

(D) Sigmoid diverticulitis

(E) Ventral hernia

67. Optimal treatment for the patient whose chest x-ray is (Fig. 14–3) depicted below would be:

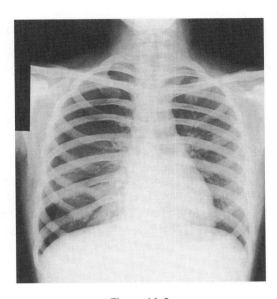

Figure 14–3.
Spontaneous pneumothorax on right side. *(Reproduced, with permission, from Doherty GM: Current Surgical Diagnosis and Treatment, 12th ed. 36. McGraw-Hill, 2006.)*

(A) Endotracheal intubation, mechanical ventilation, and PEEP

(B) Diuretics

(C) Metered dose inhalers using bata agonist drugs

(D) IV antibiotics

(E) Needle decompression

68. A 45-year-old woman who smokes is found to have a splenic artery aneurysm. It was most likely caused by:

(A) Atherosclerosis

(B) Trauma

(C) Medial dysplasia

(D) Pancreatitis

(E) Protal hypertension

69. A patient receiving total parenteral nutrition for a month is noted to have elevated aspartat aminotransferase (AST), alanine aminotransferase (ALT), and alkaline phosphatase levels. A percutaneous liver biopsy shows fat vacuoles. This finding is most commonly secondary to excess administration of:

    (A) Glucose
    (B) Fat
    (C) Protein
    (D) Selenium
    (E) Insulin

70. A 73-year-old man has ischemic rest pain of the left calf. Workup reveals occulsion of the left superficial femoral artery. He is scheduled for an elective femoral-popliteal bypass. A good way to reduce the risk of infection would be to:

    (A) Irrigate the wound with bacitracin during the operation
    (B) Start cefazlin 1 gIV 4 hours before the surgery
    (C) Use a plastic adherent drape
    (D) Not shave the leg
    (E) Finish the case in under 5 hours

71. A 44-year-old woman is found to have an elevated serum calcium of 11.3 mg/dL during a routine physical examination. It remains elevated after 3 months and serum parathyroid hormone (PTH) levels are also high. You suspect a parathyroid adenoma. The best test to localize the lesion preoperatively is:

    (A) Ultrasound of the neck
    (B) Sestamibi scan
    (C) I^{131} scan
    (D) CAT scan of the neck
    (E) MRI of the neck

72. A 75-year-old man is admitted with epigastric pain, anemia, and weight loss. On upper gastrointestinal endoscopy, a large ulcer is found in the distal antrum. The biopsy report shows adenocarcinoma of the stomach. CAT scan of the liver shows no metastasis. You would recommend:

    (A) Whipple procedure (pancreaticoduodenectomy)
    (B) Vagotomy and antrectomy
    (C) Subtotal gastrectomy
    (D) Vagotomy and pyloroplasty with wedge resection of the ulcer
    (E) Total gastrectomy

73. A 12-year-old perpubertal female has a painless 2.5-cm firm mass in the left subareolar area upon examination in the clinic. The right side has no palpable masses. The patient's mother is quite concerned. You recommend:

    (A) Excisional biopsy
    (B) Ultrasound
    (C) Fine needle aspiration
    (D) Incisional biopsy
    (E) Observation

74. A 30-year-old alcoholic is admitted with severe epigastric pain. He has hypoxemia, dehydration, and an elevated amylase and lipase. CAT scan shows probable hemorrhagic pancreatitis. An antibiotic shown to reduce the incidence of pancreatic sepsis in this type of pancreatitis is:

    (A) Ampicillin/sulbactam
    (B) Aztreonam
    (C) Imipenem/cilastatin
    (D) Cefotaxime
    (E) Gentamicin

75. A 51-year-old man presents with recent onset of what appears to be a large left varicocele. He should be investigated for possible:

    (A) Infertility
    (B) Testicular tumor
    (C) Renal tumor
    (D) Portal hypertension
    (E) Torsion of the appendix testis

76. A 23-year-old baseball player falls on his outstretched hand while attempting to catch a ball. He complains of persistent wrist pain. Although the initial wrist x-rays are read as normal, pain on palpation of the anatomic snuffbox suggests fracture of the:

(A) First metacarpal

(B) Hook of the hamate

(C) Pisiform

(D) Proximal phalanx of the thumb

(E) Scaphoid

77. A 12-year-old boy with sickle cell disease presents with pain and swelling of the right lower extremity. A bone scan reveals osteomyelitis of the tibial diaphysis. An organism found more commonly than in the general population in these cases is:

(A) *H. influenzae*

(B) *Salmonella* species

(C) *Klebsiella* species

(D) *Bacteroides* species

(E) *Aspergillus*

78. A 57-year-old woman presents with vague abdominal pain. After a course of treatment with H_2-blockers failed and abdominal ultrasound was negative, she underwent a CAT scan of the abdomen. The scan was negative except for the presence of a 3-cm mass in the left adrenal gland. Her pain disappeared. Urine and serum biochemical studies for a functioning adrenal tumor are negative. Her past medical history is negative. The next step should be:

(A) Adrenalectomy

(B) CT-guided percutaneous core needle biopsy

(C) Arteriography

(D) MRI

(E) Repeat CAT scan in 6 months

79. A 79-year-old man had a chest x-ray because of a history of smoking. However, a calcified gallbladder was noted. This was confirmed by CAT scan. The patient is asymptomatic and has no medical illnesses. The next step in the management of this patient should be:

(A) Cholecystectomy

(B) CT-guided percutaneous core needle biopsy

(C) Cholecystectomy with pancreaticoduodenectomy

(D) Cholecystostomy

(E) Repeat CAT scan in 6 months

80. A 62-year-old man presents with epigastric pain for 3 weeks. He had undergone a vagotomy and antrectomy 18 years ago for a bleeding duodenal ulcer. On examination, he does not appear ill and has no significant physical findings. The patient should now be:

(A) Treated with a proton pump inhibitor

(B) Endoscoped

(C) Treated with a prostaglandin E1 analog

(D) Prepared for an exploratory laparotomy

(E) Worked up with a CAT scan of the abdomen

81. A 42-year-old woman presents with a swollen, painful, erythematous left breast which does not repond to a 10 day course of oxacillin. Ultrasound reveals no abscess. The next step in management should be:

(A) Begin a 10-day course of vancomycin

(B) Workup the patient for an immunosuppressive disease

(C) Incise and drain the area

(D) Biopsy the skin and parenchyma of the breast

(E) Begin a 5-day course of prednisone in decreasing doses

82. An aid in the prevention of aspiration of gastric contents prior to endotracheal intubation in patients about to undergo general anesthesia is:

(A) Insertion of a nasogastric tube

(B) Administration of an emetic agent 30 minutes before intubation

(C) External pressure on the cricoid cartilage

(D) Placement of a Blakemore tube

(E) Administration of ondansetron 15 minutes before intubation

83. A 68-year-old woman is admitted with an acute surgical abdomen. After resuscitation with crystalloids IV fluids and administration of antibiotics, she is taken for an immediate laparotomy. Perforated diverticulitis of the sigmoid colon is found. The sigmoid colon is inflamed but mobile and the mesentery contains a perforated abscess. The best operation for this patient would be:

(A) Insertion of a sump drain in the abscess and a transverse loop colostomy
(B) Sigmoid resection including the abscess and colon-to-colon anastomosis
(C) Sigmoid loop colostomy
(D) Abdominoperineal resection
(E) Sigmoid resection and end sigmoid colostomy and oversew the rectum (Hartmann procedure)

84. Five days after a craniotomy for a brain tumor, a patient in the ICU suffers a massive upper gastrointestinal bleed. On arrival to the unit, you note bright red blood in the nansogastric tube. The patient has a BP off 85/50 mm Hg and a heart rate of 126 bpm. Laboratory tests and type and crossmatch were sent, but the results are still pending. The first therapeutic option you would choose is to:

(A) Lavage the nasogastric tube with cold saline.
(B) Give norepinephrine starting at 0.5 mcg/kg/min and titrate to BP of 120/80 mm Hg.
(C) Infuse 2 L of Ringer's lactate IV as fast as possible.
(D) Call for a gastoenterology consult and request upper gastrointestinal endoscopy.
(E) Give recombinant protein C.

85. The most commonly used drug in the immunosuppression of renal transplant patients is cyclosporine. A major side effect of this drug is:

(A) Pancytopenia
(B) Constipation
(C) Nephotoxicity
(D) Amenorrhea
(E) Peripheral neuropathy

86. A 40-year-old man was admitted with severe acute pancreatitis. He was noted to have a pH of 7.29, $PaCO_2$ of 65, and HCO_3 of 16. He was intubated and placed on mechanical ventilation. After aggressive fluid resuscitation, peak airway pressure was 55 cm H_2O and abdominal pressure measured via the bladder was 32 mm Hg. The best therapeutic option at this point is:

(A) Apply PEEP
(B) Tracheostomy
(C) Use inverse ratio ventilation
(D) Decompressive laparotomy
(E) Insert bilateral chest tubes

87. A 10-month-old boy has recently been weaned and placed on solid food. He develops colicky abdominal pain with vomiting. Examination of the abdomen shows emptiness in the right iliac fossa and a mass in the epigatrium. Intussusception is suspected. Following adequate hydration, this condition should be treated by which of the following?

(A) Laxatives
(B) Gastrojejunostomy
(C) Laparotomy and manual reduction
(D) Radiologic reduction by barium with measured pressure control of column of barium
(E) Right hemicolectomy

Question 88 and 89

A premature infant is noted at birth to have mild abdominal distention. There are no abnormal pulmonary findings on auscultation.

88. A plain x-ray of the abdomen shows intramural air (Fig. 14–4), which is attributed to which of the following?

(A) Choledochojejunal fistula
(B) Perforation of bowel caused by colon cancer
(C) Perforated gastric ulcer
(D) Gangrene of the small bowel
(E) Pneumatosis cystoides intestinalis

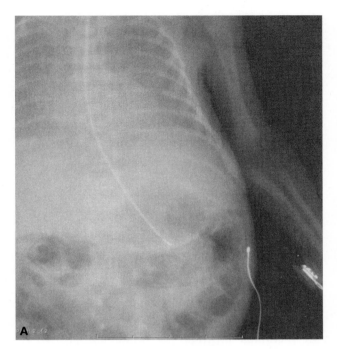 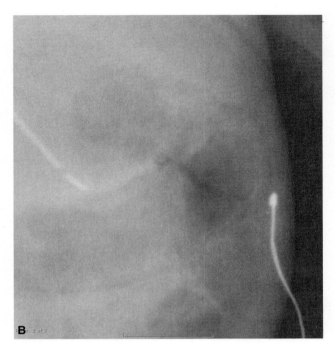

Figure 14–4.

Abdominal x-ray of premature infant. Intramural air is evident.

89. What is the most appropriate treatment?

(A) Urgent laparotomy

(B) Treatment for *E. coli* species

(C) Treatment for intestinal gangrene

(D) Reassurance and no intervention, in most cases

(E) Charcoal

90. With regard to the injured pregnant patient, which of the following is true?

(A) Hematocrit, blood volume, and BP all decrease with advancing pregnancy.

(B) CT scan is the diagnostic test of choice in pregnancy.

(C) Amniotic fluid analysis has a very low sensitivity in detecting viability of the fetus.

(D) The ideal position of transport of a pregnant patient is on her right side.

(E) Pregnant patients who are injured are at high risk for the development of disseminated intravascular coagulapathy (DIC).

91. Which of the following is a contraindication to nonoperative management of splenic injury?

(A) Prior hematologic disorder

(B) HIV-positive patient

(C) Hemodynamic instability

(D) Multiple other solid-organ injuries

(E) Pediatric patient

92. A 60-year-old man with no significant past medical history is scheduled for elective cholecystectomy. He has been taking aspirin daily. Preoperative recommendations should include which of the following?

(A) Determination of prothrombin time (PT)

(B) Estimation of platelet count

(C) Discontinuation of aspirin 2 days before surgery

(D) Discontinuation of aspirin at least 1 week before surgery

(E) Determination of bleeding time

The responses for questions 93–95 are the same. you will be required to select one answer for each item in the set.

(a) Glucagonoma

(b) Insulinoma

(c) Zollinger-Ellison syndrome (ZES)

(d) Watery diarrhea, hypokalemia, and achlorhydria (WDHA) syndrome

(e) Somatostatinoma

(f) Multiple endocrine neoplasia type-1 (MEN)-1

(g) MEN-2A

(h) MEN-2B

For each patient below, select the most likely diagnosis.

93. A 50-year-old woman complains of weakness, profuse watery diarrhea and crampy abdominal pain. She reports a 10-lb weight loss. Her serum potassium is 2.8 mEq/L.

94. A 45-year-old man presents with an upper gastrointestinal bleed. An upper endoscopy reveals multiple duodenal ulcers and an enlarged stomach.

95. A 35-year-old woman with epigastric pain, which did not improve on ranitidine, is found to have a nonhealing pyloric channel ulcer on upper endoscopy. Her serum calcium level is 12 mg/dL.

The response options for items 96–98 are the same. you will be required to select one answer for each item in the set.

(a) Thalassemia

(b) Hereditary spherocytosis

(c) Sickle cell disease

(d) Idiopathic autoimmune hemolytic anemia

(e) Thrombotic thrombocytopenic purpura

(f) Idiopathic thrombocytopenic pupura

(g) Systemic lupus erythematosus

(h) Myeloid metaplasia

(i) Non-Hodgkin's lymphoma

(j) Felty's syndrome

96. A 30-year-old man is noted to be anemic, with clinical jaundice and a palpable spleen on abdominal exam. Splenectomy is the only treatment for this patient's automsomal dominant disorder.

97. The peripheral smear of a child with anemia shows hypochromic microcytic anemia with target cells. What is the child's diagnosis?

98. A woman with longstanding rheumatoid arthritis has neutropenia on routine labs and splenomegaly is noted on physical examination. Which is the most likely diagnosis?

The response options for items 99–100 are the same. you will be required to select one answer for each item in the set.

(a) Nonparasitic cyst

(b) Hydatid cyst

(c) Hamartoma

(d) Adenoma

(e) Focal nodular hyperplasia

(f) Hemangioma

(g) Hepatocellular carcinoma

(h) Metastatic carcinoma

Select the most likely diagnosis for the patients below.

99. A 50-year-old woman underwent wide excision of a 2.5-cm infiltrating ductal carcinoma of the breast with axillary lymph node dissection followed by radiation and chemotherapy 2 years ago. The patient now complains of RUQ abdominal pain. A CAT scan reveals two masses in the right lobe of the liver.

100. A 35-year-old woman complains of RUQ pain after meals with nausea and vomiting. An ultrasound reveals cholelitiasis and an anechoic 3-cm mass on the inferior surface of the right lobe of the liver.

Answers and Explanations

1. **(B)** The CT scan findings of this patient plus the history of prolonged use of oral contraceptives are characteristic in hepatocellular adenoma. Because the tumor extensively involves both the right and left lobes of the liver, oral contraceptive use must be discontinued, and the patient must be observed for 3–6 months. Significant reduction in size of the adenoma has been noted in many cases after cessation of oral contraceptive use. If there is no regression of lesions, then liver transplantation should be recommended.

2. **(B)** Fever, jaundice, RUQ pain with tenderness, and leukocytosis are symptoms common to both cholangitis and liver abscess. Elevation of the right diaphragm on chest x-ray favors a diagnosis of a liver abscess. Because of the popularity of treating patients with cholangiocarcinoma with long-term indwelling stents, the incidence of complications due to pyogenic abscess has also increased.

3. **(D)** Administration of antibiotics and CT-guided percutaneous drainage of a liver abscess (consequent to biliary stenting) can be achieved with lower morbidity and mortality. Most pyogenic liver abscesses harbor multiple organisms (*E. coli*, *Klebsiella*, *Proteus*, *Streptococcus*, and anaerobes). Broad-spectrum antibiotics should be empirically started before the specific organism has been identified and before sensitivities are known. Closed aspiration of a liver abscess without drainage is inadequate in providing a more rapid resolution of the condition.

4. **(D)** For the patient who is unstable and has a pyloric or duodenal ulcer, oversewing the ulcer and closing the pyloric incision as a pyloro-plasty and performing a vagotomy is the procedure of choice because of its low operative mortality. However, this procedure carries a higher-recurrence rate. Major resections, such as antrectomy and subtotal gastrectomy are contraindicated in the unstable patient. At endoscopy biopsies for *H. pylori* should be taken and, if positive, treatment designed to eradicate *H. pylori* should be started. Eradication of *H. pylori* reduces the recurrence rate of bleeding.

5. **(C)** It is unclear why patients develop overwhelming infection at certain times. A surgical wound must be examined if a high fever occurs.

6. **(A)** Ceftizoxime (Cefizox) is not effective against many strains of *Pseudomonas*. If the drug is used, a higher dosage may be indicated, and the antibiotic should be changed if a quick response does not occur. Complications may occur in patients who are allergic to penicillin.

7. **(D)** He has a history of biliary tract disease. Pyogenic abscess occurs after abdominal sepsis, biliary tract surgery, and septicemia. Amebic liver abscess is not commonly encountered in the United States. Amebic liver abscess should be considered, however, if the patient has recently visited a tropical country or if abdominal pain and diarrhea are present. Metronidazole (Flagyl) is most effective in treating amebic abscess, and laparotomy should be avoided when possible unless complications specifically indicating intervention are present.

8. **(C)** *Candida sepsis* is an important clinical problem in burn units and ICUs and in patients with immunosuppression. *Candida albicans* is

dimorphic, and both yeast and mycelial forms are seen in infected tissues. Ketoconazole is given by mouth; it cannot be given in liver disease or in a nonacid environment. The main treatment of *Candida sepsis* is administration of amphotericin B. Actinomycin is an antibiotic that has antineoplastic action.

9. **(A)** The lumbrical muscles arise from the flexor digitorum profundus tendons at a level distal to the small bones in the hand. The hypothenar muscles are on the ulnar side, and the thenar muscles are on the thumb side of the hand. The medial two lumbrical muscles are paralyzed, and this leads to the typical deformity.

10. **(D)** The distal radial metaphysis is displaced dorsally. This fracture was described by Colles over 150 years ago. The impact is caused by a fall on the flexor surface of the wrist. The distal segment is displaced dorsally. The reverse injury, involving a fall on the extensor surface of the wrist and flexor deformity, is a Smith fracture. Colles's fracture occurs more commonly in older women. The styloid of the ulna—not the shaft of this bone—is fractured.

11. **(A)** The single most serious prognostic sign for adverse changes after vascular surgery is the presence of congestive cardiac failure. Every effort must be made to correct pulmonary congestion and improve left ventricular function before undertaking elective procedures. MI occurring within 3 months before operation carries a high mortality rate.

12. **(E)** Sickle-cell disease typically affects small arterioles and causes acute and chronic clinical manifestations. After an interval of a few days, an ophthalmologist should reexamine the patient to determine the next step in treatment.

13. **(A)** Treatment of sickle-cell disease is aimed at minimizing the precipitating factors, such as hypoxemia and alkalosis. Analgesics are required to treat the acute attack.

14. **(D)** If this method is unsuccessful, then fluid drained into the peritoneal cavity by a shunt could be considered.

15. **(D)** The common fibula (peroneal) nerve divides into the superficial fibula (peroneal) nerve, which supplies the fibula (peroneal) compartment, and the deep fibula (peroneal) nerve, which supplies the extensor compartment of the leg. This injury may occur because of a fracture of the proximal fibula or because of compression of the nerve by a tightly applied plaster cast in this region.

16. **(B)** In multiple myeloma, pamidronate calcium biphosphonate has been found to be useful as an adjunctive treatment, reducing the incidence of skeletal fractures.

17. **(E)** During the operative procedure, care must be taken to avoid spilling fluid from the cyst, which contains daughter scoleces. Perioperative treatment with albendazole should be started to help protect against any operative spillage of cyst contents. Recommended course is albendazole (10 mg/kg) for 1 week. If spillage occurs, treatment should continue for 1 month postoperatively.

18. **(C)** The distal ileum is the site of absorption of vitamin B_{12} following release of intrinsic factor from the gastric mucosa.

19. **(B)** The most common causes of gastric varices in patients with splenic vein thrombosis occur following pancreatitis and malignancy.

20. **(E)** The clinical finding of a positive family history suggests autosomal dominant hereditary spherocytosis. The diagnosis is confirmed by the presence of spherocytes in the peripheral blood and the abnormal osmotic fragility of their RBCs in dilute saline. In childhood, pigmented biliary tract stones and hemolytic anemia may be present.

21. **(D)** The Schilling test is performed by giving radiolabeled B_{12} orally (after saturating the B_{12} stores by intramuscular B_{12}). In pernicious anemia, less than 3% of the label is found in the 24-hour urine collection (N >7%). Hemoglobin electrophoresis will detect defects in α- or β-globin chain synthesis, as seen in thalassemia (Mediterranean anemia).

22. **(C)** Eight percent of American blacks have the HbS gene and 1 in 400 have the disease. Symptoms may appear in the first year of life if associated infection or hypersensitive drugs are administered.

23. **(A)** Laparoscopy in abdominal trauma is indicated in the management of select patients with intra-abdominal injuries. It may minimize intraoperative intervention in select patients with penetrating wounds to the abdomen.

24. **(A)** In general, a needle biopsy or needle aspiration cytology is performed as an out-patient procedure. Establishment of the diagnosis before hospital admission enables the surgeon to discuss surgical options before anesthesia is given. Excision biopsy is performed if the biopsy fails to confirm the diagnosis of a suspicious lesion.

25. **(D)** Blunt trauma to the neck is the most frequent cause of injury to the larynx. Rapid accumulation of blood, usually in supraglottic portions, can produce rapid laryngeal obstruction. A tear in the mucosal lining of the larynx and pharynx causes subcutaneous emphysema. The initial treatment is establishment of an adequate airway. Physicians should familiarize themselves with this technique. All clinics and doctor's offices should have the essential equipment required to perform this procedure when such an emergency arises.

26. **(C)** Among all causes of renovascular hypertension, FMD responds best to angioplasty. Results of PTA for FMD are similar to those of bypass. PTA has lower morbidity, causes less discomfort, and is less expensive. Recurrence can be treated by repeated PTA.

27. **(C)** Spinal anesthesia induces venous vasodilation because of sympathetic blockade. Venous pooling can seriously impair venous return. It is the sympathetic blockade and not somatic nerve blockade that is responsible for the vasomotor and respiratory changes. It is important to ensure that volume depletion is corrected before induction of spinal anesthesia, because venous return and, hence, cardiac output are diminished. These changes are aggravated by keeping the head raised.

28. **(C)** This is paradoxical rhinorrhea. CSF leaks through a fracture in the temporal bone (with a local dural laceration) into the mastoid air cells and middle ear. Because of the communication of the middle ear with the nasopharynx through the eustachian tube, CSF enters the nasopharynx and may exit through the nose. In the case of a small leak, there may be no more than the complaint of a postnasal drip or an unusual salty taste in the back of the mouth. In more severe cases, one can experience a frank constant drip of CSF through the nose. In this case, the evidence for the site of the leak being the temporal fracture is compelling—the presence of a petrous fracture, the opacification of the normally aereated mastoid air cells, and the presence of air in the middle fossa.

29. **(E)** After the facial nerve leaves the brainstem, it exits the skull through the internal acoustic meatus. Subsequently, it has a long and tortuous intraosseous pathway through the petrous bone that makes it particularly vulnerable to injury when the petrous bone itself had undergone a fracture. Nondisplaced fractures can result in a contusion of the nerve; whereas, displaced fractures can result in a complete transection of the nerve before it exits the skull through the stylomastoid foramen. Hyperacustism occurs if the hyperacustism facial nerve lesion is proximal to innervation of the stapes muscle. Severance of the accompanying chorda tympany nerve will result in loss of taste sensation in the anterior two-thirds of the tongue.

30. **(C)** Upward of 95% of CSF leaks that are caused by nonpenetrating trauma will heal without the need for surgery. Optimal conservative management in these cases consists of head elevation geared toward reducing the pressure of CSF and, thus, its tendency to leak out of the head. In the case of more persistent leaks, serial spinal taps or a lumbar drain can be employed. A lumbar drain places a small silicone tube into the lumbar subarachnoid space through a spinal needle. CSF can be drained through it in

a controlled fashion. Only a minority of patients with nonpenetrating CSF leaks will develop meningitis or eventually need surgery to repair the leak.

31. **(B)** In congenital absence of the vas deferens, mutation of the cystic fibrosis transmembrane receptor gene (CFTg) occurs. The epididymis vas deferens, seminal vesicle, membranous urethra, part of the trigone of the bladder, and ureter arise from the mesonephric duct. In the presence of a normal FSH level, testicular biopsy would most likely confirm normal sperm formation. In the presence of a Sertoli cell tumor, spermatozoa are unlikely to form, and the FSH level is elevated.

32. **(C)** The breast tissue extends over the medial margin of the serratus anterior muscle. The nerve to the serratus anterior lies on the lateral aspect of this muscle and may be accidentally injured during breast surgery.

33. **(E)** Secretions drain from the nipple by multiple openings. The most common cause of a bloody nipple discharge is intraductal papilloma (approx. 45%), but malignancy must be excluded. In about 10% of cases, an underlying carcinoma is detected. Prolactinoma of the pituitary gland may be responsible for clear or milky discharge (frequently bilateral). This may be diagnosed by an elevated prolactin level. Fibrocystic disease is not associated with bloody nipple discharge.

34. **(D)** Symptoms, although not always perfectly symmetric, are almost invariably bilateral. Symptoms are usually accompanied by diminished tone and reflexes and the absence of upper motor neuron features of spasticity, hyperreflexia, and upgoing toes.

35. **(E)** Ketamine is a neuroleptic agent (it suppresses psychomotor activity). It often provides adequate analgesia without respiratory or cardiorespiratory depression. It may increase laryngospasm and raise intracranial pressure (ICP). In adults, its main disadvantage is that it may induce hallucinations (emergence reactions), which occur in 12% of patients, manifesting as

dreamlike states, confusion, excitement, and possible irrational behavior.

36. **(B)** Patients with metastatic bone disease from prostatic cancer may survive for several years after diagnosis is established.

37. **(C)** The superior mesenteric artery will supply the inferior pancreaticoduodenal branch, which will form collateral branches with the superior pancreaticoduodenal branch from the celiac axis branch (gastroduodenal).

38. **(D)** Hepatic arterial ligation is often well tolerated. It reduces hepatic blood flow and, thus, decreases portal pressure. As in many other sites, the effect of proximal ligation is less drastic than that of distal ligation, because collaterals beyond the obstruction supply the definitive organ. Hepatic artery ligation should be avoided in the presence of obstructive jaundice or portal vein obstruction.

39. **(C)** After gastrin or histamine administration, there is an increase in acid secretion to between 20 and 60 mEq/h, with a mean value in this group significantly higher than in normal individuals or gastric ulcer patients. The rise in acid secretion after injection of gastrin is known as the augmented value. Basal acid output is usually 0.5–15 mEq/h.

40. **(A)** In burns, the Parkland formula is used to calculate initial fluid management. Fluid requirement = 4 × weight (kg) × % second and third degree BSA. Half this volume is given over the first 8 hours from time of the burn and the other half over the next 16 hours. After the initial 24-hour period, clinical parameters are used to guide fluid management.

41. **(E)** Both the right and left vagi contribute to the cephalic, gastric, and intestinal phase of acid secretion. The left vagus contributes predominantly to the anterior and the right to the posterior vagus nerve as they enter the abdominal cavity.

42. **(C)** The mandibular branch of the facial nerve may pass below the margin of the mandible

(15% of cases). Injury to the nerve will result in considerable deformity of the lower facial muscles including paralysis of those acting on the angle of the mouth and lower lip.

43. **(B)** The numerous causes of gout can conveniently be divided into overproduction of uric acid and undersecretion of uric acid by the kidneys. Hyperuricemia results from increased cellular turnover in patients with lymphoma.

44. **(A)** Osteoarthritis is characteristically a noninflammatory condition with normal WBC count in joint fluid; rheumatoid arthritis causes a symmetrical polyarthritis and marked inflammatory synovitis with an increase in the fluid WBC count.

45. **(C)** *S. aureus* infection is likely to be present. Osteomyelitis may also be caused by compound fractures and infection of the soft tissues surrounding the periosteum.

46. **(D)** The palpebral portion of the orbicularis oculi muscle closes the eye. Damage to the facial nerve causes inability to close the eye, and serious dryness of the conjunctiva may cause blindness.

47. **(C)** The physis is the growing cartilaginous portion of the bone. The diaphysis is toward the center and the epiphysis toward the ends of the bone.

48. **(C)** It is important to recognize this entity on x-ray. Treatment must be carried out to avoid further slipping of the joint epiphysis, because arthritis may result in neglected cases. Unlike fractures of the head of the femur occurring in older persons, the condition is unlikely to lead to necrosis of the femoral head.

49. **(I)** The patient has typical features of hyperparathyroidism. The other conditions do not have these three features.

50. **(C)** A corpus luteum cyst is functional and usually regresses within one menstrual cycle. If a cyst is smaller than 5–6 cm, reevaluate the patient in 4–6 weeks before suggesting laparotomy. Dermoid cysts are benign variations of teratomas. They usually are cured by simple excision, but the opposite ovary may be involved in 10% of cases.

51. **(C)** Survival rates are increased in patients with gastric ulcer. The 5-year survival rate for all types of gastric carcinoma is about 12%, but it is 35% if the nodes are clear and 7% if the nodes are involved. It is important that the cut edges are clear of tumor to avoid almost certain recurrence.

52. **(B)** The test of choice is ultrasound. It is quick, noninvasive, and accurate for the diagnosis of gallstones and acute cholecystitis. When present, signs of acute cholecystitis such as pericholecystitic fluid and a thickened gallbladder wall can easily be seen on ultrasound. CAT scan often does not show gallstones if the density of the stones is similar to that of bile. HIDA scan is usually reserved for patients in whom ultrasound is negative but suspicion of gallbladder disease is high. MRI is expensive and not studied for the diagnosis of stones. ERCP is usally done to rule out common duct stones.

53. **(A)** A large amount of seroanguinous drainage from the abdominal wound that occurs 5 to 7 days post-op is usually the result of dehiscence of the abdominal wound closure. A wound infection is heralded by erythema, swelling, and thick pus. Leaks from either enteric suture line would probably be bilious. Ascites is not commonly blood tinged.

54. **(A)** Rapid institution of full nutritional support can cause "refeeding syndrome" in malnourished patients. The hall mark of this condition is hypophosphatemia. Phosphate is taken up by phosphate-depleted cells trying to metabolize the nutrition and levels of ATP fall precipitously. This leads to respiratory failure. Refeeding syndrome can be avoided by starting nutritional support at low levels and increasing slowly. The other substances listed are not associated with respiratory failure after starting nutritional support.

55. **(E)** The patient almost certainly has a noninfectious reason for his early postoperative fever. There is no evidence that this is so. Most fevers

of this type resolve without any specific cause being found. Clostridial myonecrosis is always accompanied by cardiovascular instability, obtundation, and severe pain. UTI, pneumonia, and wound infection are unlikely so early in the postopertive period.

56. **(B)** In keeping with the current recommendation of lung protective ventilation with tidal volume of 5–7 mL/kg, answer B is correct. Low to moderate levels of PEEP should also be applied. This strateg of low tidal volume plus PEEP is thought to prevent overdistension of normal alveoli and limit secondary injury to the lung.

57. **(A)** Aztreonam is effective against gram-negative aerobic organisms. Clindamycin and metronidazole cover gram-negative anaerobic bacteria. Vancomycin and methicillin are effective drugs against gram-positive organisms.

58. **(A)** Recombinant activated protein C (drotrecogin) was shown to reduce mortality in severe septic shock, but not mild septic shock. The major side effect of recombinant activated protein C is bleeding. Anti-TNF antibody, IL-1 receptor antagonist, and antiendotoxin antibody have failed to change outcomes in randomized, prospective trials. Sodium nitroprusside is a vasodilator and would worsen septic shock.

59. **(C)** Minute ventilation (abbreviated Ve and the product of tidal volume x rate) of <10L/min suggests the patient is ready for weaning. A PaO_2/FiO_2 ratio of >300 is normal and would be helpful inconfirming the patient's readiness for weaning. A rapid shallow breathing index (frequency/tidal volume) of <105 if favorable as is a negative insipatory force of >−20 cm of H_2O. Mean airway pressure does not predict successful extubation.

60. **(A)** In the absence of significant contamination or devitalized tissue in a stable patient, the wound should be repaired without having to resort to a colostomyor a resection. This represents a change in the philosophy of managing colon injuries from 20 years ago. It is based on solid evidence-based medicine and experience with such patients.

61. **(B)** First described by Marjolin in 1828 and known as Marjolin's ulcers, malignant degeneration arising in a chronic wound is nearly always squamous cell carcinoma. These lesions are most commonly seen in burn scars but have been associated with osteomyelitis, radiation therapy, hidradenitis suppurativa, and diabetic ulcers.

62. **(D)** The approximate ratio of anaerobic organisms to aerobic organisms in the colon is 300:1. *Pseudomonas* and *C. difficile* are not normally found in large quanitites in the colon.

63. **(E)** Warm water immersion is the preferred method of rewarming extremities suspected of suffering from frostbite. Vigorous massage is contraindicated as it may cause trauma to the tissues. IV fluids warmed to 37°C would take a very long time to have an impact even if the circulation to the skin of the hand was adequate, which is not likely in frostbite. The other two choices would not provide a consistent temperature.

64. **(A)** The nonsteroidal anti-inflammatory drug, indomethacin, is the drug of choice for closure of a patient ductus arteriosus in a premature infant with an isolated patient ductus arteriosus. For complex cardiac anomalies, which require a patient ductus arteriosus to sustain life until corrective surgery can be done, prostaglandin E_1 can be administered to keep the ductus arteriosus open. The other choices are not indicated in patient ductus arteriosus.

65. **(C)** Radiation and chemotherapy are indicated for squamous cell carcinoma of the anus. Surgery is used only for biopsy and for selected cases of recurrence after radiation and chemotherapy.

66. **(D)** The most likely cause of the finding depicted, which is air in the bladder, is a colovesical fistula secondary to acute sigmoid diverticulitis. A renal stone, if visible at all, would be a calcific density and would be in the dependent portion of the bladder. There is no motion visible. A bladder tumor would appear as a filling defect with the density of soft tissue. It is not a hernia.

67. **(E)** The x-ray shows a tension pneumothorax. Insertion of a needle in the second intercostal space, midclavicular line can be a lifesaving procedure. The diagnosis of tension pneumothorax should be made on the basis of clinical findings such as decreased breath sounds and tympany to percussion on the affected side. Neck veins may be destended if the patient is not phyovolemic. The patient will be short of breath and hypotensive. The other answers are incorrect, especially A, which would exacerbate the problem by introducing positive pressure into the airways.

68. **(C)** Splenic artery aneurysms in women are almost always caused by medial dysplasia of the artery. It may be the cause of rupture in pregnancy and can be life-threatening if not treated promptly by laparotomy. Aneurysms may be caused by atherosclerosis, trauma, and pancreatitis (when complicated by pseudocyst formation). Portal hypertension is not a cause of aneurysm.

69. **(A)** Adminstration of excess glucose will lead to hepatic steatosis with 3–4 weeks. Liver function test will become abnormal and a liver biopsy will show fat vacuoles. Excess glucose administration can also lead to overproduction of CO_2 and difficulty in weaning patients from mechanical ventilation. Excess administration of intravenous fat may cause suppression of the immune system. Excess protein administration may lead to elevated levels of urea nitrogen in the blood.

70. **(D)** Shaving is associated with an increased incidence of wound infection compared to the use of electric clippers or depilatories, as well as compared to no hair removal at all. Prophylatic antibiotics should be started within 60 minutes of the incision time. Plastic adherent drapes and antibiotic wound irrigation have not been proven to reduce wound infection rates. Wound infection rates increase as duration of surgery increases beyond 2 hours due to the reemergence of skin flora.

71. **(B)** The best study for localizing parathyroid adenomas is the sestamibi scan I^{131} is used occasionally to work up thyroid disease. The other three test will often show the location of the parathyroid adenoma, especially if it is large. However, they are not as accurate as sestamibi for this problem.

72. **(C)** A subtotal gastrectomy with negative margins is appropriate treatment for gastric carcinoma. Vagotomy adds nothing as patients with gastric cancer are invariably achlorhydric. A Whipple procedure is done for panccreatic carcinoma. Total gastrectomy is rarely indicated for a distal gastric carcinoma.

73. **(E)** In a 12-year-old prepubertal female, the overwhelming likelihood is that the mass is budding breast tissue. The patient and her mother should be reassured and told to return in a few months if the other breast has not begun to develop. The other answers are incorrect because they will not help in the diagnosis and in the case of the two biopsies, they may actually cause harm in the breast may not develop normally.

74. **(C)** Imipenem/cilastatin has been reported in several randomized, prospective studies to decrease the risk of infecious omplications in severe pancreatitis. The other antibiotics have not been subjected to such rigorous investigation.

75. **(C)** Because of the fact that the left testicular vein empties into the left renal vein, a renal cell carcinoma of the left kidney, which occludes the renal vein, may also occlude the testicular vein. The right renal vein empties into the inferior vena cava. A variocoele will not occur in right renal cell carcinoma.

76. **(E)** The scaphoid or carpal navicular bone can be palpated in the anatomic snuffbox, which is formed by the abductor pollicis longus and the extensor pollicis brevis tendons on the lateral or radial side and the pollicis longus tendon on the medial or ulnar side. Scaphoid fractures are not always clearly visible at the time of initial injury. Pain in the anatomic snuffbox should heighten suspicion that a scaphoid fracture is present. The patient should be splinted and repeat x-rays should be taken a few days

later. These fractures are prone to nonunion, especially if the diagnosis is delayed.

77. **(B)** Although *S. aureus* is the most common organism found in osteomyelitis associated with sickle-cell disease, nontyphoid *salmonella* species are often found. *Salmonella* bacteria are thought to escape from the colonized colon due to microvascular infarcts secondary to sickle-cell disease. They then seed the bone via hematogenous spread.

78. **(E)** So-called adrenal "incidentalomas" have been reproted in up to 3% of people over the age of 50. Nonfunctioning masses <3 cm in diameter are almost never malignant. Lesions of >4 cm should probably be removed as the incidence of carcinoma rises as the size of the masses increases. MRI and arteriography are unlikely to change the management of this patient's lesion. Biospy is not indicated. She should have a repeat CAT scan at 6 months and if the lesion is stable be ovserved with yearly CAT scans.

79. **(A)** Due to the high rate of carcinoma (up to 50% of cases) found in patients with calcified gallbladders, cholecystectomy is indicated. A biopsy would not be helpful because of the possibility of missing the tumor. A negative biopsy would not rule out cancer. A pancreatioduodenectomy is not part of the treatment of gallbladder cancer. Cholecystostomy (tube drainage of the gallbladder) would not help the patient.

80. **(B)** Carcinoma in the gastric remnant has been reported in up to 19% of patients who have undergone partial gastrectomy. It usually takes more than 15 years to develop but has been reported in as few as 5 years after surgery. It is thought to be caused by either bile reflux into the gastric remnant or relatively low gastric acid output in the operated stomach. Some have advocated routine surveillance endoscopy in patients who have had gastric resectional sugery. The other answers are not appropriate. Although CAT scan might reveal some changes in the stomach, it would be difficult to differentiate them from surgical scarring in most cases, and endoscopy has the advantage of providing the means to obtain a biopsy.

81. **(D)** The patient should have a biopsy of the skin and breast tissues. The most likely diagnosis is inflammatory breast cancer. The skin should be included in order to assess for invasion of the dermal lymphatics. Dermal lymphatic invasion is not mandatory for the diagnosis of inflammatory breast cancer. Incision and drainage is not indicated as no abscess was seen on ultrasound. This is not likely to be caused by methicillin-resistant *S. aureus*; therefore a course of vancomycin would not be indicated. The other answers are not appropriate even if the problem was an infection.

82. **(C)** External pressure on the cricoid cartilage (the Sellick maneuver) helps prevent aspiration of gastric contents. An emetic would be contraindicated as aspiration might occur during vomiting. A nasogastric tube almost never empties the stomach completely, and it keeps the cardioesophageal junction open which promotes aspiration. A Blakemore tube is used for the treatment of uncontrolled bleeding esophageal varices. Aspiration is common with its use. Onndansetron is an antiemetic used for the treatment of nausea in chemotherapy patients. Vomiting during intubation is due to mechanical stimulation of the gag reflex, not nausea.

83. **(E)** Whenever possible, the inflamed colon should be resected. Since the patient had peritonitis, the safest procedure would be to avoid an anastomosis of the colon. Performing just a loop colostomy would subject the patient to two more operations, one to resect the sigmoid and another to close the colostomy. Abdominoperineal resection is removal of the rectum which is not indicated in diverticulitis. The rectum does not contain diverticula.

84. **(C)** The first choice for almost all hypotensive emergencies is the rapid infusion of crystalloid IV fluid. Cold saline lavage is useless and will render the patient hypothermic, which is detrimental to the clotting cascade. Vasoactive α-adrenergic agents such as norepinepehrine may raise the BP but will decrease perfusion to the vital organs. A gastroenterology consult would take too long to accomplish. Recombinant protein C causes bleeding and would be contraindicated.

85. **(C)** Ironically, nephrotoxicity is the major problem associated with the use of cyclosporine. Despite this fact, it is the most commonly used immunosuppressive drug in renal transplant patients.

86. **(D)** The patient has secondary abdominal compartment syndrome. The correct option is to perform a laparotomy and leave the abdomen open to relieve the pressure. Adjusting the ventilator might help temporarily but the root of the problem is the increased intra-abdominal pressure. A tracheostomy or insertion of chest tubes would be of no value.

87. **(D)** Treatment in infants is by controlled radiologic reduction initially, with surgery reserved for cases in which ischemia is expected or reduction is unsuccessful. The leading part of the intussusception is the apex. The outer sheath is the intussuscipiens, which receives the inner intussusceptum. The outer intussuscipiens elicits peristalsis, which forces the intussusceptum to extend distally.

88. **(E)** Pneumotosis cystoids intestinalis results from diverse causes. In most instances it does not in itself indicate a serious complication. In premature infants, initial feeding results in mucosal damage with tracking of intramural air (pneumotosis cystoides intestinalis). In adults, it may result from emphysema or rupture of a pulmonary bulla, which tracts below the diaphragm and encircles the bowel wall.

89. **(D)** Pneumatosis cystoides intestinalis may be associated with other conditions in the intestines or elsewhere. The finding of this condition as an incidental finding requires no further treatment other than that of the underlying cause. In newborns pneumotosis cyctoides intestinalis must be differentiated from the more serious and critical entity of necrotizing enterocolitis.

90. **(E)** Hematocrit, blood volume, and BP all increase with pregnancy. Ultrasonography is the preferred method to evaluate the abdomen and can also determine fetal viability. Aspiration of amniotic fluid and determination of lecithin/sphingomyelin ratio is helpful in the determination of fetal prematurity. The pregnant patient should be placed on her left side so that the full-term uterus will not compress the inferior vena cava and interfere with venous return.

91. **(C)** Hemodynamic instability is the most pressing indication for operative treatment in a patient with splenic injury. In all other situations listed a trial of nonoperative management may be continued.

92. **(D)** Discontinuation of aspirin at least 1 week before surgery. Aspirin inactivates platelet cyclo-oxygenase and thus inhibits platelet aggregation. The effect of aspirin is irreversible and lasts for the entire life span of the platelets. Therefore, aspirin should be discontinued for at least 1 week before surgery.

93. **(D)** WDHA, or VIPoma (vasoactive intestinal polypeptide) is characterized by voluminous diarrhea, 5 L or more daily, rich in potassium, which looks like watery tea. The diarrhea is secretory and if refractory to antidiarrheal agents. Patients are weak, with metabolic acidosis and hypokalemia. Octreotide decreases diarrhea volume. The pancreatic tumor should be excised. Secretory diarrhea also occurs in some patients with ZES, and is the only complaint in <10% of ZES patients. More than 90% of ZES patients have peptic ulcer disease. Unlike the diarrhea associated with ZES, the diarrhea of WDHA continues with fasting and continuous nasogastric tub suctioning. 15% of patients with glucagonoma have diarrhea; glucagonoma is associated with migratory necrotizing dermatitis.

94. **(C)** Gastrinoma, or ZES, should be suspected in patients with peptic ulcer disease refractory to medical treatment, or in patients with multiple ulcers or ulcers in uncommon locations. Gastrin secretion by the tumor, most commonly found in the pancreas, results in hypersecretion of gastric acid. Common patient complaints are epigastric pain, melena, hematemesis, diarrhea, and weight loss. ZES may occur as part of the MEN-1 syndrome; this patient presents with only atypical peptic ulcer disease. Omeprazole is the treatment of choice for control of peptic ulcers in ZES.

95. **(F)** MEN-1, or Werner's syndrome, and autosomal dominant disorder, involves tumors or hyperplasia of two or more glands, most commonly parathyroid, pancreas, and pituitary glands. Hyperparathyroidism is most common, followed by various pancreatic isle cell tumors and pituitary adenomas. MEN-2A (Sipple's syndrome) consits of pheochromocytoma, medullary carcinoma of the thyroid, and often hyperparathyroidism. MEN-2B is characterized by medullary carcinoma of the thyroid, pheochromocytoma, neuromas and marfinoid body habitus. MEN-2A and -2B are also autosomal dominant.

96. **(B)** Hereditary spherocytosis is the most common symptomatic familial hemolytic anemia, and is transmitted as an autosomal dominant trait. A defect in the red cell membrane causes increased trapping in the spleen and hemolysis. Anemia, jaundice, and splenomegaly are clinical findings. Splenectomy is the only treatment. Thalassemia is transmitted as a dominant trait; anemia is the result of a defect in hemoglobin synthesis. Thalassemia major, or homozygous thalassemia, is associated with anemia, icterus, splenomegaly, and early death. Transfusions are usually required. Splenectomy may reduce hemoloysis and transfusion requirements. Sickle-cell anemia is hereditary hemolytic anemia. Serum bilirubin may be mildly elevated. Splenomegaly often precedes autoinfraction. Splenectomy may be indicated for chronic hypersplenism or acute splenic sequestration.

97. **(A)** In thalassemia, intracellular hemoglobin precipitates, or Heinz bodies, damage red cells and contribute to early destruction. Cells are small, thin, misshapen, and resistant to osmotic lysis. Diagnosis is made by peripheral smear. Nucleated red cells, or target cells, are present. Distorted red cells, or target cells, are present. Distorted red cells of different shapes and sizes are found. In sickle-cell disease, characteristic sickle cells are seen on peripheral smear. In hereditary spherocytosis, the peripheral smear shows small, thick, nearly spherical red cells. Cells have increased osmotic fragility.

98. **(J)** The triad of rheumatoid arthritis, splenomegaly, and neutropenia is known as Felty's syndrome. Gastic achlorhydria is common. Thrombocytopenia and mild anemia are sometimes seen. Splenectomy is sometimes used to treat the neutopenia in patients with serious infections, anemia requiring transfusions, or severe thrombocytopenia.

99. **(H)** Breast cancer commonly metastasizes to bone, lung, soft tissues, liver, and brain. The patient should be worked up for local recurrence as well as other distant metastasis.

100. **(A)** Benign liver cysts can be single or multiple. Solitary nonparasitic cysts usually contain clear, watery fluid. These cysts are more common in the right lobe. They are most likely congenital and most are asymptomatic; many are found incidentally. An anechoic area on ultrasound is suggestive. Hydatid cysts, caused by *Echinococcus*, are also more common in the right lobe. The colorless fluid in the cyst is under high pressure, unlike parasitic cysts. Ultrasound will show internal echoes. Hemangiomas can have a variable echogenic pattern on ultrasound; focal nodular hyperplasia is often hypodense. Hepatocellular carcinoma and metastasis have a characteristic sonographic appearance different from benign nonparasitic cysts.